www.harcourt-international

Bringing you products from all Harcourt companies including Baillière Tindall, Churchill Livingstone, Mosby and W.B. Saunders

▶ **Browse** for latest information on new books, journals and electronic products

▶ **Search** for information on over 20 000 published titles with full product information including tables of contents and sample chapters

▶ **Keep up to date** with our extensive publishing programme in your field by registering with **eAlert** or requesting postal updates

▶ **Secure online ordering** with prompt delivery, as well as full contact details to order by phone, fax or post

▶ **News** of special features and promotions

If you are based in the following countries, please visit the country-specific site to receive full details of product availability and local ordering information

USA: www.harcourthealth.com

Canada: www.harcourtcanada.com

Australia: www.harcourt.com.au

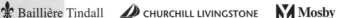 Baillière Tindall ⬧ CHURCHILL LIVINGSTONE Ⓜ Mosby 🅆🅢 W.B. SAUNDERS

Public Health in Policy and Practice

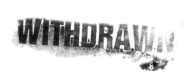

For Baillière Tindall:

Senior Commissioning Editor: Ninette Premdas
Project Development Manager: Karen Gilmour
Project Manager: Gail Murray
Designer: George Ajayi

Public Health in Policy and Practice: A Sourcebook for Health Visitors and Community Nurses

Edited by

Sarah Cowley BA PhD PGDE RGN RHV HVT

Professor of Community Practice Development, Public Health and Health Services Research Section, Florence Nightingale School of Nursing and Midwifery, King's College London, London, UK

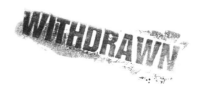

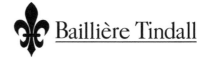

Baillière Tindall

EDINBURGH   LONDON   NEW YORK   PHILADELPHIA   ST LOUIS   SYDNEY
TORONTO   2002

BAILLIÈRE TINDALL
An imprint of Harcourt Publishers Limited

© Harcourt Publishers Limited 2002

✤ is a registered trademark of Harcourt Publishers Limited

The right of Sarah Cowley to be identified as editor of this work has
been asserted by her in accordance with the Copyright, Designs and
Patents Act 1988

First published 2002

ISBN 0 7020 2317 5

British Library Cataloguing in Publication Data
A catalogue record for this book is available from the British Library

Library of Congress Cataloging in Publication Data
A catalog record for this book is available from the Library of Congress

Note
Medical knowledge is constantly changing. As new information
becomes available, changes in treatment, procedures, equipment and the
use of drugs become necessary. The editor, contributors and the publishers have taken care to ensure that the information given in this text
is accurate and up to date. However, readers are strongly advised to
confirm that the information, especially with regard to drug usage,
complies with the latest legislation and standards of practice.

The
publisher's
policy is to use
**paper manufactured
from sustainable forests**

Printed in China

Contents

for health improvement – Identifying need – Community-based needs assessment – Difference between need and want – A strategic plan for health – Values in public health – Health promotion and public health – User involvement – Methods of obtaining the views of local people – Commissioning and needs assessment – Teamwork – Clinical effectiveness – Audit – Outcomes-measuring – Research – Development – Preparing a proposal or a bid for a research project – Public health professionals – Conclusion – Discussion questions – Further reading – References

Contributors

Jane V Appleton   BA(Hons) MSc RGN RHV PGCEA
Principal Lecturer in Research Education, Oxford Brookes University, School of Health Care, John Radcliffe Hospital, Oxford, UK

Christine Bidmead   RGN RHV
Training Facilitator, Centre for Parent and Child Support, South London and Maudsley NHS Trust, Munro Centre, Guy's Hospital, London, UK

Jennifer Billings   BSc(Hons) MSc RGN PGDipHV DipN
Research Programme Coordinator, East Kent Hospitals NHS Trust, Trent and Canterbury Hospital, Canterbury, UK

Jill Clemerson-Trew   RGN RSCN RHV
Bank Health Visitor, Tower Hamlets Healthcare NHS Trust and Researcher, Tower Hamlets Social Services, London, UK

Sarah Cowley   BA PhD PGDE RGN RHV HVT
Professor of Community Practice Development, Public Health and Health Services Research Section, Florence Nightingale School of Nursing and Midwifery, King's College London, London, UK

Pauling Craig   BSc(Hons) MSc RGN RHV
Health Visitor/Senior Health Promotion Officer, Greater Glasgow Health Board, Glasgow, UK

Yvonne Dalziel   BA MPhil RGN RHV FWT
Community Development Programme Manager, Lothian Primary Care NHS Trust, Edenhall Hospital, Musselburgh, UK

Anne Graney   MSc Dip Health Sciences RHV RGN
Regional Teenage Pregnancy Co-ordinator (Northern and Yorkshire), NHS Executive, Durham, UK

Peter Griffiths   BA(Hons) PhD RGN
Lecturer, Primary and Intermediate Care Section, Florence Nightingale School of Nursing and Midwifery, King's College London, London, UK

Sally Kendall   BSc(Hons) PhD RGN RHV
Professor of Nursing, Faculty of Health and Human Sciences, University of Hertfordshire, Hatfield, UK

Pauline Pearson   BA PhD DipSocRes RN RHV
Senior Lecturer in Primary Care Nursing, Department of Primary Health Care, Medical School, University of Newcastle, Newcastle upon Tyne, UK

Jean Rowe   MSc(SocRes) RGN RHV PGCEA
Acting Director for Health and Organisational Development, Lambeth, Southwark and Lewisham Health Authority, London, UK

Susan Walters   BA(Hons) MSc RMN RGM HV
Project Manager, Surviving Homelessness Project, St Anns, Nottinghamshire, UK

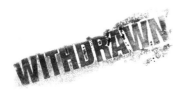

Preface

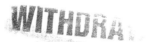

This book has had a relatively long gestation: it was commissioned shortly before the election of a new Labour government in 1997. At that time, it would have been difficult to predict the huge impact that the new government would have on public health policy and practice. A key part of the Labour party's electoral platform was its vision of an end to what was seen as tremendous unfairness in society, characterised by widespread inequalities and social exclusion. This is nowhere more evident than in the field of health and health care. Public health is based on the science of epidemiology, which involves the careful surveying and collation of statistics and disease patterns. That habit of rigorous data collection provided the incoming government with clear evidence of the link between inequalities in health and socioeconomic position, and a strong basis for its evolving policies.

For the first time, a Minister for Public Health was appointed, who set in train a whole series of projects and events designed to develop and enhance the public health function and capacity. An independent inquiry into inequalities in health was commissioned (Acheson 1998) to identify an evidence base for policies to improve this situation. The Chief Medical Officer (CMO) set up a multi-faceted project to strengthen and develop the public health function. In the initial report, this project highlighted a need for more attention to be paid to education, training and organisational development. It described different needs at the following three levels of public health functioning:

1. Most professionals, including managers in the NHS, local authorities and elsewhere, for example teachers, would benefit from a better basic understanding of public health. Knowledge of how to gain access to more specialist input would be useful to strengthen their role in furthering health improvement goals in their daily work, a role they may not recognise as contributing to public health.
2. A smaller group of hands-on public health practitioners spend a substantial part of their working practice furthering health by working with communities and groups. They need more specialised knowledge and skills in their respective fields. This group includes public health nurses, health promotion specialists, health visitors, community development workers and environmental health officers.
3. A still smaller group are public health specialists, who come from a variety of professional backgrounds and experience and need a core of knowledge, skills and experience. This core is in urgent need of definition so that generic public health specialists can be fully acknowledged for their contribution. This group includes professionals from backgrounds such as the social sciences, statistics, environmental health, medicine, nursing, health promotion and dental public health.

(Department of Health 1998 p 15)

The nursing professions are represented at each of the three levels and subsequent policies have been developed to map and enhance the public health capacity across nursing, midwifery and health visiting. This book contains much of interest across the levels, but it is particularly directed at the middle one of these three groups: the grass roots public health practitioners, especially those public health nurses and health visitors who spend a substantial amount of their time furthering health improvement by working with groups and communities. The text is based on a belief that the skills and knowledge needed to operate at this level have much in common with those identified for public health specialists, but also include additional, practice-specific abilities. As suggested by the CMO, these groups 'need more specialised knowledge and skills in their respective fields'; they also need the ability to network and contribute to the public health functions at the other two levels.

The first section of the book opens with three chapters to set the scene for these roles by looking at grass roots practice in public health. A feature of practice at this level is that the division between clinical treatments and population-wide strategies is less clear-cut than in the traditional medical model of public health. The idea in that view is that one group of workers (typically the public health specialists) consider only populations and never encounter individuals with clinical needs in their work. Conversely, the traditional view suggests that treatments for individuals are only ever delivered on the basis of the clinical need identified in that person; population needs are not considered. This traditional division now represents a rather outdated view, with the World Health Organization (WHO 1999) representing the services as a continuum rather than a dichotomy. Public health directors may, for example, point to the individual requests for funding they receive when particular treatments are not encompassed in a local service agreements; general practitioners continue to treat individual patients on their lists whilst carrying out commissioning roles within primary care groups and trusts.

The new agenda for public health offers some exciting opportunities, but also makes a number of fresh demands on practitioners who need to adapt to different ways of thinking and new roles. At the same time, there is much continuity in the principles, the underlying philosophy and the knowledge base that inform grass roots practice. The opening two chapters examine in some detail the shifts and similarities in these principles and philosophies as roles change in nursing and in health visiting, while the third chapter considers the overall place of health promotion in the field of public health.

The changing policy agenda that has given rise to these new functions and the increased emphasis on public health are considered in more detail in the second section of the book. Public health requires an ability to plan and develop practice-based strategies to meet identified needs. Chapter 4 explains the organisational changes and developments that have been designed to create innovations and a more equitable approach to service delivery, with a clear focus on health improvement, rather than on maintaining services in their traditional form and place. Next, primary care is considered, as it has long been seen as the key to enhancing the public's health; policies to make this a reality have led to enormous organisational upheavals in the way health improvement strategies are planned and delivered. The process of needs assessment is essential to discover where priorities should lie, and suitable approaches are explained in the middle chapter of this section. Once needs have been identified, sound research evidence to support the implementation of preferred strategies is fundamental in determining directions for practice. A strong quality agenda has focused renewed attention on the importance of effectiveness; services and strategies can be planned meaningfully only where there is sufficient knowledge of 'what works' to be clear about future planning. One chapter explains how 'clinical effectiveness' is determined and used in order to inform treatment and commissioning decisions, whilst a second emphasises the importance of understanding and using different types of evidence when considering the effectiveness of empowerment practice or community-wide strategies.

The final section returns to the paradox highlighted in the first. As a sphere of activity and interest, public health cannot function at a single, individual level; yet it cannot progress without involving those people who make up the population, and whose individual states of illness or well-being are collectively described as the 'public health'. The work of grass roots public health practitioners is characterised by their operating at the point where individuals and populations meet and cross over – in the local community. They may work with individuals in order to achieve a collective benefit, as in community development work, or across communities to improve facilities and knowledge used by individuals, as when promoting breastfeeding. There is clear evidence to show that a focus on family support is essential to begin to tackle the most fundamental root causes of health inequalities. Likewise, looked-after children or those in need of protection are amongst the vulnerable and disadvantaged groups who need to be regarded as a public health priority in many areas.

The chapters in the final section explore the practicalities of working in each of these four priority areas, an example of how public health is implemented at this grass-roots level. In contributing to the public health, the overall good of the population, rather than the specific needs of individuals, is always considered paramount. However, this apparently simple approach can create enormous tensions in the practice situation, which are not easily resolved. This text does not claim either to resolve those tensions, or to provide all the answers needed to work at the grass roots in public health. Overall, it does aim to unravel the source of some of the difficulties, to explore the new policy agenda and provide readers with a sound evidence base from which to examine the different approaches to practice. It is offered as a sourcebook for those health visitors and community nurses who are either struggling to understand the new public health agenda, or who are already enthusiastic but would appreciate a collection of material relevant to their practice.

Tunbridge Wells 2001   Sarah Cowley

REFERENCES

Acheson D 1998 Independent inquiry into inequalities in health. The Stationery Office, London

Department of Health 1998 Chief Medical Officer's Project to Strengthen the Public Health Function in England: a report of the emerging findings. Department of Health, London

World Health Organization 1999 Health 21: Health for all in the 21st century. European Health for all series No. 6. World Health Organization, Copenhagen

Acknowledgement

Special thanks to Karen Gilmour of Harcourt Publishers who has kept this project going from start to finish.

1 'GRASS ROOTS PRACTICE' IN PUBLIC HEALTH

INTRODUCTION TO SECTION I

Sarah Cowley

The whole idea of 'public health' has created considerable discussion and confusion, perhaps because it is an immensely complex concept that encompasses many different, often contested views that have changed a great deal over time. The same might be said of both nursing and health visiting. The first section of the book is intended to open these issues out for examination and to explore how they operate in practice. It begins by confronting a debate that is often considered a taboo subject: the links in practice between health visiting and nursing. In statute, the two are distinct professions, yet since both began to be regulated by the same body (the United Kingdom Central Council for Nursing, Midwifery and Health Visiting (UKCC)), there has been an increasing tendency to treat them as if they were a single entity (Cowley et al 2000). Chapter one deconstructs the practice of both groups, exploring the important differences and, equally important, similarities in the ways both contribute to public health. Four polarised concepts are described that need negotiating in practice:

- whether individual or population needs dominate service provision
- whether the focus of care belongs in the public or private domain
- whether to focus on determinants of health or treating established problems
- if a social or biomedical model of health is prioritised.

These are used to explain how nursing and health visiting set out to emphasise different aspects in the delivery of their service; each may be frustrated in their intentions or not, but both can make a significant contribution to public health. The chapter also considers the changing nature of practice in primary care, and the increasing breadth of the community nursing role, in relation to public health.

It is interesting to note that the Chief Medical Oficer's project (Department of Health 1998), cited in the preface, distinguishes between health visitors and public health nurses, listing both as having a hands-on role in contributing to public health. The UKCC (1998), on the other hand, conflates the two titles, inferring that 'public health nursing: health visiting' are one and the same. In Chapter 2, Craig challenges this kind of conceptual slurring, unravelling the relationships between health visiting, nursing and public health, both historically and internationally. She concludes that, over time, 'public health health visiting' has come together with 'public health nursing' in the UK; she particularly notes the similarities between health visiting and school nursing. Although both have maintained separate roles since the nineteenth century, there is a new policy suggestion that the two should be merged into a single discipline in Scotland (Scottish Executive Health Department 2000). Further details are promised early in 2001, when a report of the review of the contribution of nurses, midwives and health visitors to improving the public's health is promised. In England, too, those two groups are closely linked in a single health visiting/school nursing development project, which is intended to develop the public health focus of the services in line with functions spelt out in an earlier strategy document (Department of Health 1999).

Craig further identifies the significance of different political perspectives on the practice of public health nursing and health visiting, as collectivist, community approaches are supported or not by successive governments. Twinn (1991) has noted the extent of unresolved contradictions in health visiting over the years; she links this with long-standing professional and philosophical dilemmas about how health promotion is best achieved. These debates are picked up in the final chapter of this introductory section, which looks at health promotion, and its relationship to health, public health and primary care. Pearson illustrates how adopting different philosophical perspectives can have a clear impact on the way work is approached. An illness perspective is very different from one that emphasises positive health (salutogenesis). Also, lay people may hold views that differ from those adopted by professionals, but their perspectives are important in their own right. Social, medical and lay forms of knowledge are all explored in depth. Pearson shows how these different theoretical perspectives underpin health promotion work in practice, whether the practitioner is working with individuals, groups, organisations or at policy level in pursuit of public health.

Being a politically charged, multiprofessional endeavour with a very long history, it is, perhaps, inevitable that public health will provide a great deal of food for thought, debate and discussion. Taken together, these three chapters are intended to set the scene for the rest of the book, introducing the reader to the variety of different views and contradictions. Hopefully, they also begin the illustrate the extent to which there are enduring principles and areas of agreement in the field of public health.

REFERENCES

Cowley S, Buttigieg M, Houston A 2000 A first steps project to scope the current and future regulatory issues for health visiting. Florence Nightingale School of Nursing and Midwifery, King's College, London (Unpublished report to United Kingdom Central Council for Nursing, Midwifery and Health Visiting)

Department of Health 1998 Chief Medical Officer's Project to Strengthen the Public Health Function in England: a report of the emerging findings. Department of Health, London

Department of Health 1999 Making a Difference: strengthening the nursing, health visiting and midwifery contribution to health and healthcare. Department of Health, London

Scottish Executive Health Department 2000 Our National Health: A plan for action, a plan for change. The Stationery Office, Edinburgh.

Twinn S 1991 Conflicting paradigms of health visiting: a continuing debate for professional practice. Journal of Advanced Nursing 16:966–973

United Kingdom Central Council for Nursing, Midwifery and Health Visiting 1998 Standards for specialist education and practice. UKCC, London

1 Public health practice in nursing and health visiting

Sarah Cowley

KEY ISSUES

- Nursing, health visiting and public health are three occupational groups that have much in common as well as a number of clear differences. This gives rise to many contradictions in practice, although the contribution made by each group is important in its own right.
- An increase in inequalities in health has given rise to a new political focus on public health approaches as a way of reducing them. In turn, this has led to an expansion in the scope and meaning of 'public health' and to its development as a distinctive, multidisciplinary profession.
- The implications of these developments and the complementary public health contributions that can be made by nurses and health visitors in practice are unravelled in some detail.
- Some key concepts are prioritised differently according to the public health purpose being served by each occupational group. Examples are given to show how decisional control, professional and client autonomy, empowerment and consumer choice are all influenced by whether:
  - the priority focus is on individuals or whole populations
  - the service is mainly about the determinants of health or caring for people with established health problems
  - the social or biomedical model of health is prioritised
  - matters are considered the legitimate interest of publicly funded health services or should remain private.
- Their diversity and the wide range of different health needs mean there are many ways that nurses and health visitors can contribute effectively to public health.

INTRODUCTION

Both public health and nursing encompass a huge and rapidly expanding body of knowledge. In each case, the knowledge and related policies are intertwined and inseparable from a range of other, equally vast and highly respected theoretical perspectives. Health visiting is a practice discipline that has an interest in both nursing and public health, yet it fits neatly in neither. This dual allegiance gives rise to a multitude of contradictions and competing demands on practitioners; as well a range of opportunities that may be lost or gained in all three professional areas of interest and, more importantly, on the public whose health is under consideration. Nursing, as Johnson points out, is a social construct; he describes (Johnson 1999 p 68) it as:

'A mode of social organization for the delivery of (mainly) care, comfort and treatment to the ill.'

By and large, people would recognise this familiar description of the sphere of practice engaged in by nursing, but the 'mainly' in brackets is important, because of course there are exceptions. We might debate the extent to which people with profound disabilities are actually 'ill' for example, or insist that the term 'treatment' be extended to encompass rehabilitation and some preventive care. However, the *organisation of nursing* in various health care systems – such as in the NHS, for example – mostly assumes that nurses not only deliver care, comfort and treatment, but (notwithstanding the presence of relatives, family rooms and occasional group therapy) that they do so on a basis that recognises each ill person as a significantly important individual, who will usually have a medically defined condition of some kind.

Specialist public health, on the other hand (Lessof et al 1999 p 3):

'...addresses the totality of issues that interact to determine the public's health and carries responsibility for it. It is inherently multidisciplinary and denotes a determined focus on issues that impact on the health of populations at a complex strategic or managerial level.'

Public health is also a social construct; it is based on a population perspective and is concerned (mainly) with ensuring that the health of the public as a whole is sufficiently strong to ensure that society is able to function in a manner that is socially and politically determined as appropriate. Placing 'mainly' in brackets again serves as a warning against stereotypical assumptions about social control or abstract managerialism. Public health has a very clear history of personal compassion, social concern and philanthropy directed at individuals, but the key message is that public health is about collectives and populations, and that it is as much about social and political concepts as medical ones.

So, at first glance, nursing and public health appear quite at odds with each another: one is individually focused, one is about society as a whole. This introductory chapter will explore those contradictions through four phases. First, it will explain the expanding scope of public health and why it has risen so high on the government's agenda, and second, how it is being developed as a distinctive, multidisciplinary profession. Third, the implications of these developments and the complementary public health contributions that can be made by nurses and health visitors in practice will be unravelled in some detail. Finally, some brief concluding comments will consider the opportunities arising from these diverse issues for the three practice disciplines of nursing, public health and health visiting.

EXPANDING SCOPE OF PUBLIC HEALTH

The root causes or main 'determinants' of health have now been clearly identified: Figure 1.1 is much cited as a framework for action in planning national and international strategies. Nursing sits mainly within the 'health service' sector, and it is salutary to acknowledge how small that seems when viewed from a multiagency public health perspective. The government appointed a Minister for Public Health for the first time in 1997; this minister had

FIGURE 1.1   *Determinants of health (Dahlgren & Whitehead 1999).*

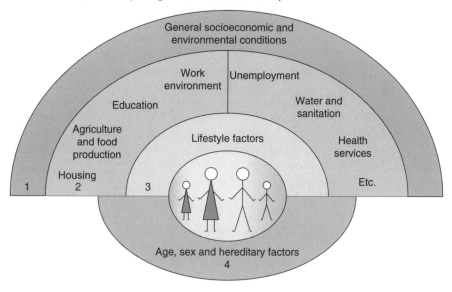

cross-departmental responsibility to coordinate issues across government. The English public health strategy (Department of Health 1998a, 1999) recognises the importance of all these other services in determining health, and the importance of collaboration is mirrored in policies across the United Kingdom (Department of Health and Social Services 1999, Scottish Assembly 1999, Welsh Office 1998).

Early work in identifying the 'determinants of health' tended to regard age, sex and hereditary factors as fixed and unchangeable. Developments in the science of genetics look set to challenge this perception quite dramatically over the next century. Parallels might be drawn with an exciting, new, but then ill-defined theory discovered in the second half of the nineteenth century, that indicated the importance of germs as the cause of many diseases. That revelation changed our whole understanding of disease processes; public health and nursing services changed to reflect the therapeutic interventions that became available in ways that could not have been predicted a hundred years ago. Likewise, at the end of the twentieth century:

> 'The breathtaking and rapidly expanding technology of the 'new genetics' has the potential to revolutionize the way we conceptualise the prevention and management of disease.' (World Health Organization 1999 p 68)

We cannot generally presume to change our biological heritage, sex or age just yet. However, there is a new emphasis on postponing the age at which disability or dependence occurs: in an ageing society, instead of seeking only to extend life-expectancy, the main aim now is to promote independence for longer. Personal and private interpretations of what counts as 'independent' and how that can be achieved are immensely varied, but autonomy is a central feature of health that potentially outweighs the significance of many behavioural, so-called 'lifestyle' factors (Rijke 1993).

These personal perceptions are mediated by the cultural, psychological and social environment in which individuals live. So, the outer 'ring' of Dahlgren and Whitehead's diagram (Figure 1.1) could, perhaps, be further sub-divided. The physical environment was one of the first determinants of health to be recognised and it continues to be highly significant. In addition, the 'social environment' is beginning to recognised as very important mediator of health (Marmot & Wilkinson 1999). The term 'social environment' is not explained or defined in policy, but it is held to include some key features (Listed in Box 1.1).

The inclusion of 'crime' in a policy about health seems unlikely at first glance, but being a victim of crime, or indeed a criminal – at least one that is convicted and imprisoned – is clearly bad for health. Also, Kennedy et al (1998) have shown significant correlations between increases in violent crime and widening inequalities in health.

These authors, among others, use the terms 'social environment' and 'social capital' interchangeably. 'Social capital' is increasingly promoted as an important mediator of health in highly unequal societies like Britain (Campbell et al 1999, Gillies 1998, Wilkinson 1996). The term itself is contentious, but it refers to the norms of reciprocity and networks of civic engagement that become embedded and enacted through moral resources such as trust and cooperation, across the whole social system and not only by individuals. A cohesive society is one that has a demonstrably high level of these resources, which are cumulatively described as social capital. They are affected by styles of government, democratic structures and involvement in local organisations (Putnam 1993).

This has implications for public health, for policy initiatives and for the people whose daily living experiences reflect what it is like to live in a socially cohesive society or one that offers residents stress, violence and social exclusion. Three residents interviewed for a family health needs project (Cowley & Billings 1997) describe the stresses:

> 'You get a gang come up at sort of 7 o'clock at night ... you can't tell them to go away 'cos they'll put a brick through your window.'

> 'In [estate] they're f ...-ing and blinding, they're screaming at their children, they're having screaming matches at one another all the time.'

> 'The seven year old, she'll be invited out by a friend, and then you invite them back here, as soon as they find out it's this estate, well, they won't come.'

That final, stigmatising rejection illustrates that the stresses arising from a poor social environment are not only about poverty; although the first two of these

BOX 1.1	Key features of the 'social environment' (Department of Health 1998a paras 2.15–2.17)
	1. Quality of life in the community
	2. Social exclusion
	3. Social isolation
	4. The extent to which people respect and support each other
	5. Neighbourhoods where people know and trust each other
	6. Neighbourhoods where people have a say in the way the community is run
	7. Crime, fear of crime in the community, youth crime

informants were single parents living on welfare benefits. A positive social environment clearly encompasses a more varied range of resources for health, but material resources can help to compensate for other difficulties, as some other quotes suggest:

> 'Everybody gossips like frantic but I think that's fairly good because then you do know what's going on, which is helpful. People will come and tell you when your children are doing wrong things!'

> 'There is a great community spirit; this unseen underground network where everybody helps each other because everyone is in a similar position.'

> 'Playgrounds and that sort of thing are, I think, pretty poor and play, open play areas for children here are not very good [but] there's a country park that lays just over there but I suppose it's about ten minutes in the car.'

These examples are all drawn from the same town; they illustrate the kind of inequalities that exist in the UK, which is in many ways a typical example of a 'developed society'.

Public health records of deaths and health treatments show that most developed countries have passed through what Wilkinson (1996) terms an 'epidemiological transition'. This point marks the change from infectious disease as the biggest health hazard, to a situation in which most people die of degenerative disorders. Traditionally, the accompanying increases in life-expectancy have been attributed to economic gain and improvements in the physical environment, but this explanation fails to account for changes in population health once countries have passed through the epidemiological transition.

Epidemiological studies suggest that the psychosocial liberalisation that accompanies economic development may be a major determinant of health. This refers to the collective increase in personal freedoms and individual choices for people as their material situation improves. However, if these improvements are unequally spread across societies, the inequalities seem, themselves, to be a cause of disease. The biological impact of absolute poverty is not questioned, but Wilkinson (1996) shows that the psychosocial and emotional stresses that accompany material insecurity and relative disadvantage are additional, major health hazards. The causal pathways are not clear, but a growing number of studies about health inequalities show that whatever it is that produces these variations affects the whole of society, not just people living in poverty.

This propensity to spread across society explains the public health interest in the phenomena of social exclusion and the opposite, preferred, state of social cohesion that occurs when a rich store of social capital exists. All of this emphasises that by its very nature, public health is interlinked with policy and is, therefore, a very contested and political sphere of action.

Even definitions can be contentious, but the most widely accepted one suggests that public health is:

> '…the science and art of preventing disease, prolonging life, promoting, protecting and improving health and well-being through the organised efforts of society.' (Acheson 1988)

The public health paradox

It is the focus on the 'organised efforts of society' in the above definition that demonstrates the essential link to policy, whether at a national, international or local level. Public health has implications for every person, and each individual's health has an effect on the accumulated health of the public. This gives rise to a profound paradox:

■ As a sphere of activity and interest, public health cannot function at a single, individual level; yet it cannot progress without involving those people who make up the population, and whose individual states of illness or well-being are collectively described as the 'public health'.

This paradox inevitably creates tensions and contradictions about whether supremacy should be afforded to the clinically-based or population-based activities, and the extent to which these should fall within public or private spheres of action. A further contradiction is inevitable. Independence, autonomy and empowerment are significant and provide a necessary basis for individual health, yet decisions made to protect the health of the public as a whole may sometimes, of necessity, seem to limit the extent of personal choice. However, given the potential damage to society as a whole from increasing inequalities in health, and the need to reduce social exclusion, when a new government was elected in the UK in 1997 they considered that a stronger public health orientation was needed.

DEVELOPING THE PUBLIC HEALTH FUNCTION

The government set in train a series of enquiries and projects intended to redefine and strengthen the public health function under the auspices of the Chief Medical Officer (CMO). His initial project report (Department of Health 1998b) identified three levels of contribution to the public health function:

1. 'Most professionals,' including Local Authority and National Health Service (NHS) managers, teachers and health workers, whose daily work involves 'furthering health improvement goals' but who may not recognise this as a contribution to public health.
2. A smaller group of 'hands-on' public health practitioners who spend a substantial part of their working practice furthering health by working with communities and groups – includes public health nurses, health promotion specialists, health visitors, community development workers and environmental health officers.
3. A still smaller group of 'public health specialists' who come from a variety of professional backgrounds and experience, and who need a core of knowledge, skills and experience.

A feasibility study was carried out to establish agreement about the core of knowledge and skills needed, and to establish national standards required by a public health specialist from any background (Lessof et al 1999). These standards have been accepted in principle as a marker for a new profession; the government signalled their acceptance of this multiprofessional approach by accepting that, in future, it will not be necessary for Directors of Public Health to be drawn exclusively from the ranks of the medical profession (Department of Health 1999). The first steps toward setting up a register for public health professionals are underway and degree programmes are being developed so that school leavers can have the option to go straight into a public health career.

Nurses have a contribution to make to public health at each of the three levels highlighted by the CMO's project. Around 8% of the staff employed in the public health departments of commissioning authorities currently hold a nursing qualification (Baker 1999). In future, they will need to meet the nationally agreed standards to progress in their careers, but some are already acknowledged as public health specialists, along with colleagues from other disciplines.

The middle-sized group contains those singled out as 'hands-on' public health practitioners; these include health visitors, school and occupational health nurses, communicable disease nurses and possibly infection control nurses (see Standing Nursing and Midwifery Advisory Committee 1995). There is a debate in some quarters about the extent to which these practitioners can really be regarded as wholly public health workers, because their activities are not always directed solely at a 'population level', although those who work in community development and mainly with groups tend to be granted approval. Pauline Craig (Chapter 2) details the history and background to these debates.

Community development workers and those who provide an outreach function to particularly vulnerable groups are singled out for 'public health approval' because their primary responsibility lies with the entire population of the particular community (which may be defined as a locality, a school or workplace), rather than with individuals who have reached their caseload through referral from other sources, as is the case with most other community nurses. So, it is important to recognise that the distinction between 'individually-focused' and 'population-based' work relates to the scope of responsibility and focus for prioritising decisions, not to the specific task or type of activity engaged in.

Many terms are altogether too poorly specified, under-theorised and interlinked in practice to serve as categorical markers through which to assign any particular activity as being 'public health work' or not. There is no reason to suppose that the individual learning that occurs in a group is any more about public health than that which occurs in a one-to-one setting, for example. It makes no sense for a health visitor whose work is exclusively focused on a homeless population to be considered more legitimately concerned with public health than one who addresses the same issues about homelessness as one problem among others faced by an individual. And community development work requires practitioners to engage with individual members of the local population in order to activate any projects that are deemed necessary (see Chapter 10).

It is easy to understand why nursing, an occupation that prides itself on its ability to deliver individualised care, personally tailored to the needs of each particular patient, may find a great deal of difficulty in engaging with a practice philosophy that appears to raise questions about whether that is always the right approach. Recognising this philosophical dilemma, the World Health Organization (1999) challenges the usefulness of maintaining a division between individually focused clinical practice and public health, suggesting that health care should, instead, be seen as a continuous link of actions that all contribute in different ways to enhancing health.

Such a collaborative stance cannot be questioned, but it runs the risk of fudging the difficult issues rather than confronting and solving the dilemmas in practice. More usefully, Hicks reminds us that health services, themselves, constitute one of the determinants of health, particularly in developed societies. He suggests that:

> 'The *goal* of public health practice is to maintain and improve the health of populations. The *practice* of public health involves identifying determinants of health and effective means of influencing them, and then applying that knowledge in practice. ... To be *effective*, a public health practitioner must influence at least one determinant of health.' (Hicks 1999 p 224; my emphasis)

This begins to offer a way in which to clarify the contribution made to public health in different practice spheres, by offering a conceptual basis to explain the work. The next section will use these ideas and the concepts identified so far to analyse the slightly different approaches to practice in nursing and in health visiting, to explain the contribution each makes to public health.

NURSING AND HEALTH VISITING IN PUBLIC HEALTH PRACTICE

There is a huge range of nursing titles in use around the world that each reflect something of the health care systems in which practitioners work, even if they provide little guidance about differences or similarities of the services they deliver, or the actual type of work undertaken. A 'public health nurse' in one country may undertake a very similar role to a 'community nurse' or 'primary care nurse' in another, for instance. The importance attached to education, qualification or regulation is immensely varied internationally, as is the extent to which practitioners are expected, or permitted the power, to engage in public health activities.

Multiple titles exist within the UK too. In 1999, the government affirmed their commitment to maintaining health visiting as a separate qualification and profession regulated alongside, but not within, nursing (NHS Executive 1999). Health visiting does not exist in many countries in the same form as in the UK, but where it does, the title always signifies a priority focus upon public health and prevention, rather than the delivery of clinical interventions. Health visiting developed within the burgeoning public health movement in Victorian England, precisely because of the need to bridge the gap between individual and population-wide policies (Symonds 1991), and between the ever-contested and contradictory concepts outlined above.

By the beginning of the twentieth century, most health visiting was undertaken by women sanitary inspectors who, unlike their male colleagues, could gain entry to the private sphere of the home (Davies 1988). However, also unlike the men (who were to evolve into today's environmental health officers) women in those days were forbidden from requiring male landlords to improve the slum dwellings that caused so much ill-health. From the start, therefore, health visiting required practitioners that were able to work in a contradictory domain. As the twentieth century progressed, these more radical ties diminished as links were made with midwifery and then nursing (Dingwall 1977). This connection means that health visitors have increasingly been managed, educated and their service organised as if their role and purpose was, like nursing, (mainly) concerned with the provision of individualised care to particular clients with established problems. That approach fails to recognise that there are as many contradictions in the sphere of health visiting practice today as there were over 100 years ago. It remains extremely difficult for health visitors to maintain public health values in practice because of the way their service is organised (Cowley 1997).

Experiences in public health practice

There are four polarised constructs summarised in Box 1.2, in which nursing and health visiting each have different emphases or priorities, and which each create different dilemmas in practice stemming from their basis in public health. Making a choice that favours one option or the other does not lead to any better or more virtuous approaches in practice. As the World Health Organization (1999) point out, different ways of operating and prioritising each have their place across the totality of service provision, and each require a particular ability to implement successfully. However, the way a service is constructed, the way practitioners are educated and the way they are managed will, at any one time, privilege the implementation of some approaches in practice and inhibit others. It follows from this that 'success' depends largely upon getting those constructs right for each occupational group or team. Depending upon traditional views of 'nursing,' 'health visiting' or 'public health', or insisting on conformity to one style or another across the board, is bound to lead to difficulties in practice.

The rest of this section will use excerpts of data taken from three studies (Cowley 1991, Bergen et al 1996, Cowley & Billings 1997) to illustrate points and explain how these contradictions affect real people; both members of

BOX 1.2	*Polarised concepts and priorities in public health*	
	Individual/population	Encompasses not only service responsibilities, but also points to the dilemmas inherent in choosing between personal rights and collective responsibilities within society as a whole
	Public/private	Access and use of public services such as health and nursing care is related to both personal perceptions and wider social views about what they should be for, and what remains 'properly' private
	Determinants/treatments	Services may be designed to directly target the determinants of health ('root causes') or to treat established problems by offering clinical treatments to affected individuals
	Social/biomedical model	Views are changing and contested about whether a social or biomedical view of health is considered paramount in promoting the public health

the public whose health is the focus of attention and the practitioners contributing to public health. These data are used to put a 'human face' on an otherwise abstract and conceptual analysis and to unravel some of the differences in nursing and health visiting practice.

Speaking of the emergency care her baby received, for example, one mother said:

> '...she fell back and smacked her head on the concrete ... she was admitted to hospital. Yes and I actually stayed up there with her, and she was in there for a couple of days ... I thought they were really good, I mean, they actually sort of like come in every ten, twenty minutes checking on her and stuff like that, it was good, I liked that.' (Cowley & Billings 1997)

This description highlights the kind of emergency services that we take for granted in the UK and in developed societies. They are, of course, a significant part of the 'civic community' and the formal resources that contribute to social capital. At the height of the Kosovo conflict in 1999, a television report illustrated what happens when this is missing. A very confused and elderly Serb lady had been shown to a journalist by worried neighbours. When he entered the flat he found the decomposing body of her husband who had died, apparently of natural causes, some days earlier. But there were no emergency services, no one to help her and no trust because the local population was divided. The war had resulted in a breakdown and complete loss of the civic community.

Just knowing that a service will be there when it is needed is hugely significant in terms of health – while knowing that such help cannot be relied upon is immensely harmful. So the very existence of acute, high-dependency and emergency services makes a major contribution to the social environment and thence to the public health. Embedded within the above examples too, are the assumption and expectation that it is socially acceptable and correct to seek hospital care when these kinds of emergency arise.

There is an increasing expectation that high-dependency and acute care should be equally available at home, and community nursing services all reach into an essentially private setting. When people think of 'health services' and 'nursing', it is often this kind of high-intensity care that comes to mind:

> 'I did have a problem a couple of weeks ago where this gentleman was coming home and was only given a couple of days, but he wanted to come home to die ... He's got three days and he did last three days ...
> I pleaded on the phone and social services got a reclining chair for him.'
> (District nurse cited in Bergen et al 1996)

This description fits with the social construct of nursing mentioned at the start of the chapter, as a mode of social organization for the delivery of (mainly) care, comfort and treatment to individuals who are ill. Delivery of such care in the home is promoted as a way of allowing people to maintain greater control over their own health, even in the face of high needs. Enabling and allowing individuals and families to develop a capacity for coping with their own health needs in their own way is a mechanism for promoting independence, autonomy and, ultimately, health.

However, family-based care leads to increasing complexity and a need for greater skill on the part of the practitioner, as this excerpt suggests:

'During the observation period a district nurse described a situation where she had to balance a mother's anxiety about the child's ability to eat whilst undergoing chemotherapy with the child's need for the cytotoxic agent, and the resultant lack of appetite. Explanations, negotiations and reassurance were not enough to prevent the mother from withdrawing the child from treatment if his appetite became suppressed beyond the mother's ability to cope ...' (Bergen et al 1996)

Given the complexity of this situation, the polarised and contested concepts listed in Box 1.2 allow the identification of some clearly defined aspects to help decide how the service should be constructed and the effectiveness of care evaluated. The individual child is clearly the patient; medical treatment is a priority but the nurse must also consider and provide for the concerns of the mother. Timing is of the essence. Treatment cannot be delayed to explore societal norms and maternal expectations surrounding a child's appetite, although they may be relevant. Choices for immediate action are limited, because there is a clear, overriding priority shared between client and practitioner, that treating the child's disease must come first. Using Hicks' (1999) proposition that effective clinical care is a significant determinant of health, this kind of sensitive care is clearly contributing to the public health overall.

To support his strong defence that individual clinical interventions make a major contribution to the public health, Hicks cites studies that have shown their collected impact upon whole populations. Potentially, three of the extra 7 years of life-expectancy since 1950 can be attributed to the accumulated effect of clinical interventions. Also, medical care may be expected to provide around 5 years of partial or complete relief from the poor quality of life associated with chronic disease (Bunker et al 1994, Bunker 1995).

Health visiting services, too, provide immediate acute care if required; prior arrangements might have to be reorganised to deal with this kind of situation, for example:

'There are crises that have to be sorted out. I can't say to someone who 'phones me up and says: "Please come, I'm DESPERATE", "I can't come because I'm ...", you would go, and it depends on what you saw. If the child is being battered or the mother was going to have – or had – a nervous breakdown, you would have to do all the emergency things that any other professional would do ...' (Health visitor cited in Cowley 1991)

The timing and immediate availability of care-delivery is of the essence here. Indeed, in this tranche of data, 'timing' appeared to be what distinguished an approach that the health visitors almost universally called 'crisis work'. There were no parallels with the psychiatric theories of crisis intervention in these data, nor did the severity of a case decide whether it was considered 'a crisis'. In many examples there were no diagnosed diseases, illness or disability, despite perceived and expressed distress, but the sense of immediacy was always present as a defining feature. Most health visitors expressed a degree of resignation, accepting that such needs required an immediate response, so they would have to reorganise other planned activities. Even so, once this type of approach became dominant in an area, a number made similar remarks, in apparent contradiction:

'We were all doing crisis visiting, and we were all so demoralised
because that's not health visiting, just crisis visiting ...' (Health visitor
cited in Cowley 1991)

The difficulty in assimilating this kind of crisis work into a public health role
lies in the fact that the underlying causes of the problem are not being tackled.
There is little clarity about whether the client is the mother, the child or the
family as a whole, which inevitably inhibits clear evaluations. Furthermore, the
determinants of health that create the crisis situations lie in the wider social
environment, even if they are manifest within a single family. Effective health
services only help the individuals they reach, and many people need help with
recognising that such a service might be useful for them, for example:

'It turned out there were all sorts of problems in her [client's] own life
which were impacting on her relationship with her husband and their
relationship with the children and she had not realised but she thought it
was one of those things and she just had to live with it ... it has to be
done very gently, because we want to work with clients and we need to
maintain their trust.' (Health visitor cited in Cowley 1991)

Often, when health visitors begin working in such complex situations, there are
few identifiable points of clarity; it is clear only that there is suffering of some
kind, and that there is an unspecified risk. Something may go wrong with someone's health, perhaps the child's development will be adversely affected by the
mother's depression; child abuse might be a risk. Or there may already be an
underlying problem that has not yet been identified: perhaps the person's
marriage is abusive, domestic violence affects people from all walks of life.
While there is a clear need to relate to the person concerned in a positive and
therapeutic way, the prospect of reaching any kind of official, medical diagnosis remains quite distant, if indeed one is possible. Adverse childhood experiences or domestic disharmony are rarely revealed at the first encounter and
may never be specified. Similar sensitivities surround interpersonal and family
relationships which are, after all, intimate and intensely personal, as this
informant revealed in interview:

'I remember seeing my notes down at the surgery one time and a couple
of remarks on there were "marital problems" and I was incensed ... you
don't want it down on paper necessarily. You know, they, when people
have lots of problems that they don't necessarily want somebody to
write down they – she has that because of that; because it could be
fleeting, it could be a lot of other things that were affecting it as well,
not just that one thing say ...' (Mother cited in Cowley & Billings 1997)

Unlike the life-and-death needs of an injured child or someone with a diagnosed
illness, the kinds of sensitive issues mentioned here are extremely private,
and there is no social agreement that the public domain of the health service
exists to help with such situations. Indeed, once a difficult time has passed,
people may not want to be reminded that it happened; that does not mean
that they wanted to be left without help at the time when they were suffering.
And if practitioners do not maintain at least minimal records, their work
remains invisible, unaccountable and open to charges that their practice is
ineffective.

Extensive involvement of family members in such complex situations is almost universal. At times, the high levels of sensitivity and lack of clarity may be such that it is not even possible to be sure who, within a family, has the most pressing needs. What if there are suspicions that a child is currently vulnerable to the kind of abuse experienced by the mother in this example?

'I had someone who had an awful lot – was troubled by a lot of depression, and couldn't really cope, not managing with the family. So once I sat down with her a lot came out, like she was abused as a child and that was why, or might be why she couldn't cope with things. Also the sexual relationship with her husband wasn't right ...' (Health visitor cited in Cowley 1991)

Whose rights should be paramount – is the mother's privacy more important than the child's protection? The family focus of the service in such cases means that health visitors can assess, care, offer support and sensitivity; timing interventions and referrals to other services according to professional judgement and careful negotiations with the family. Indeed, the professional skill of the practitioner might make the difference between whether or not such disadvantaged people are ever able to access effective medical, social or psychological care. As with emergency care for a physically or mentally ill person, the existence of such facilitating services increases the sense of civic community, and confidence that society as whole can be trusted to care for its most vulnerable members.

Yet to ignore the wider determinants and the whole social environment is to severely limit the public health contribution and risk unending increases in such family dilemmas. When the data were collected for this study, about 10 years ago, it was still unusual for health visiting services to be offered in any form other than by individual, face-to-face contact. But there was a growing realisation that such an approach was insufficient to challenge or change the underlying determinants of health and a still-familiar frustration about the difficulty practitioners face in trying to find time to undertake a meaningful level of work directly targeting the community.

'I think maybe it'll mean that some health visitors should maybe specialise in – so there isn't this terrible conflict between trying to do some community development and the needs of your own caseload ... In theory, yes; even in practice I'm saying yes, but I'm not saying it's compatible with a caseload.' (Health visitor cited in Cowley 1991)

The terms 'social environment' and 'social capital' were not in general use in 1991, but a great deal was known about the importance of social networks, of social support and building self-esteem; there was a growing awareness of the importance of working to develop networks across the community. The idea that 'individual needs' are located within the caseload is borne of long experience. The accountability of practitioners to individuals accepted on their caseload (Cowley & Andrews 2001) and inflexible contract specifications combine to create an overriding view that the treatment of existing, established needs must take priority within health service provision over the prevention of future problems.

In the Family Health Needs Project, Cowley and Billings (1997) began by compiling a profile of health needs in the local area; the extent of deprivation was measurably high and revealed the root causes of the problems. The summary (Box 1.3) might apply to any deprived area.

No one denied the accuracy of the root causes of ill-health identified in the profile, which was extensive. Indeed, the issues were so apparent that it was obvious they were correct. Even so, it took around 18 months of lobbying, negotiating, bargaining, networking and persistence before a coalition of funding agencies was formed through which a single post was established, initially for 2 years (Cowley & Billings 1999a). The post-holder was to direct attention to the community as a whole, to change the underlying social causes of the measured health problems. This meant that more emphasis would be placed on issues common to the whole community, than to concentrating on individuals and their problems in isolation.

Getting even limited funding felt like a major achievement, but most community development posts are funded similarly on a short-term basis and come into being only after a considerable struggle (Billingham & Perkins 1997). After all, such activities do not fit with the social construction of health services and clinical practice, which are concerned with the provision of individualised nursing care to particular clients with established problems. There were plenty of these. In that locality, there was never an option to substitute community development work for the kind of sensitive, individualised care required to deal with the problems encountered on a daily basis by the health visitors (Cowley & Billings 1999b). These were pressing and urgent, echoing the 'terrible dilemma' identified by the health visitor trying to develop a community approach alongside her caseload work some 10 years earlier.

The social environment is emerging as a key determinant of health, and looks set to be as significant in the future as the physical environment has been shown to be in the past. Trust is a key component in establishing the 'civic community'

BOX 1.3	Patterns of deprivation (Cowley & Billings 1997)	
	Poor physical environment	■ Chronically high levels of unemployment ■ Poor housing: high levels of private rented accommodation ■ Low income levels; low car ownership ■ Poor mortality rates
	Poor psychosocial environment	■ Illicit drugs readily available ■ High levels of juvenile crime ■ Changing family structures creating instability ■ Lack of social support in local area
	Problems reflected on health visiting caseloads	■ Excessive rates of long-term, limiting illnesses ■ Poor mental health, rising depression rates: pre- and postnatal mothers ■ Twice the national incidence of detected child abuse ■ Commonly reported behavioural problems ■ Self-mutilation/attempted suicide among young people ■ High levels of family tensions and bullying ■ School bullying, truancy and classroom disruption ■ Increasing numbers of single parents; difficulty in coping

and the networks of reciprocity that are needed to mediate health in local areas or neighbourhoods; one part of that is knowing that effective health and nursing services will be available when needed. Equally important is the need for autonomy and individual independence; yet the need to develop social capital and tackle the root causes of inequalities in health may mean concentrating on issues common to the whole community rather than prioritising individual needs. Overall, this agenda represents a need for a vast range of services and skills to promote, enhance and maintain the health of the population – the public health.

OPPORTUNITIES FOR THE PRACTICE DISCIPLINES

This chapter began by linking together and distinguishing between three practice disciplines: nursing, public health and health visiting. The diversity of the whole public agenda is huge and expanding; the planning of strategies and services to meet them across the board is a clear challenge. Dahlgren and Whitehead (1991) created their diagram (Figure 1.1) of the determinants of health partly to serve as a guide to such planning at the level of national, or at least regional, service provision.

However, as noted above, despite being so large in terms of its members and potential contribution to the public health, nursing is embedded within the single sector labeled 'health services'. While this is quite justified in terms of the whole, it does not help with planning services at a local level, or with organising the education or management of such provision. Health visiting is a smaller occupational group that is, all too often, lumped together with nursing as if the two were indistinguishable. If health visitors are educated and their services managed as if they were nurses and nothing else, it is likely their distinctive contribution to the public health will be lost.

As Hicks (1999) has noted, the term 'public health' signifies both its goal and its practice; this can lead to some very tautological statements like, 'the goal of public health is achieved through public health practice'. Furthermore, the helpful distinction of three groups, or 'levels' at which public health operates (Department of Health 1998b) is relatively new. Much attention has been paid to the skills and knowledge needed to operate as a public health specialist, which is the smallest (if the most powerful) of the three levels. Far less attention has been paid to the skills and knowledge needed by the middle-sized group of 'grass roots' public health practitioners. As this chapter has suggested, applying the defining features of specialist public health to this more grounded level of practice is not particularly helpful in identifying the skills that are needed or the best way to organise such services at a local level. There is, therefore, a great deal of work still needed to clarify and develop public health at this practitioner level.

Figure 1.2 was developed to offer a guide to the public health contribution of nursing and health visiting services within a primary-care-focused NHS. The idea that primary health care is the mechanism through which public health can be best achieved was first promoted by the World Health Organization (WHO) with the publication of the Alma-Ata Declaration (WHO 1978). The WHO view of primary health care encompasses a far wider field than the traditional

FIGURE 1.2   *Primary healthcare.*

	Preventive care	Intermediate care	Acute care

Other agencies – not NHS hospitals	• Environmental health
	• Housing
	• Education
	• Social services
	• Crime prevention
	• Community
		• Nursing homes
		• Voluntary sector:
		  residential care
			• Hospices; palliation
			• Ambulances/emergency
			  services

PRIMARY HEALTH CARE	• Public health • Health promotion • Therapeutic prevention • Primary prevention	• Chronic disease management • Rehabilitation • Long-term care at home • Family care • Secondary prevention • Screening	• 'Hospital at home' • Acute and terminal care • Post-hospital recovery • Severe/enduring illnesses

NHS hospital sector	• Infection control
	• Communicable
	  diseases
		• General wards; respite
		  care; OPD treatments;
		  ambulatory care
			• Critical care; high
			  dependency; post-trauma
			  care; surgical recovery

UK interpretation, that has tended to associate primary care almost exclusively with general practitioner services. However, the UK health services began, tentatively, to change during the 1980s. Legislation about primary and community care increased the pace of the shift throughout the 1990s, culminating in the passage of the Health Act 1999 and major changes to the way services are commissioned.

This shift has been accompanied by various other developments that challenge any simple division between 'community nursing' and 'hospital nursing'. If it ever was, primary care is certainly no longer only a site for people with either chronic disabilities or mild self-limiting disorders. Indeed, in primary care, there is the need to care for the profoundly ill and people with acute disorders, with attendant demands on nurses from across the disciplines. Service provision across the primary care field is, therefore, at least as complex and diverse as in hospitals. Figure 1.2 illustrates how it cuts across three domains of acute care, intermediate care and preventive care; all are needed to achieve the goal of public health, but the work of 'public health practitioners' is mainly located within the preventive field.

It is noteworthy that the collaborative interface differs in each of those domains, too. An increasing amount of care is delivered to acute and seriously ill patients in the home. The collaborative interface for practitioners involved in this field is most clearly focused on NHS hospitals and emergency services, although joint working with the voluntary sector represented by charitable hospices are a significant feature of palliative care. Nurses caring for an acutely ill child receiving chemotherapy in the home or someone dying at home, such as in the examples cited above, will need to maintain close links with the hospital teams involved in the whole treatment package. Different problems confront practitioners, but the range of possible actions and decisional control are inevitably and usefully limited by a focus on specific problems and varying clarity about shared priorities in treatment aims and knowing exactly who the patient is.

The 'intermediate care' domain also involves much collaboration between home and institutional care, especially for the classic 'care in the community' groups of elderly people, those with enduring and severe mental illnesses and those with learning disabilities. Because so much care for these groups is delivered in the voluntary sector and in conjunction with social services, the proportion of collaboration outwith the NHS is larger in this domain than for 'acute care'. However, there is a growing need to develop links with NHS hospitals ·and their specialist services, given the increase in rapid discharge, portable technologies and chronic disease management within primary care. The availability of effective individual treatments across this range of services, and the nursing contribution involved, is one essential part of the whole of public health.

The preventive care domain is the field in which the public health practitioners are located. These include health visitors, occupational health and school nurses who operate across the wider primary care field, and infection control and communicable disease nurses who mainly operate from NHS hospitals. However, this domain has a collaborative interface that is largely outwith the NHS hospital sector. Instead, practice in preventive care involves networking with various different departments in the local authorities (education, social services, housing, environmental health), social security, police and criminal justice services, as well as with local community provision from voluntary or commercial sectors (playgroups, support groups, after-school networks, etc). The diversity of this collaborative interface means that its practitioners are especially well-placed to contribute to the NHS strategic planning, through primary care groups, local health groups or other commissioning arrangements (see Chapter 5).

In the practice of preventive care multiple problems abound, but clarity of diagnosis is largely and usefully absent; this lack of bounded-ness allows decisional control to remain within the 'private sphere,' under the control of the individual concerned, rather than the professional. Thus, preventive services need to remain loosely specified at the point where they encounter individuals, to safeguard private citizens from over-zealous intrusions by professional services. The trade-off is that the services need to maintain a clear focus on changing the wider determinants of health. For nurses and health visitors, there is a specific focus on determinants located within the social environment, on enabling individuals with identified needs to access services established within the other spheres of action and on promoting self-empowerment so that people can control their own health-creating potential. Once supposedly preventive services devote more time to meeting established needs than avoiding them in the first place, the public health purpose of influencing the determinants of health is lost.

CONCLUSION

This chapter has explored the expanding scope and purpose of public health, and the way it is being developed as a new, multidisciplinary profession. The details of the different, equally important roles in public health practice were explored through a focus on health visiting and nursing, culminating in a summary of the diversity of the roles across primary health care. 'Multidisciplinary professions' are beginning to develop in response to the complexity of health care needs and the skills required to operate them. To sieze the opportunities and contribute most positively to the public health agenda, nursing may need to cast itself as a multidisciplinary profession. This would mean not just encompassing, but valuing and using the plurality of disciplines, skills and practice, so that the distinctive contributions of each can be brought to bear in different ways to contribute to the wider goal of improving the public health.

<table>
<tr><td>DISCUSSION QUESTIONS</td><td>

- Reflect on your practice with a single client or group of clients. How have your actions contributed to public health?

- In what ways do 'hands-on' public health practitioners differ from public health specialists? How are they similar?

- Is it possible to combine 'caseload work' with 'public health work'? How?

- What benefits or problems would arise for public health if all nursing and health visiting activities in primary healthcare (across acute, intermediate and preventive spheres) were combined into a single role?
</td></tr>
</table>

FURTHER READING

Acheson D (chair) 1998 Inquiry into Inequalities in Health. The Stationery Office, London
Outlines the extent of health inequalities and reviews the evidence to show what can be done about them. Health visitor home visiting is singled out as one approach that has a sound evidence base to show that it can be expected to reduce inequalities in the long term.

Cowley S 1997 Public health values in practice: the case of health visiting. Critical Public Health 7:82–97
Unravels aspects of organisational requirements that militate against a public health approach in health visiting practice.

Department of Health 1998 Chief Medical Officer's Project to Strengthen the Public Health Function in England: a report of the emerging findings. The Stationery Office, London
Brief report that sets out the different public health functions that are needed and lists areas of development required to meet those needs.

Griffiths S & Hunter D (eds) 1999 Perspectives in Public Health. Radcliffe Medical Press, Abingdon, Oxon
Explains public health from a range of different perspectives, illustrating the multifaceted, multiprofessional, multiagency nature of the work.

Pearson P, Mead P, Graney A, McRae G, Reed J, Johnson K 2000 Evaluation of the developing specialist practitioner role in the context of public health. English National Board for Nursing, Midwifery and Health Visiting, London
All community health care nurses are now educated through a 'specialist practitioner framework'. This research focuses on three groups: district nurses, health visitors and practice nurses, to show how the new education is

preparing students for the public health role asked of them. It illustrates the varied perceptions, and hurdles and levers in learning about public health.

Standing Nursing and Midwifery Advisory Committee 1995 Making it happen. Public health: the contribution, role and development of nurses, midwives and health visitors. HMSO, London
Still relevant, despite being produced before the change of government in 1997. Good, clear examples.

REFERENCES

Acheson D 1988 Public Health in England. HMSO, London

Baker J 1999 Public health scientists. In: Griffith S & Hunter D (eds) Perspectives in Public Health. Radcliffe Medical Press, Abingdon p 250–260

Bergen A, Cowley S, Young K & Kavanagh A 1996 An investigation into the changing educational needs of community nurses with regard to needs assessment and quality of care in the context of the NHS and Community Care Act, 1990. English National Board, London

Billingham K & Perkins E 1997 A public health approach to nursing in the community. Nursing Standard 11(35):43–46

Bunker J P, Frazier H S & Mosteller F 1994 improving health: measuring effects of medical care. The Millbank Qarterly 72:225–258

Bunker J P 1995 Medicine matters after all. Journal of the Royal College of Physicians 29:105–112

Campbell C, Wood R & Kelly M 1999 Social Capital and Health. Health Education Authority, London

Cowley S 1991 A grounded theory of situation and process in health visiting. Unpublished PhD thesis, CNAA, Brighton Polytechnic, Brighton

Cowley S 1997 Public health values in practice: the case of health visiting Critical Public Health 7:82–97

Cowley S & Andrew S A 2001 A scenario based analysis of health visiting dilemmas. Community Practitioner 74(4): 139–142

Cowley S & Billings J 1997 Family Health Needs Project. Department of Nursing Studies, King's College/South Thames Primary Care Development Fund, London

Cowley S & Billings J 1999a Implementing new health visiting services through action research: an analysis of process. Journal of Advanced Nursing 30:965–974

Cowley S & Billings J 1999b Identifying approaches to meet assessed needs in health visiting. Journal of Clinical Nursing 8:527–534

Dahlgren G & Whitehead M 1991 Policies and strategies to promote social equity in health. Institute for Future Studies, Stockholm

Davies C 1988 The health visitor as mother's friend: a woman's place in public health, 1900–1914. Social History of Medicine 1(1):39–59

Department of Health 1998a Our Healthier Nation: a contract for health (Cmnd 3852). The Stationery Office, London

Department of Health 1998b Chief Medical Officer's Project to Strengthen the Public Health Function in England: a report of the emerging fndings. Department of Health, London

Department of Health 1999 Saving Lives: Our Healthier Nation. The Stationery Office, London

Department of Health and Social Services 1999 Fit for the future: a new approach. Department of Health and Social Services, Belfast

Dingwall R 1977 Collectivism, regionalism and feminism: health visiting and British social policy. Journal of Social Policy 6(3):291–315

Gillies P 1998 Effectiveness of alliances and partnerships for health promotion. Health Promotion International 13: 99–120

Hicks N 1999 Public health and clinical practice. In: Griffiths S & Hunter D (eds) Perspectives in Public Health. Radcliffe Medical Press, Abingdon p 192–197

Johnson J 1999 Observations on positivism and pseudoscience in qualitative nursing research. Journal of Advanced Nursing 30(1):67–73

Kennedy B, Kawachi I, Prothrowstith D, Lochner K & Gupta V 1998 Social capital, income inequality and firearm violent crime. Social Science and Medicine 47(1):7–17

Lessof S, Dumelow C, McPherson K 1999 Feasibility study of the case for national standards for specialist practice in public health. Cancer and Public Health Unit, London School of Hygiene and Tropical Medicine, London

Marmot M & Wilkinson R (eds) 1999 The social determinants of health. Oxford University Press, Oxford

NHS Executive 1999 Review of the Nurses, Midwives and Health Visitors Act 1997: Government response to the recommendations (Health Service Circular No. 1999/030). NHS Executive, London

Putnam R 1993 Making democracy work: civic traditions in modern Italy. Princeton University Press, Princeton; New Jersey

Rijke R 1993 Health in medical science: from determinism towards autonomy. In: Lafaille R & Fulder S (eds) Towards a New Science of Health. Routledge, London p 74–83

Scottish Assembly 1999 Towards a Healthier Scotland. The Stationery Office, Edinburgh

Standing Nursing and Midwifery Advisory Committee 1995 Making it happen. Public health: the contribution, role and development of nurses, midwives and health visitors. Department of Health, London

Symonds A 1991 Angels and interfering busybodies: the social construction of two occupations. Sociology of Health and Illness 2(13):249–264

Welsh Office 1998 Better Health Better Wales. Welsh Office, Cardiff

Wilkinson R 1996 Unhealthy Societies: The Afflictions of Inequality. Routledge, London

World Health Organization 1978 The Alma-Ata Declaration. Primary Health Care. World Health Organization, Geneva

World Health Organization 1999 Health 21: Health for all in the 21st century. European Health For All series No. 6. World Health Organization, Copenhagen

2 The development of public health nursing

Pauline Craig

KEY ISSUES

- Development of community nursing in the UK from public health roots.
- Relationship between nursing and public health, historically and currently.
- Legitimacy of health visiting as public health nursing.

INTRODUCTION

In order to provide a context for the current theory and practice of public health nursing in the UK, this chapter will explore the historical development of the modern public health movement. Both public health and nursing practice have met with a number of controversies and changes in direction in relation to national policy over the years. The implications of their tortuous paths through the last century are considered in this chapter with regard to the health of the public and to the real and implied relationship between nursing and public health. The term 'public health nursing' has been introduced into the UK fairly recently and is being snapped up by nurses working in a variety of fields, creating some confusion over its meaning and adding to the international confusion over its definition. Health visiting in the UK is often regarded as having a particular public health role, partly due to its roots in the public health movement of the nineteenth century, and partly due to its focus on needs assessment and prevention. The legitimacy of applying the title of public health nursing to contemporary health visiting is explored in this chapter in a historical context.

THE EARLY PUBLIC HEALTH MOVEMENT

British towns grew rapidly in the nineteenth century as a result of industrialisation. Living and working conditions for the unskilled labouring classes were overcrowded and unsanitary, and had dramatic consequences for health. Employers took advantage of the lack of social controls and the large pool of unskilled labour, while workers fell prey to mental and physical exhaustion with extended working hours and inadequate nutrition, sanitary and safety arrangements. Consequently, working-class families became particularly susceptible to infectious diseases (Doyal & Pennell, 1979).

The cholera epidemics that swept through Europe are often credited with providing the greatest force for public health reform. The first cholera epidemic in Britain in 1831–1832 spread dramatically through the middle and upper classes, as well as the working classes. The high mortality rate created public hysteria and an unprecedented threat to commerce which helped to spur on the fledgling sanitary movement (Hamilton 1987). However, cholera epidemics came and went rapidly, while typhus, tuberculosis and childhood diseases were the main endemic causes of death in the early part of the nineteenth century. Some industrial districts had mortality rates of around 40 per thousand population, with half of all infants dying before the age of 5 years (Webster 1990). In the 1830s tuberculosis was overwhelmingly the major cause of death but typhus followed close behind. Typhus, known then as 'fever', was recognised in the 1830s as the 'poor man's disease' and was directly related to squalor, overcrowding and insanitary conditions (Flinn 1965). Then, as now, there were marked differences in mortality rates between poor and affluent areas. For example, in 1901 in Glasgow the overall infant mortality rate per thousand births was 149, ranging from 69 in the 'best' areas to 217 in the 'poorest' areas (McGregor 1967).

In the early part of the nineteenth century the government took little responsibility for safeguarding the health of the population. Elizabethan legislation from the sixteenth century set a compulsory 'poor rate' for prosperous members of the community to support the poor. This included medical care as part of a social welfare programme. The Poor Law Amendment Act of 1834 replaced the Elizabethan welfare framework (Webster 1993). The New Poor Law aimed to reduce public expenditure and stressed deterrence against claiming, rather than entitlement. It was harsh and unpopular and set a trend for long-stay institutional care for vulnerable groups (Webster 1990).

Government involvement in disease prevention began with the sanitary movement, which was first launched in the 1820s (Webster 1993). Edwin Chadwick's radical document of 1842, 'Report on the Sanitary Condition of the Labouring Population of Great Britain' laid the foundation of the Victorian public health movement and led to the first Public Health Act in 1848 (Flinn 1965). The Act stimulated a steady growth in sanitary reform and increased powers for public health doctors with new acts passed for improving water supply, sewage removal and food production, and the creation of Medical Officers of Health (MOsH) in local authorities (Webster 1990).

In considering the part that medicine has played in combating illness and disease, it is interesting to note that the mortality rate began to fall dramatically in the UK during the nineteenth century, before major scientific advances were made such as anti-tuberculin drugs (Doyal & Pennell 1979). McKeown and Record (1963) argued that the medical establishment played only a small role in the major decline in mortality levels. Instead, they identified a combination of public health legislation and improvements in living standards, which accompanied higher wages, as the overriding factors responsible for the decrease in mortality.

DEVELOPMENT OF PUBLIC HEALTH SERVICES

Towards the end of the nineteenth century, opinion about the causes of ill-health began to change, with increasing bacteriological understanding and the development of the germ theory of disease (Webster 1993). Public health began to move away from its environmental focus on housing and sanitation, taking on a more individualistic approach based on personal preventative services (Ashton & Seymour 1988). Responsibility for health began to be levelled at the individual, particularly at mothers, with maternal inefficiency deemed a major influence on the health of the working class (Webster 1993). Recognition of the poor physical state of young male recruits to the Boer War at the end of the nineteenth century highlighted the need for improving general health, and this prompted the development of advice for mothers, child welfare services, ante-natal clinics and free school meals (Berridge 1995). Public health, housed within local authorities, led the campaign to educate mothers, with the development of maternal and child welfare services such as infant welfare centres and better maternity services.

By the 1920s, health education was now central to public health and this led to antagonism between public health doctors and medical practitioners (Berridge 1995). During the 1920s, the focus on individual preventative work made public health difficult to distinguish from curative medicine, and led general practitioners (GPs) to accuse public health doctors of encroachment (Lewis 1991). Public health departments were further weakened in the 1930s by the shift of power and resources towards hospitals that came with the develop-ment of therapeutic medicine (Ashton & Seymour 1988). Despite the rift with GPs, public health practice had enough support from elsewhere to continue to grow, particularly with regard to their administration of a range of medical and welfare services.

By the Second World War, local authority public health departments were responsible for providing the following services:

- Maternal and child welfare services including obstetrics and gynaecology
- School medical service
- School meals and milk
- Dentistry
- TB schemes including sanatorium treatment clinics
- Health centres
- Administration of Poor Law hospitals (Lewis 1991).

In addition, MOsH collected and analysed medical statistics, although figures such as mortality and birth rates had been collected since the sixteenth century (Webster 1993). Up until the 1940s, a number of reports were produced by MOsH showing an association between poverty, unemployment and over-crowding with, e.g. death rates among the poor (Webster 1993) and infant mortality (Womersley 1987). However, public health doctors neglected to bring these issues to public notice, concentrating instead on their administrative func-tions (Lewis 1991). At this time, public health was criticised for not responding to the general dangers of the time to the population, such as unemployment or malnutrition in depressed areas, with MOsH unwilling to challenge the dominant orthodoxies (Berridge 1995).

There was a view that public health doctors expected to continue their administrative 'empire' within the NHS from 1948, but found themselves considerably weakened when control of the NHS did not go to local authorities (Berridge 1995). McKeown (1965) argues that the public health movement was compromised at this time because it lacked a clearly defined philosophy, as it had been introduced initially to control infectious disease but was subsequently extended to make up for deficiencies in other medical services. Attempts were made to establish a philosophy for public health through academic departments of social medicine in the 1940s, and later, the development of the concept of community medicine in the 1970s (Lewis 1991). However, social medicine was soon rejected on the grounds of being too clinical and too ready to dismiss the local authority public health departments (Lewis 1991). Community medicine was understood to comprise epidemiology and medical administration, but was criticised for the lack of clear guidelines as to how these would operate in practice (Webster 1993). The responsibilities of MOsH were divided between prevention, family practitioners and hospital services and this led to difficulties in ensuring coverage of the whole population (Department of Health 1988).

Public health doctors finally became responsible for planning health services in the 1970s when public health (in the form of community medicine) moved to the NHS from the Local Authorities under the 1974 NHS reorganisation. The aim of the reorganisation was to integrate the tripartite NHS, but Lewis (1991) argues that public health doctors were unsure of their role within the management structures, which led to further confusion rather than successful integration. The Department of Health (1988) review of public health renamed the specialty 'public health medicine' and couched its function in terms of prevention and promotion within the context of the World Health Organization (WHO) definitions of public health, Health for All and the Ottawa Charter for Health Promotion. This in itself has raised conflict between public health and other health-related services over two main issues. First, despite the emphasis on prevention, NHS public health departments focus on the analysis of health service needs (Lewis 1991). Secondly, other specialisms, such as environmental health, general practice, and health promotion also have a role in developing policies that prevent illness and disease (Webster 1993).

The nurse's contribution to the early public health movement was mostly in the form of school nursing and health visiting, although originally health visitors were not all trained nurses. Contemporary health visiting is often regarded as public health nursing, perhaps due to its public health roots or the notion that health visiting is designed as a population-based service rather than an individualised one. The development of health visiting has mirrored the development of public health, particularly with regard to conflicts with other health and local authority departments. The next section describes the development of health visiting in relation to the public health movement in the UK and to public health nursing in other countries, in order to explore the links between health visiting and public health nursing.

THE EARLY DEVELOPMENT OF HEALTH VISITING

Dingwall (1977) notes that antecedents of health visiting have been recorded as far back as 1769, but it is widely believed that the recognisable form of current health visiting appeared at the same time as the early development of the public health movement. A number of diverse origins of health visiting in the UK have been described, but in general the UK system of health visiting towards the end of the nineteenth century arose from the sanitary movement's 'volunteer visiting of the poor' (Webster 1993) gradually adapting to maternal instruction on the care of infants (Davies 1988).

Volunteer visitors in the last half of the nineteenth century were usually middle-class women, often from temperance movements and the Charity Organisation Society (McGregor 1967). They were said to be acting out of concern for the high mortality and dreadful living conditions of the urban poor and their aim was to promote independence and self-reliance, in line with the philosophy of the New Poor Law of 1834 (Robinson 1982). For the 'Lady Visitors', philanthropic work offered a socially acceptable opportunity to work outside the home, but in a way that did not challenge men's positions as providers for the family. It also led to a place for both middle-class and working-class women in the public health movement. For local authorities, philanthropic and religious work provided a framework for accessing and influencing working class families. (Davies 1988).

The most frequently repeated account of the first health visitor is that of the Manchester and Salford Ladies Sanitary Reform Association who employed a 'respectable' working-class woman in 1867 to assist the lady volunteers of the sanitary reform movement (Dingwall 1977). In 1867, duties of the volunteer visitors included teaching hygiene and child welfare, social support, and teaching mental and moral health (Robinson 1982). Assisting doctors at child welfare clinics was added to the duties of health visitors at the turn of the century (McGregor 1967). Davies (1988) argues that health visiting developed not only from the work of women philanthropists, but also from male sanitary inspectors objecting to women taking on their work and effectively blocking women from equal pay and employment status. At the same time, MOsH supported the 'mothers' friend' role of health visitors as a means of addressing high infant mortality rates (Davies 1988). For example, McGregor, MOH for Glasgow in the 1920s, recognised that for health visitors working with mothers:

> 'Time was required to create a friendly atmosphere in which to insinuate new ideas and practices and to discuss domestic difficulties, common in these years of recurring poverty and privation.' (McGregor 1967 p 111)

In 1907 the Notification of Births Act was passed as a result of lobbying of the Government by the powerful pressure group, the National Association for the Prevention of Infant Mortality (McGregor 1967). This Act enabled a direct approach to be made to all mothers of newly born infants and, for the first time, accurate information could be gathered about all births. Under the Act, every birth had to be notified to the MOH within 36 hours and this led to the expansion of paid and voluntary family visitors. For example, in 1908 in Glasgow (population 678 000) there were 300 voluntary helpers working with a handful of paid health visitors to visit families and give advice on infant care (Chalmers 1930). Compared to more recent figures, Glasgow's families were well-served. In 1997, there were 270 health visitors employed in Glasgow – population 908 000.

In July 1910, a Health Visitor's Bill was introduced into parliament, which was to give powers to local authorities to appoint health visitors under the Notification of Births Act and to decide on appropriate qualifications in conjunction with MOsH. It was subsequently withdrawn after much protest from a number of women's organisations who voiced concern that the proposed

Bill would lower the status of women working in public health. However, a number of local authorities around the UK had already started to employ health visitors in place of sanitary inspectors at lower salaries, focusing their work on women and children and leaving the legislation-based activity to male sanitary inspectors (Davies 1988).

The early employed health visitors were drawn from a range of occupations including medicine, sanitary inspection, midwifery, teaching and nursing, and separate training courses were established for nurses and non-nurses (White 1985). By the beginning of the First World War, most large cities had some form of health visiting training in place. For example, in Scotland the training course for nurses consisted of six months theory in the School of Social Study at Glasgow or Edinburgh University and practical training under the Senior Medical Officer of the Maternity and Child Welfare Department (McGregor 1967).

By the 1920s health visiting was part of the expanding public health departments within local authorities, accountable to and fully supported by MOsH (Davies 1988). The most common role for health visitors at that time was with maternity and child welfare services. During the 1920s health visiting gradually extended to middle class families, enabling health visiting to become a universalist, non-stigmatising service (Dingwall & Robinson 1993). Between the wars, nurses began to make up the largest group of recruits to health visiting, although entry to health visiting training remained open to non-nurses until 1962 (Robinson 1982). A review of nursing registration in 1998 maintained the status of health visiting as separate from nursing, although a first-level nursing qualification continues as a requirement of entry to health visiting (RCN Personal Communication 1998).

HOME CARE IN THE UK AND USA

Health visiting in the UK developed quite separately from domiciliary nursing of the sick, despite some of the early health visitors being expected to care for any sick family members they encountered. District Visiting Societies emerged from the Victorian Christian practice of visiting the sick poor, preceding the trend towards home visiting at the end of the nineteenth century (Webster 1993). Florence Nightingale is usually associated with the development of hospital nursing and education in the 1860s but was also committed to public health and home care (Baly 1991). Nightingale is credited with suggesting that Liverpool Infirmary should train some of its nurses for home care, leading to the development of the first state-run district nursing service in Liverpool in 1863 (Baly 1991).

Such specialism in home-care nursing as developed in the UK was unusual. At around the same time as the development of public health services in the UK, many countries developed public health nursing to provide both nursing care of the sick and preventative services. For example, in the United States, Lillian Wald, the American nursing visionary, is said to have coined the term 'public health nursing' in the 1890s (Frachel 1988). Wald's vision for public health nursing was as an all-inclusive service to patients in their homes, addressing the family situation, hygienic housing and living conditions, providing both direct care and health teaching (Boschma 1997). The early public health nurses in

America developed a specialised nursing method which incorporated an ability to relate to people, scientific knowledge and the freedom to work for the good of society (Frachel 1988). In this way, Wald was able to use her experiences in caring for the sick poor in the New York slums to convince policymakers about the social, economic and environmental causes of ill-health she encountered (Frachel 1988).

The early UK health visitors shared some of the concerns of the first US public health nurses, for example, the recognition of the need to address social and environmental factors in improving health. Where their underlying principles differed was that health visiting aimed to educate mothers in order to reduce infant mortality (Lewis 1991) whereas US public health nurses were said to have targeted communities in order to improve community health (Frachel 1988). In the UK, health visitors worked in a system that was dominated by male and medical dogma. It conspired to maintain the lower status of women in general and to undermine the contribution of women to the public health movement despite holding their 'womanly' qualities in high esteem (Davies 1988). Health visiting was said to be linked to radical and feminist movements in its early days but this declined after the First World War as health visiting became less political (Dingwall 1977).

In the USA, the early public health nurses worked for lay organisations, outside of the supervision of medical practitioners (Frachel 1988). The early American nursing leaders were ambivalent about the increasing authority of medicine and were said to be influenced more by the progressive politics of the feminist movement and social reform (Boschma 1997). They were able to develop a more autonomous role in prevention which emphasised empowerment and advocacy for people living in poverty (Erickson 1996). Public health nursing in the USA was therefore founded on the recognition of poverty and the need for public services to be responsive to diverse socioeconomic and cultural groups (Erickson 1996). Frachel (1988) argues that Lillian Wald's successful welding of 'womanly' qualities with a scientific knowledge of epidemiology and politics gave public health nursing status and power. However, competing views on whether sick nursing and health teaching should be separate or combined impeded the development of a unified infrastructure for public health nursing (Boschma 1997).

The gender issue was very different for the early health visitors in the UK. Davies (1988) argues that it was the gendering of public health activity into relationship-building for women and legislation work for men that led to health visitors developing lower status and lower wages than male sanitary inspectors. There was a blurring of public and private life for women in public health that did not apply to men. Middle-class women could work in public health, but on a voluntary basis; working-class women were paid for their public health work, but had to be accessible at all times and were expected to act as role models for their neighbourhoods. Women acted on a private sphere relying on personal qualities, but not in a public sphere, where there were officials and inspectors backed by scientific spirit and legal sanctions (Davies 1988). While the debate in America centred on the separation or fusion of sick nursing and health teaching, the debate in the UK for health visitors focused on gender issues, the balance between individualised and collective responses to health problems (Dingwall 1977) and later, the relationship between health visiting and other providers of health and social care.

FROM PUBLIC HEALTH INTO NURSING

Health visiting remained under the MOsH in local authorities until 1974 when health visitors were moved from public health to become accountable to hospital nurses at divisional level (Robinson 1982). The divisional nursing structure had been created by the Salmon Report in 1966 to cope with technological developments in hospitals and was based on an industrial model of professional management (Carpenter 1977). Community nurses did not fit easily into this structure for two main reasons; their work was in carrying out direct care rather than supervising other staff; and they were seen as being resistant to the bureaucracy (Carpenter 1977). In addition, few of the nurse managers had community experience, and health visitors found themselves in the position of having to compete with hospital nurses for resources (Robinson 1982). Health visitors also had to fight to maintain the higher education basis for their training, but by doing so, were successful in preserving their separate identity within the main body of nursing (Robinson 1982).

As with public health medicine, health visiting had met with conflict. One issue was the relationship between health visiting and social work, which had historically been fraught (Robinson 1982). The NHS Act in 1946 had given local authorities responsibility for providing health visiting services, but the Children Act in 1948 transferred responsibility for child protection from health visitors to social workers (White 1985). The Children Act created children's officers who were to be educated to degree level and have a remit for the care of deprived children (Robinson 1982). These new officers crossed boundaries with health visitors' child welfare work, and, as graduates, had higher status. The contention that health visiting was a female occupation providing a service predominantly for women compounded health visitors' low status, particularly among those controlling the welfare services (Orr 1981).

The relationship between health visitors and GPs was also difficult, with GPs criticised in the 1950s for their lack of cooperation with health visitors (White 1985). Since 1948, GPs had become more accessible to patients for consultations on minor ailments, which would have previously been dealt with by health visitors. However, GPs were divided in their views. Some wanted health visitors to be made redundant, others were asking for more to be employed. By this time, local authorities had been given statutory duties to visit all new babies within one month of birth. This then became the health visitor's priority and prevented further extension of their duties (White 1985).

Enquiries into health visiting and social work in the 1950s did not rectify the rift between health visiting and social work. The Jameson report in 1956 established the university base for health visiting training but recommended that health visitors should be seen as 'casefinders' with the more specialised social workers as 'caseworkers' (White 1985). By the 1960s, two major reviews by the Younghusband and Seebohm Committees had analysed the function of social work, and while they had recognised the existence of health visiting, they failed to clarify the relationship between social work and health visiting (Sachs 1990).

More recently, another potential area of conflict between social work and health visiting in addition to childcare responsibilities are the principles underpinning community work. The Younghusband and Seebohm reviews identified community work as integral to social work with the Younghusband report (1959, in Sachs 1990) defining community work as, 'helping people within a local community to identify social needs and consider the most effective ways of meeting these ... (within) ... available resources'.

The four principles of health visiting which were developed independently in 1977 by the Council for the Education and Training of Health Visitors (1977) show some similarity to the definition of community work. The principles are as follows:

- Search for health needs
- Stimulation of awareness of health needs
- Influence on policies affecting health
- Facilitation of health-enhancing activities.

In the 1980s, community work was endorsed as a method of working appropriate to effective health visiting by both the Royal College of Nursing and the Health Visitors' Association (Robinson 1982). A reappraisal of the health visiting principles in 1992, by a working group of practitioners and managers throughout the UK, concluded that the principles continue to be relevant to current and future health visiting practice (Twinn & Cowley 1992).

HEALTH VISITING: FOR INDIVIDUALS OR POPULATIONS?

Dingwall (1977) argues that health visiting has its roots in collectivist public health philosophies of the early twentieth century. As health visiting developed, health visitors became more middle-class and less political, and more focused on individualism as recruits were increasingly being drawn from hospital-trained nurses. From the 1940s, political reforms began to move away from a collectivist ideology towards individual remedies for social problems such as poverty and unemployment. In the 1960s, social services began to shift from individuals to individual families, and health visiting began to abandon district visiting, adopting casework philosophies and selective visiting of those in proven need (Dingwall 1977).

The policy context until the late 1990s continued to emphasise the individualistic approach for health visiting, with NHS reforms placing health visiting firmly within GP-led primary care service provision. The 1997 NHS White Papers (Box 2.1) suggested that health visitors and other community nurses may have the opportunity to work across primary care practice boundaries and have a greater voice in commissioning local health services.

In practice, health visiting continues to be identified primarily with child health surveillance, although authors have highlighted a lack of confidence within health visiting since the 1970s regarding the child health role (Goodwin 1988; Robinson 1985). Despite the restrictive policy context of the recent past, professional nursing organisations such as the Health Visitor's Association (Twinn 1991) and the Royal College of Nursing (1994) repeatedly espoused the need for health visiting to adopt a collective approach, with a growing body of health visitors developing collective responses to health problems (Cowley 1996).

The lack of policy support for collectivism meant that health visitors working in this way remained on the margins of health visiting practice (Craig 1998). However, the 1999 public health White Papers may provide the policy context

---

| BOX 2.1 | *NHS White Papers, 1997* |

Some implications for public health nursing in primary care from the white papers, 'The New NHS' (Department of Health 1997a) and 'Designed to Care' (Scottish Office Department of Health 1997):

- Local doctors and nurses ... will be in the driving seat in shaping services. (The New NHS, p 11)

- Co-operation will replace competition. GPs and community nurses will work together in Primary Care Groups. (The New NHS, p 13)

- In Scotland: Primary Care Trusts will build on the strengths of general practice and give a voice to community nursing and other primary care professionals managing and delivering care to their local communities. In this way primary care will be able to pool resources, work across organisational boundaries and develop shared aims and objectives. (Designed to Care, p 19)

- Primary Care Groups will ... share expertise such as public health skills. (The New NHS, p 38)

- Primary Care Groups ... will be encouraged to play an active part in community development and improving health in its widest sense. Health visitors and health promotion professionals will have a strong contribution to make in identifying health needs and implementing the programmes that best address them. (The New NHS, p 40)

---

required to support health visitors working with a population approach. For example, the Scottish public health White Paper 'Towards a Healthier Scotland' (Scottish Office Department of Health 1999) recognised the potential for health visitors to be more involved in promoting public health and called for a review of the public health roles of health visitors, school nurses and practice nurses. The English public health White Paper, 'Saving Lives: Our Healthier Nation' (Department of Health 1999a), provided a more detailed description of health visitors' public health function. It echoed the 1999 nursing, health visiting and midwifery strategy (Department of Health 1999b) and the 'Supporting Families' consultation document (Home Office 1998) in focusing the public health function on a family-centred role, with some additional work with special needs groups and general health promotion programmes.

A family-centred role is, without doubt, relevant to some of the priority health issues in communities, as well as to existing health visiting skills and experience. However, this interpretation of the health visiting public health function may be too narrowly defined, with the focus on prescribed current issues and specified populations preventing real flexibility in addressing health priorities of communities or populations.

WHAT IS A PUBLIC HEALTH NURSE?

The term 'public health nursing' appears to have been introduced to the UK in the 1990s without much discussion about its relationship to current UK nursing practice. Consequently there has been some confusion about the roles or potential roles of nurses in relation to public health. The Standing Nursing and Midwifery Advisory Committee (1995) stated that all nurses, midwives and health visitors have a contribution to make to public health, playing a key role in improving the health of the population, rather than just providing a service to individuals. The examples they gave of nurses' public health roles were nurses working in infection control, commissioning health promotion, and health visitors taking on specialist roles in needs assessment and homelessness.

The Royal College of Nursing (1994) also outlined the issues for nurses taking on public health activity but did not specify which nurses, and under what circumstances they might be able to fulfil a public health function. In addition, health visitors, district nurses, midwives and practice nurses have been described as 'all nurses working within public health' (Smith 1997), while Caraher and McNab (1996) suggest that the 'so-called' public health nursing posts that do exist in the UK may have no more than an extended health visitor or district nurse role. Adding to the confusion is a lack of consensus for describing nurses who are working across populations. For example, a study of 26 health visitors with community-focused remits identified no less that thirteen job titles including: health visitor, public health nurse, public health health visitor, community development health visitor, community health development worker and community health worker (Craig 1998). There are therefore a multitude of ways in which to interpret 'public health nursing' in the UK and the muddle is far from being resolved.

In addition, 'public health nursing' has a variety of meanings across the world and is apparently a source of confusion in a number of countries. For example in the USA, public health nurses are one group of nurses within the umbrella term of 'community health nursing', used to describe all nurses working outside of health institutions (Scruby & McKay 1991). The main distinction between public health nurses and other community health nurses appears to be that, in general, public health nurses focus on populations or communities, whereas community health nurses target their services towards individuals and families (Deal 1994). In Canada, the terms 'public health nursing' and 'community health nursing' are also confused (King et al 1995). A public health nursing service based in public health departments was first used in Alberta in 1918 to provide health education for schoolchildren and families. The term 'community health nursing' was introduced in the 1970s when the public health nursing service expanded to cover nursing the sick and disabled in the community, ironically very similar to Lillian Walds' vision of public health nursing in the late nineteenth century as described by Boschma (1997).

While 'community health nursing' is the umbrella term in some countries, it is 'public health nursing' that is used as the umbrella term in Ireland to describe all nurses working in the community. The current Irish public health nursing service was set up in 1956 as an amalgamation of local authority nurses concerned with public health and the voluntary district nursing service (Hanafin 1997). In general, Irish public health nurses focus on individualised care and health promotion mostly with children and elderly people. However, they work in geographical areas and have a mandate to include work at the community level, although community participation work is often not supported by their line managers (McDonald and Chavasse 1996).

In a review of the international literature Khan and Landes (1993) found that public health nurses in the UK, Finland, Sweden, Canada and the USA share a number of common features:

- They focus on a defined community rather than individuals or families
- There is an emphasis on disease prevention and health promotion as well as curative medicine
- They perform an outreach function involving case finding and consultation, and
- They have professional autonomy.

Health visitors in the UK certainly share some of these features, although it could be argued that the medically defined role within primary care prevents them focusing on communities or populations (Symonds 1997). Despite lack of policy support for health visitors working beyond individuals and families, the Standing Nursing and Midwifery Advisory Committee (1995) identified that health visitors are 'public health workers in the entirety of their role'.

PUBLIC HEALTH HEALTH VISITING IN PRACTICE

Billingham (1994a) described a public health approach for health visitors as taking a population perspective. This could be interpreted as either a role in commissioning or as working in a community with a community focus. With regard to commissioning, nurses in general are scarce in senior positions within commissioning and purchasing (Standing Nursing and Midwifery Advisory Committee 1995) and there are no established career pathways for nurses to increase their numbers at decision-making levels (Salvage 1993). At the time of writing it is too early to tell if the NHS reforms of 1997 will provide a platform for nurses to establish an effective public health role at a commissioning level.

At a fieldwork level, it has been noted that the community-focused aspect of health visiting appears to be becoming more visible (Cowley 1996). Health visiting activity with groups or communities tends to take place in areas of disadvantage, addressing inequalities in health and recognising the wider factors affecting health, such as poverty, housing, environment, education and social networks (Billingham 1994a). Community development methods of working are often used for health promotion by health visitors in areas of disadvantage, emphasising a holistic approach and the importance of personal and community empowerment in improving health and well-being (Box 2.2).

HEALTH VISITING AND HEALTH INEQUALITIES

The issue of health inequalities is now recognised in government policy as a major public health problem and one that the NHS must address (Department of Health 1997b). As one in three children in the UK (1994 figures) is born into

BOX 2.2	*Health visiting in Drumchapel Community Health Project (Craig 1996)*

- Project based on HFA principles
- Collaborative community health profile
- Supporting Community Health Volunteers Scheme to facilitate health forums such as the Women's Health Network, a community drugs forum and Food Action Drumchapel, and groups for asthma, breastfeeding, postnatal and bereavement support
- Developing new projects, e.g. complementary therapies, men's health and a child safety equipment loan scheme
- Health promoted through participation and involvement
- Community development approach central

a family which qualifies for social fund payments (Laughlin & Black 1995), few health visitors can avoid the need to respond to poverty and health issues.

Blackburn (1991) identified that health visitors can take action with regard to families living in poverty with three broad types of response:

- Profiling and monitoring to gather information which can be used for planning and working for social change
- Prevention and alleviation for families coping with the material and health affects of poverty, and
- Social change responses – directly challenging team, local and national policies.

Health visiting responses to families in poverty are comparable to Whitehead's (1995) findings regarding policy responses to inequalities in health. Effective policies were found to act at one of the following four levels: strengthening individuals, strengthening communities, improving access to essential facilities and services, and encouraging macroeconomic and cultural change; with the most powerful focus for change being at level four (Whitehead 1995).

Examples can be demonstrated of health visiting developments acting at each of the four policy levels, as shown in Box 2.3.

Areas where health visitors can be visible in addressing health inequalities were also highlighted by 'The Acheson Inquiry into Inequalities in Health in England' (Acheson 1998). The recommendations from the Inquiry included specifying that the role of health visitors should be developed, particularly in relation to the social and emotional support of parents as part of an increased range of neighbourhood services, and more intensive home visiting within children's first two years.

A NEW FRAMEWORK FOR PUBLIC HEALTH HEALTH VISITING

It is clear that health visitors potentially have a major role to play as 'public health nurses' if the main elements of public health nursing are taking a

BOX 2.3	*Examples of health visiting at the four policy levels*

1. Strengthening individuals

Maximising material income, e.g. through helping to claim benefits (Billingham 1994b) or child safety equipment loan schemes (Boyd et al 1993), or by counselling, support or developing self-esteem and skills as in the community mothers programme (Whitehead 1995).

2. Strengthening communities

Collecting and using information at community level, for example, through community profiling and community development.

3. Improving access to essential facilities and services

Advocacy at an individual or community level for example, in pursuing adequate housing or social services, and 'fringe work' including providing food, clothes or money, and setting up support groups (De la Cuesta 1994).

4. Encouraging macroeconomic and cultural change

Challenging local and national policies that create and maintain family poverty. For example, supporting local health campaigns or raising awareness about the links between poor housing and health; or lobbying managers and decision makers within health services to address poverty and health issues (Blackburn 1991).

population perspective on a public health issue, focusing on case-finding and prevention. However, health visitors' community-focused activity and their role in challenging policy are both far from being accepted within the mainstream of health visiting practice. In a study aiming to develop a description of health visitors' public health role, health visitors with remits for community-focused activity found that they had little support from nursing management. Although most of the respondents in the study had legitimate, funded health visiting posts, support usually came from outside community nursing, such as community health projects or public health departments (Craig 1998).

The lack of nurse management support for health visitors' public health activity can be explained using Robinson's (1982) examination of health visiting practice within the social policy framework of legitimacy, feasibility and support. Health visiting had originally achieved legitimacy through its association with the infant welfare movement. There is currently no equal movement, although if the movement to address health inequalities gathers momentum there is arguably the potential for achieving legitimacy through the health visitor's role in poverty and health work. Feasibility of early health visiting was due to its status as a low-cost service to disseminate health education knowledge, and support came initially from Medical Officers of Health and subsequently through the family-centred philosophy of post-war social policy. Health visiting could again be utilised as a cost-effective entry into communities for public health departments and as a means of bridging the public health/primary care gap, with support coming from public health departments and from the new primary care structures. There is currently renewed policy support for health visiting in general, as well as for a public health role, but it is not yet clear how health visitors and other nurses adopting public health roles will relate to the main body of public health theory and NHS practice.

NURSING, HEALTH FOR ALL AND THE NEW PUBLIC HEALTH

The definition of public health medicine from 1988, as noted previously, was based on the World Health Organization (WHO) definitions of public health, Health for All and the Ottawa Charter for Health Promotion, as follows:

'The science and art of preventing disease, prolonging life and promoting health through the organised efforts of society.' (Department of Health 1988)

The definition alone does not help to clarify nurses' roles in relation to public health, but there has been some discussion about nurses' roles in relation to Health for All.

The Health for All by the Year 2000 (HFA) movement began in 1977 when the WHO adopted a resolution for citizens to attain a level of health by the year 2000 that would allow a socially and economically productive life (Salvage 1993). In 1981 a global strategy was adopted by many governments who produced local targets for achieving the goal of HFA (Salvage 1993). HFA also acted as a springboard for developing the concept of health promotion and the Ottawa Charter for Health Promotion was adopted in 1986 (Ashton & Seymour 1992). The Ottawa Charter provided the basis for the WHO Healthy Cities Project which was set up to develop policy processes in cities to enable people to live healthier lives (Curtice 1993).

The WHO also defined a role in HFA for all nurses, midwives and health visitors in Europe (Salvage 1993). The key concept was to create a nursing role that is responsive to people's health needs rather than to the needs of the health care system. The principles of the HFA nurse should be in line with the European policies of HFA and primary care, as follows:

- Positive health promotion
- Participation of individuals, families and communities in care
- Working towards equity
- Collaborative working
- Assurance of quality of care.

It was recommended that education, management and planning of nursing services should take account of HFA principles and that nurses should be more involved in debating health policy (Salvage 1993). While it appears that nurses across Europe have been unwilling or unable to adopt the HFA principles, health visitors using community development approaches in isolated projects have demonstrated that these principles serve community nursing well in responding to community health issues (Craig 1996).

It could then be argued that the point at which nursing and public health meet is at the new public health movement, which combines environmental change – i.e. physical, socioeconomic and psychological circumstances – with personal preventive measures. The new public health movement was supported by the development of HFA and the Ottawa Charter for Health Promotion and recognises the importance of the social and policy aspects of health problems (Ashton & Seymour 1992). However, neither the new public health movement nor the HFA nurse have been able to enter the mainstream of NHS practice.

NURSING, HEALTH VISITING AND PUBLIC HEALTH PRACTICE

Current practice of nurses in public health departments appears to be patchy across the UK, with nurses rarely having a lead role in needs assessment or commissioning. Bhopal (1993) suggested that improvements in public health would be more likely to occur if public health doctors collaborated with other health service employees to 'inspire' them to analyse determinants of health and health service needs, and to carry out health promotion. It could be argued that health visitors have already been 'inspired' to work in this way through training and experience, and that public health doctors appeared to have overlooked the potential of health visitors as allies in improving public health. One public health doctor appeared to recognise the preventative potential for health visiting when he argued that the NHS was recruiting inexperienced and untrained health promotion workers directly at the expense of health visiting (Stone 1996). However, another group of doctors writing in the same journal at around the same time, used health visiting as an example of an 'untested assertion' that should not be purchased by the NHS until hard evidence could be produced as to their effectiveness (Roberts 1996). It appears that until health visiting can be evaluated in a 'scientific' way, there may be little scope for closer involvement with public health departments.

CONCLUSION

It is clear that the development of public health nursing in the UK has not been straightforward. Like public health, public health nursing has drawn on a number of disciplines and sets of principles to underpin theory and practice. Consequently, the scope of public health nursing is very broad. On one hand, such a broad scope inevitably attracts competing viewpoints about theory and practice. On the positive side however, the broad base engenders flexibility in responding to complex health problems.

Public health nursing in the UK is therefore a term that can describe the work of nurses from a number of specialties. The common thread appears to be that they focus on a population or community, dealing with public health priorities from a top-down and/or bottom-up approach. Health visitors have a specific contribution to make to the improvement of public health, based on the body of experience built up over the last hundred years. They are also in an ideal position to take a population approach to promoting health, but the issue of whether they should be targeting individuals or populations still needs to be addressed at policy and practice level. While health visiting may have been singled out as having a particular public health role, it should not be assumed that health visitors have more of a claim over the public health nursing title than other nurses. There are many examples of all kinds of nurses who are able and willing to take up the challenge of working beyond an individual level. Public health nurses must support each other in meeting this challenge.

DISCUSSION QUESTIONS	<ul><li>To what extent do current policies support a public health model in primary care?</li><li>Should the title of health visiting be changed to public health nursing?</li><li>To what extent should other community nurses be adopting a public health approach?</li></ul>

FURTHER READING

Townsend P and Davidson N (eds) 1988 Inequalities in Health – The Black Report and Whitehead M, the Health Divide. Penguin, London
Although written 20 years ago, the Black Report stands up as a classic text on health inequalities. It goes into detail on many issues around poverty and health that remain pertinent today, in this climate of worsening health inequalities.

Davies C 1996 Gender and the Professional Predicament in Nursing. Open University Press, Buckingham
Some of the problems identified in this chapter, regarding recognition of the nursing contribution to public health, are not dissimilar to those highlighted by Celia Davies in this enlightening book about the position of nursing in general within the male, medically-dominated NHS.

Public Health Alliance 1998 A Public Health Model of Primary Care – From Concept to Reality. The Public Health Alliance, Birmingham
This is the report of a project which developed a public health model for primary care and tested the model in four sites in Scotland, England and Wales. It identified a theoretical framework for public health in primary care, as well as practical barriers and drivers for public health to be integrated with primary care practice.

REFERENCES

Acheson D 1998 Report of the Independent Inquiry into Inequalities in Health. The Stationery Office, London

Ashton J & Seymour H 1988 The New Public Health. Open University Press, Milton Keynes

Baly M E 1991 As Miss Nightingale Said ... Scutari Press, London

Berridge V 1995 The social and historical development of public health and public health nursing. Presentation to Standing Nursing and Midwifery Advisory Committee Workshop

Bhopal R S 1993 Public health medicine and purchasing health care. British Medical Journal 306:381–382

Billingham K 1994a Beyond the individual. Health Visitor 67(9):295

Billingham K 1994b The challenge for practice. Nursing Times 90(39):43

Blackburn C 1991 Family poverty: what can health visitors do? Health Visitor 64(1): 368–370

Boschma G 1997 Ambivalence about nursing's expertise: the role of a gendered holistic ideology in nursing, 1890–1990. In: Rafferty A M, Robinson J & Elkan R (eds) Nursing History and the Politics of Welfare. Routledge, London

Boyd M, Brummell K, Billingham K & Perkins E 1993 The public health post at Strelley: An Interim Report.

Nottingham Community Health NHS Trust, Nottinghan

Caraher M & McNab M 1996 The public health nursing role: and overview of future trends. Nursing Standard 10(51):44–48

Carpenter M 1977 The new managerialism and professionalism in nursing. In: Stacey M, Reid M, Heath C & Dingwall R (eds) Health and the Division of Labour. Croom Helm, London

Chalmers A K 1930 The Health of Glasgow 1818–1925. Greater Glasgow Health Board, Glasgow

Council for the Education and Training of Health Visitors 1977 An Investigation into the Principles and Practice of Health Visiting. Council for the Education and Training of Health Visitors, London

Cowley S 1996 Reflecting on the past; preparing for the next century. Health Visitor 69(8):313–316

Craig P 1996 Drumming up Health in Drumchapel: community development health visiting. Health Visitor 69(11):459–461

Craig P 1998 A Description of the Public Health Role of Health Visitors. Unpublished MSc Thesis, University of Glasgow

Curtice L 1993 Strategies and values: research and the WHO Healthy Cities project in Europe. In: Davies J K, Kelly M (eds) Healthy Cities Research and Practice. Routledge, London

Davies C 1988 The health visitor as mother's friend: a woman's place in public health 1900–1914. Social History of Medicine 1(1):39–59

De la Cuesta C 1994 Marketing: a process in health visiting. Journal of Advanced Nursing 19:347–353

Deal L W 1994 The effectiveness of community nursing interventions: a literature review. Public Health Nursing 11(5):315–323

Department of Health 1988 Public health in England: the report of the Committee of Inquiry into the Future Development of the Public Health Function. HMSO, London

Department of Health 1997a The New NHS. The Stationery Office, London

Department of Health 1997b Priorities and Planning Guidance for the NHS 1998/99. Department of Health, London

Department of Health 1999a Saving Lives: Our Healthier Nation. The Stationery Office, London

Department of Health 1999b Making a Difference: strengthening the nursing, health visiting and midwifery contribution to health and health care. The Stationery Office, London

Dingwall R 1977 Collectivism, regionalism and feminism: health visiting and British social policy 1850–1975. Journal of Social Policy 6(3):291–315

Dingwall R & Robinson K M 1993 Policing the family? Health visiting and the public surveillance of private behaviour. In: Beattie A, Gott M, Jones L & Sidell M (eds) Health & Wellbeing: A Reader. Macmillan Press, Basingstoke

Doyal L & Pennell P 1979 The political economy of health. Pluto Press, London

Erickson G P 1996 To pauperize or empower: public health nursing at the turn of the 20th and 21th centuries. Public Health Nursing 13(3):163–169

Flinn M W (ed) 1965 Report on the Sanitary Condition of the Labouring Population of Great Britain, by Edwin Chadwick. Edinburgh University Press, Edinburgh

Frachel R R 1988 A new profession: the evolution of public health nursing. Public Health Nursing 5(2):86–90

Goodwin S 1988 Whither health visiting? Health Visitor 61:379–383

Hamilton D 1987 The Healers: a History of Medicine in Scotland. Canongate, Edinburgh

Hanafin S 1997 The role of the Irish public health nurse: manager, clinician and health promoter. Health Visitor 70(8):295–297

Home Office 1998 Supporting Families – A Consultation Document. The Stationery Office, London

Khan M & Landes R 1993 The Role of the Public Health Nurse – a Review of the International Literature. Public Health Research and Resource Centre, Salford

King M E, Harrison M J & Reutter L 1995 Public health nursing or community health nursing: examining the debate. Canadian Journal of Public Health 86(1):24–25

Laughlin S & Black D (eds) 1995 Poverty and Health, Tools For Change. Public Health Alliance, Birmingham

Lewis J 1991 The public's health: philosophy and practice in Britain in the twentieth century. In: Fee E & Acheson R (eds) A History of Education in Public Health. Oxford University Press, New York

McDonald A & Chavasse J 1997 Community participation within an Irish Health Board area. British Journal of Nursing 6(6):341–345

McGregor A 1967 Public Health in Glasgow 1905–1946. Livingstone, Edinburgh

McKeown T 1965 Medicine in Modern Society. George Allen & Unwin, London.

McKeown T & Record R G 1963 Reasons for the decline of mortality in England and Wales during the nineteenth century. In: Glass D V & Grebenik E (eds) Population Studies – A Journal of Demography, Vol XIV. London

Orr J 1981 Feminism and health visiting. Health Visitor 54(4):156–157

Roberts C et al 1996 The proof of the pudding. Health Service Journal 106(5494):27

Robinson J 1982 An Evaluation of Health Visiting. Council for the Education and Training of Health Visitors, London

Robinson J 1985 Health visiting and health. In: White R (ed) Political Issues in Nursing: Past, Present and Future, Vol. 1. John Wiley & Sons, Chichester

Royal College of Nursing 1994 Public Health: Nursing Rises to the Challenge. Royal College of Nursing, London

Sachs H 1990 A Brave Attempt. The King's Fund, London

Salvage J (ed) 1993 Nursing in Action: Strengthening Nursing and Midwifery to Support Health For All. World Health Organization, Copenhagen

Scottish Office Department of Health 1997 Designed to Care: Renewing the National Health Service in Scotland. The Stationery Office, Edinburgh

Scottish Office Department of Health 1999 Towards a Healthier Scotland. The Stationery Office, Edinburgh

Scruby L S & McKay M 1991 Strengthening communities: changing roles for community health nurses. Health Promotion International 6(4):263–268

Smith C 1997 Public health measurement. Nursing Management (UK) 3(9):12–13

Standing Nursing and Midwifery Advisory Committee 1995 Making it Happen. Department of Health, London

Stone D 1996 Visiting time. Health Service Journal 106(5497):28–29

Symonds A 1997 Ties that bind: problems with GP attachment. Health Visitor 70(2):53–55

Twinn S 1991 Conflicting paradigms of health visiting: a continuing debate for professional practice. Journal of Advanced Nursing 16:966–973

Twinn S & Cowley S 1992 The principles of health visiting: a re-examination. Health Visitors Association and United Kingdom Standing Conference on Health Visiting, London

Webster C 1990 The Victorian Public Health Legacy: A Challenge to the Future. Public Health Alliance, Birmingham

Webster C (ed) 1993 Caring for Health: History and Diversity. Open University Press, Buckingham

White R 1985 The Effects of the NHS on the Nursing Profession 1948–1961. King's Fund, London

Whitehead M 1995 Tackling inequalities: a review of policy initiatives. In: Benzeval M, Judge K & Whitehead M (eds) Tackling Inequalities in Health: An Agenda for Action. King's Fund, London

Womersley J 1987 The evolution of health information services. In: McGlachlan G (ed) Improving the Common Weal: Aspects of Scottish Health Services 1900–1984. Edinburgh University Press, Edinburgh

3 Public health and health promotion

Pauline Pearson

KEY ISSUES

- This chapter addresses notions of health, public health, health promotion and primary health care, and some of the important overlaps and distinctions between them.
- Distinctions between the 'medical' model of health – that health is the absence of disease – 'social health' – the ability to fulfil social roles – and lay definitions of health, are outlined.
- The ways in which public health nurses negotiate between the various views of health in practice are discussed.
- The main theoretical perspectives underpinning health promotion work in practice are described, for example, DiClemente and Prochaska's (1982) behaviour change cycle, Becker's (1974) health belief model, organisation theories of transformational change, and economic theory, locating these in relation to work with individuals, with groups and organisations and at a policy level.
- Brief examples from practice are given. These include a pilot scheme to provide warfarin-monitoring sessions through a GP practice, lunch-time health fairs to identify the health needs of young adolescents and work with a housing department.

INTRODUCTION

Since the beginning of movements to promote and maintain the public health, it has been necessary for those engaged in practical hands-on, activity to think about explanations for the situations they encounter, and to ground their responses in appropriate frameworks. There has grown up a substantial body of theory in relation to the promotion of health, which supports and can enhance public health practice, in nursing as much as in other groups. This chapter first of all looks at the notions of health, public health, health promotion and primary health care, and teases out some of the important overlaps and distinctions between them. Some of the distinctions which have been made between medical, social and lay definitions of health, and the way in which public health nurses have negotiated between the various views are investigated. Consideration is given to some of the main theoretical perspectives underpinning health promotion work in practice, locating these in relation to work with individuals, with groups and organisations and at policy level. Finally, some brief examples from practice are given, which will be developed further in Section Three.

WHAT IS HEALTH?

Before considering 'public health' or 'health promotion' it is important to briefly consider definitions of health. Ask three people the meaning of 'health', and each may give a different answer. One may say, 'It's when you're not ill'. Another may say, 'It's when you can get around and do what you have to do'. A third may suggest that it is when you feel good about yourself. Each of these views has been described in numerous research studies (Blaxter 1982, Cornwell 1984, Mayall 1986, Pearson 1991). The first is often described as the 'medical' model of health – that health is the absence of disease. It is described in this way because health is seen as the absence of pathogens and disease processes. Medical interventions are frequently geared to avoiding or destroying pathogens or arresting disease processes.

The second view can be described as the 'functional' model of health – often used in relation to people with disabilities or older people. Difficulties arise with this model in a society where the boundaries of everyday function and the technological supports available are changing rapidly, and where activists have strongly put the case for a 'social' model of disability, which makes clear that it is the product of society's inability to adapt and respond to impairments, demonstrated in function (French 1993). An extension of this idea is the notion of 'social health' – an ability to fulfil social roles. This is in many ways the obverse of Parsons' (1951) idea of the sick role, in which being 'ill' confers exemption, for a period, from social roles.

The third view suggests that how people feel about themselves is more important than impairment or a disease process. The World Health Organization (1946) in its constitution brought together these ideas when they stated that health was, 'a state of complete physical, mental and social well-being and not merely the absence of disease or infirmity'. While this has been criticised as Utopian, it has the merit of integrating the three most common conceptualisations. Health is thus not one but a number of ideas, which operate in different people's minds at different times in considering how the health of the public may be promoted and maintained.

WHAT IS PUBLIC HEALTH?

Asked where 'public health' began as a concept, many health professionals will date its birth to the days of the Broad Street pump, and John Snow's single-handed determination to find and deal with the cause of a raging cholera outbreak in 1854. Alternatively, they may point to the work of Florence Nightingale, pulling together and laboriously presenting data on the incidence of infection and death among soldiers in the Crimean War, and later in the poorer areas of her day, and suggesting strategies to bring about change, the results of which are well-known. There is no doubt that in those early days of Queen Victoria's reign, the burgeoning of the Industrial Revolution, the shift of populations into cities and the movement of patterns of work from those linked to natural cycles to those tied to supply and demand, among many other factors, all generated patterns of health experience which began to concern many people, and led them to begin to think about the way in which a society creates health.

My personal vote for the key person behind the original public health movement is Edwin Chadwick. Chadwick's Report on the Sanitary Condition of the Labouring Population of Great Britain (Chadwick 1965) was seminal. He was a civil servant who drew together the reports of a range of local informants to produce a hard-hitting analysis of the morbidity created by overcrowding, lack of sanitation, long working hours and lack of leisure space or opportunity. Presented to the House of Lords in 1842, this led to demands for change. From these emerged the first Public Health Act in 1848.

At the beginning, public health was driven by concerns about visible suffering and high death rates. In the modern context these are the concerns of the 'third' world (two-thirds of the world). In India, for example, only around 40% of households have toilet facilities even today, despite extensive government investment programmes. Provision of access to clean water has been more successful, though work now needs to be done to prevent build-up of waste water attracting mosquitoes and undermining progress on malaria. Polio is still relatively common, though intensive community education programmes and national immunisation drives are beginning to pay off.

In Victorian Britain, much less was known about the mechanisms of disease than is the case today, but careful analysis of large bodies of data enabled those who wanted to to begin to identify possible relationships. If urban death rates for all socioeconomic groups exceeded those for rural populations, then something about cities was bad for people! If a particular community was experiencing excessive morbidity from cholera, then something must make that area more susceptible, or it must be exposed to risk more often. From there it was a combination of trial and error and painstaking detective work on the ground. Theories about infection were in their infancy, but were to grow and become one of the central planks of public health workers' thinking up to the beginning of the NHS and to some extent beyond.

Towards the end of the nineteenth century lady sanitary inspectors (the forerunners of health visitors), supported by a cadre of locally recruited women, were employed in Salford to take action on the ground to improve hygiene and take all appropriate action to prevent or curtail outbreaks of disease. Despite Chadwick's recognition of the importance of leisure, which bore fruit in some major cities in the form of great public parks, public health at this time was primarily about the prevention and control of infection, to ensure that the workforce in the new factories, male and female, and the soldiers fighting in a variety of wars, would be fit enough to maintain acceptable levels of productivity. It was in essence about preventing disease (a medical model) and maintaining a level of health within society which enabled it to meet its economic obligations.

The next stage in the development of public health as a concept emerged at the beginning of the twentieth century, when difficulties were encountered in obtaining enough fit recruits to fight in the Boer War. The technology of warfare was changing, and larger numbers of men were required. Too many of those volunteering had poor eyesight, were undersized, or had deformities produced by rickets and other nutritional deficiencies. The government responded by refocusing some of its efforts into the welfare of children. In particular, if children could be adequately nourished, and mothers guided to make a point of this, then the young men of the future would be equipped to go to war. Infant welfare clinics were opened across the country during and after the First World War – some indeed served as memorials within their communities. Babies were weighed and measured regularly, and advice on nutrition and budget-management became part of the package offered by the health visitors – much as Florence Nightingale had suggested many years earlier. Screening of vision, height and weight was undertaken with school-age children, though until the advent of the NHS, visual defects were responded to according to income (could glasses be afforded), rather than need. Sanitary inspection branched out into issues about housing quality. Public health work had now expanded to include screening and the promotion of a healthy diet and housing. Its purpose now included establishing, as well as maintaining, health within society. There was some recognition of environmental and social contributions to health, though the predominant model was medical.

The NHS was born in 1948, with an underlying philosophy of equity in provision and entitlement to care, together with notions about providing cure/care for all, largely associated with a medical model of health. To some extent, *public* health lay outside this agenda, since many of those involved in its delivery – health visitors, school nurses, directors of public health – did not join the NHS, but remained within the local authority setting. At the same time, developments were occurring in ideas about behaviour and psychological theory. Skinner (1953) and other behaviourists were working on ideas about animals which would lead to new conceptualisations about human behaviour. Over the next few decades, Becker and colleagues (1974) were pulling together theories about people's health beliefs and examining the reasons why people take up or stop behaving in ways which damage health. Social theory was also developing rapidly, with sociologists looking at the development of professions, the functioning of communities and at marginal groups (Whyte 1993), while social policy was being driven forward by people such as Richard Titmuss (1970).

However, changes in patterns of service delivery were slow. In 1974, the NHS took in community health services, and at the same time set in place structures in which professionals began to be consciously 'managed'. Emphasis began to be placed on policies and protocols. Record systems were revised. The 'nursing process', a model originating in hospital settings and relating to the management of one or more problems, was widely promoted, and taken up by many community practitioners – for example in the form discussed by Clark (1986). In 1979, the political context changed. Margaret Thatcher came to power and over almost the next two decades proclaimed that there was 'no such thing as society'. Clearly, public health work had to reinvent itself to respond to the mood of the day.

In fact, two paths emerged. One, most clearly seen in the 1992 'Health of the Nation' document, took up the medical model and proceeded to look, in the main, at individuals' behaviour, focusing on the responsibility of each individual to contribute to improving health targets, and the need to provide individuals with the 'information to help make the right choices' (Department of Health 1992 p 22). Though there was a suggestion that other agencies might play a part in promoting the health of the public through the notion of 'healthy alliances', this idea was poorly developed, and little was done to follow it up, except to some extent in local authorities who picked up the idea of health-promoting schools. The other main deficit of policy at this time, again clearly seen in the 'Health of the Nation' document, was the failure to acknowledge poverty and socioeconomic factors as significant in shaping people's health experience. The second pathway followed the community development ideas, which had flourished a decade or more earlier, and built on a salutogenic model of health (Antonovsky 1996), in which the key to a healthy population is that it has the resources for health. While the first approach was dominant, and became increasingly so in government thinking, many community development projects were also set up during this time. Though many were short-lived – for example Strelley in Nottingham (Boyd et al 1993), some (such as Castlemilk near Glasgow and Meadowell on Tyneside) have survived.

Public health in general remained locked into these models, though there were some pioneers who began to look at what was known as the 'new' public health (Ashton & Seymour 1988). This rests on a model which draws on the World Health Organization's definition of health, acknowledging that health is a product of many factors, and that work to promote and maintain health requires a balance between individually focused work and work at the level of society. Like John Ashton, who was involved in the development of the Healthy Cities Initiative (Ashton et al 1986), Steve Watkins, Director of Public Health in Stockport, was a pioneer of this new way of looking at public health. Against the grain of policy at the time, he facilitated the establishment of an integrated public health service in Stockport, which offered community-based health development work, as well as large-scale intervention programmes (Watkins 1994, 1996).

By 1997, when a landslide unseated the Conservative government of the last 18 years, politicians had begun to acknowledge that the individualistic model alone was not sufficient, and that 'health variations' (inequalities in health) required attention at a more structural level. The new government set in place a range of initiatives which demonstrated that promoting and maintaining the health of the public was now a central plank of the government's policies. The appointment of a Minister for Public Health in 1997 confirmed that this was the case. The publication in quick succession of several green and white papers reinforced this, and emphasised the importance both of communities and of primary health care as a setting for public health work. The 'New NHS: Modern Dependable' White Paper (Department of Health 1997) shifted commissioning towards a health-oriented model and more firmly into primary health care. Late in 1998, the Acheson Report on 'Inequalities in Health' (Acheson 1998) and the publication by the Home Office of a green paper called 'Supporting Families' (Home Office 1998) gave further momentum to the shift to a psychosocial model of health. In the closing year of the millennium, the White Paper 'Saving Lives: Our Healthier Nation' (Department of Health 1999) highlighted the importance of community development approaches and of looking at environments (school, work and community), as well as the management of disease processes. It made clear the potential contribution of midwives, health visitors and school nurses, among others, to achieving this, building on their work with families and communities. The new public health had really arrived.

PROMOTING HEALTH

While the promotion of the health of the public is an intrinsic element of 'public health', it is often confused with other closely-related concepts. The World Health Organization (1984) suggest that it may be defined as 'the process of enabling people to increase control over, and to improve, their health'. The process of promoting health may be undertaken in a variety of ways. Most often people think of health promotion in terms of firstly health education and secondly prevention. Tannahill (1985) highlights a third, overlapping component, which he calls health protection. Each of these elements is discussed below.

Health education

Health education can be defined as giving people information about living healthy lifestyles, and the skills to understand and use this information. In the early part of the twentieth century, before the development of social and psychological theory, manuals gave detailed instruction on healthy living, with little concern about how real people might put the instructions into practice in real contexts (Board of Education 1928). In the later part of the twentieth century, through to the present day, educational theory has developed further. Health educators have become aware, for example, that different styles of presentation of information may be effective for different audiences. Ewles and Simnett (1985) describe five different approaches to health education, which are listed in Box 3.1.

Those engaged in health education can look more closely at ways of engaging their target audiences and assess the impact of their activity has, not only on knowledge and attitudes but also on behaviour. Health education programmes have also drawn increasingly on the developing theory of marketing. For example Kaner et al (1999) describe the use of a marketing approach in introducing a brief intervention programme for problem drinkers into general practice. The purpose of health education may range from purely educational through empowerment and personal growth to a more 'radical – political' approach.

BOX 3.1	*The five approaches to health education (Ewles & Simnett 1985)*

- **Medical** – the promotion of medical interventions to prevent or ameliorate ill health
- **Behaviour change** – to encourage the adoption of a 'healthier' lifestyle
- **Educational** – provision of information to underpin decision-making, exploration of values and attitudes and skill-development
- **Client-directed** – working with clients' own identified health priorities
- **The social-change approach** – involving political or social change to alter the physical or social environment

Prevention

The relationship between prevention and health promotion is more complex than it seems. The idea of prevention has been clearly linked to a pathogenic concept of health. Leavell (1953) sets out the inter-relationship clearly, identifying three levels of prevention and linking them to different levels of disease process. His model assumes that where there are no symptoms of disease, but exposure is possible, then primary preventive action is required – for example, immunisation programmes. Where early symptoms exist but disease may remain at a sub-clinical level (in other words may not have reached a point where the individual has presented it to a health professional), then secondary preventive action is required – for example through screening for cervical cancer or for glaucoma – to enable action to be taken to arrest the progress of the disease. Where disease processes are established, tertiary prevention aims to minimise further damage – for example through the provision of cardiac rehabilitation programmes for post-MI patients. However, though this model is widely used in discussions of health-promoting activity, its base in a pathogenic framework limits its usefulness. Wass (1994, after Brown 1985) has suggested a development of Leavell's model, which superimposes three further components on the original. Figure 3.1 shows that she suggests that the primary prevention level is also the primary health promotion level – geared to eradicating health risks at the individual level. She then suggests that there are two further levels of health promotion – secondary health promotion, which is concerned with raising individual quality of life, and tertiary health promotion, which is concerned with effecting enduring social change. The introduction of a level beyond the individual reflects the experience of most community nurses. An alternative model of health promotion put forward by Kelly and colleagues (1993) suggests that there are in fact four levels at which health promoting activity takes place – individual, organisational, social and environmental. While these are useful ways of conceptualising what is going on, they do not fully reflect the complexity of practice, where interventions may be made consecutively with the individual and his or her context at the same time as advocating social change. Individual practitioners may be carrying out activities which fit into several levels at once.

Health protection

Health protection is understood, within Tannahill's (1985) model, as comprising decisions by 'local, national or international government or other influential bodies', for example industrial or commercial organisations, which 'will positively promote health'. Examples might be the passage of seat-belt legislation, taxation on cigarettes or the voluntary installation by car manufacturers of additional safety features.

The building of healthy public policy formed an important element of the Ottawa Charter for Health Promotion (World Health Organization 1986). This suggested that health promotion through policy might involve legislation, fiscal measures, taxation and organisational change, to produce policies which would foster greater equity. The Charter linked health protection – the use of politics to create an environment which is safer, and in which healthier choices are

FIGURE 3.1 *Beyond disease prevention (Reproduced with permission from Wass A 1999 Promoting Health: the primary health care approach, 2nd edn. Harcourt Australia, developed from Brown 1985, pp 332–333).*

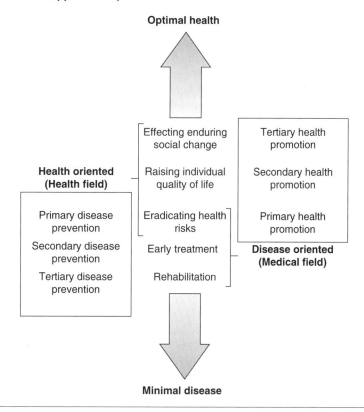

easier to make – to strengthening community action and developing personal skills. This fitted with the balance inherent in the 'new public health' agenda. Health protection alone might be seen as paternalistic, or at least imposed. Nevertheless, it is worth comparing this approach with the work of early public health pioneers such as Chadwick, who sought to make a difference to the lives of the poor through policy development.

WHERE DOES PRIMARY HEALTH CARE FIT?

Primary health care is 'essential health care made accessible at a cost a country and community can afford, with methods that are practical, scientifically sound and socially acceptable' (World Health Organization 1978). The Alma-Ata Declaration goes on to state that primary health care is based on principles of equity, participation by the community, an intersectoral approach, appropriate technology and affordable costs. Despite the inter-relationships between the notions of primary care espoused by the World Health Organization and the ideas about public health and health promotion set out above, little has been done to explore how these operate on the ground. The context in which they relate is rapidly changing. Primary care groups (PCGs) have been brought together with responsibility, in the first instance with Health Authorities, to produce a viable Health Improvement Plan (HImP) for the populations they serve. Though PCGs include a variety of disciplines, in practice it is often general practitioners and community nurses, especially health visitors, who are charged with finding ways of identifying and meeting health needs for the populations with which they work.

Bhopal (1995) advocated a much stronger public health role for general practitioners, but also identified some of the barriers to this in existing patterns of work, not least their tendency to focus on disease management. As far back as 1977 it was recognised that health visiting revolved around four key principles – the search for health needs, stimulation of awareness of health needs, facilitation of health-enhancing activities, and influence on policies affecting health (CETHV 1977). More recent reviews suggest that these principles remain valid, and could underpin the implementation of recent reforms. However, an increasingly contract-led environment has led to many health visitors being unable to do more than routine surveillance visits, with some thus losing their ability to respond flexibly to a perceived health need. Recent work (Pearson et al 2000) has examined how far programmes of education successfully prepare community nursing practitioners to carry out a public health role, and some of the factors which help or hinder this once they have qualified. Some of the key difficulties appear to be in the articulation of what public health work means at the grass roots level, and in the production of an effective model to bridge the practice-to-commissioning divide.

Primary health care is also about equitable provision and the promotion of health for *all*. Yet there is ample evidence that most inequalities in health have either remained the same or widened over recent decades. The Acheson (1998) report sets out 39 recommendations, backed by 529 references, which the committee suggest should be priority areas for action to reduce inequalities in health in England. Most do not relate directly to NHS services. However, they do highlight the importance of ensuring that communities most at risk of ill-health have good access to effective primary care, and that effective partnerships between health and social care providers are nurtured. In addition, in the White Paper 'The New NHS, Modern, Dependable' (Department of Health 1997) the importance of including 'a strong public voice' has been emphasised. It is therefore important to consider in more detail some of the ways in which medical, social and lay definitions of health differ.

DISTINCTIONS BETWEEN MEDICAL, SOCIAL AND LAY DEFINITIONS OF HEALTH

Some of the different views of health which exist have been set out above. While initially the medical perspective was dominant, an alternative set of perspectives on health, which has rather different implications for health promotion, derived from the rapidly developing social sciences over the twentieth century. The development of psychology as an academic discipline led to the conceptualisation of 'normal' and 'abnormal' behaviour. Alongside this, developmental psychology took shape, indicating 'normal' patterns of development. The notion of health as related to functional or developmental 'adequacy' was highlighted. This idea has been used in many health-related intervention studies as the basis of an outcome measurement for health promotion at some level. What proportion of the population can achieve an adequate Barthel score (Collin et al 1988) following intervention from a multidisciplinary early-discharge team (Rodgers et al 1997)? What proportion of children achieve 'normal' language development following an intensive programme of health visiting (Cox & Hill 1993)? One of the key issues here is the question of value judgements. What is adequate, or normal? For whom? Community practitioners who have transferred from inner city to outer suburb, or vice versa, anecdotally highlight the different framing which they had to develop in relation to these judgements. In one area it may be seen as developmentally normal for a child to be beginning to construct sentences by 24 months, whereas in a neighbouring area, the perceived norm may be later. In dealing with subgroups of a larger population, judgements of this sort will be common. In addition, a behaviour which is broadly harmful to health, such as smoking, may be defined, by a subgroup of society, as functional – to produce smaller babies, or to reduce stress, or both. The measures of health which emerge from this grouping of perspectives tend to relate at an individual level either to the level of independence (of function) or to the level of capacity (in terms of development towards an optimal state). Functional and behavioural problems or developmental delay can also be looked at in relation to population measures such as incidence, to determine whether particular interventions lead to significant reductions.

Promoting health in this context may link to wider debates, such as the role of parenting as an antecedent in positive or negative patterns of behaviour, and to the development of initiatives and interventions which build on this approach. The Sure Start Initiative seeks to intervene directly with young families to help them achieve effective parenting and to prevent poor literacy, child abuse and crime (DfEE 1999). Work to manage sleep problems (Kerr et al 1996) and other behaviour problems can be located within a psychological framework, though it is important to remember that low self-esteem may impact on the ability of any individual to successfully alter their behaviour, or to sustain altered behaviour.

The development of sociological theories about health and health care has been considerable, and is addressed in many other texts. Sociologists have sought to make sense of the ways in which health is understood by individuals and society as a whole. Of particular relevance to an exploration of promoting health is the literature which highlights ways in which health is socially constructed. Classically, Zola (1973) describes the way in which mental health problems are differentially presented in different ethnic groups, based on different perceptions of everyday behaviour, rather than any objective standard. This highlights both the need to review existing diagnostic and treatment standards for equity, but also more widely the need to test understandings with patients and carers as well as professionals. Cornwell (1984) interviewed a sample of people living in part of the East End of London about their health and health care. She looks at individuals' definitions of health and says that her (lay) respondents see health as 'functioning in a socially accepted way'. They perceive a moral imperative to conform, and in particular to seek relevant help or seek to avoid known risk factors. Where individuals are seen as not conforming, they are seen as blameworthy in relation to their illness. Parsons, (1951), described the notion of the 'sick role' which required an individual to take appropriate action to get better when ill. Cornwell's work appears to somewhat extend this to place an obligation to avoid risk, if possible. Using this framework, health promotion might be construed as social control, seeking to facilitate conformity. For example, Look After Your Heart classes provide information about patterns of behaviour in relation to food and exercise which are appropriate to reduce the risk of heart disease, but may be seen, at least implicitly, as disapproving of other behaviours.

Cornwell goes on to identify three lay conceptualisations of illness – 'serious illness' (for example myocardial infarction or a cerebrovascular accident), 'normal illness' (which might include measles or mumps) and 'health problems which are not illness' (a category into which many problematic aspects of child and family health might fall). Alongside this, several studies (Blaxter 1982, Mayall 1986, Pearson 1991) have highlighted three lay conceptualisations of health, touched on earlier.

Health can be seen as 'not being ill', bearing in mind the ways in which illness may be viewed. Health may also be seen as functional by lay people, being able to achieve day-to-day tasks effectively, or in relation to children achieving appropriate developmental function. Thirdly, health may be seen as related to emotional well-being. Socioemotional well-being incorporates ideas of 'happiness' and contentment, and the avoidance of the fear of crime, drugs and violence. In one survey of a local community to ascertain health needs, most lay people suggested reductions in crime and increases in shops and facilities long before exercise classes or information provision.

Because these different understandings of 'health' exist between different agencies and professional groups, and between professionals and lay people, health promotion in practice requires public health nurses (and others) to negotiate these in their work and come to a shared view, before intervention can occur. In the next section, ways in which the negotiation process works are discussed, before the theories which may underpin interventions are described, and examples given.

NEGOTIATING PERSPECTIVES

Negotiation between these ideas can arise at an individual or family level. For example, a patient who smokes and has high blood pressure may be depressed. She may be a single parent, living in vulnerable, poor-quality accommodation, harassed by violent neighbours. She may have several children, some of whom are experiencing developmental problems. Different agencies and professionals are likely to utilise different models. The GP is likely to focus on medical and behavioural ideas of health, looking at screening for and reduction of cardiovascular risk through medication or behavioural intervention. The health visitor may prioritise exploring issues to do with parenting, self-esteem and community safety, using social and psychological concepts of health, an approach which sees the family, the community and the wider environment as key players in the health of this person. Provided these models are viewed as complementary rather than in conflict or overriding each other, the GP and the health visitor can operate effectively as a health-promoting 'team'. Within the wider context, different models may also be seen to operate. The local school or nursery would probably build on a behavioural approach and prioritise intensive work with the children to facilitate their development. The housing department might take a risk-based approach to this family's housing needs, possibly looking at this in relation to severe psychological or physical risk only. If these different perspectives are recognised, they can be used to build up an action plan addressing health holistically.

At a community level agencies and professionals may also negotiate health promotion activity from different perspectives on health. In looking at the health needs of a community, local GPs may work from the traditional medically-focused base of identifying specific morbidity and mortality figures for that area. Health visitors may use social and behavioural approaches to prioritise access to healthy food choices, parenting problems and community-safety concerns. School nurses may build on behavioural ideas to highlight high school exclusion rates and incidence of bullying. All of these ideas may be negotiated in the primary care group or local health group, prioritised, and appropriate action planned, within the construction of the Health Improvement Programme.

One important issue in the debates around health promotion is the question of targeting. What is the evidence on the relative effectiveness and feasibility of targeting individuals or population groups? In practice a judicious combination may be best. Where an intervention is specific and has a clear value, whole population groups can appropriately be targeted. For example, it is now commonplace to offer all babies immunisations against diphtheria, tetanus and polio, among others, at an early age. The protective effect of this is well described, and side-effects are few. However, there has been more debate about other interventions. One example of targeting populations for health promotion is the routine 'over 75 check' which became mandatory for practice teams to offer during the Thatcher government. This was offered to everyone in the relevant age-group but was rapidly found to be of questionable value. There was an initial positive effect, particularly in relation to services such as chiropody, and in increased morale (echoing Luker 1982, who demonstrated a positive psychological impact of health visitor visits to older people). However, longer term, morbidity and mortality effects reduced the impact of the check, and further resources were required to provide an effective longer-term service, essentially with regular follow-up (McEwan et al 1990).

Attempts to develop effective postal screening tools also had mixed success. Targeting individuals for health promotion interventions requires not only an effective intervention, but also an initial screening exercise to highlight people as appropriate recipients of an intervention. One study which has looked at health promotion in relation to alcohol use (Kaner et al 1999) relies on the use of a validated screening tool to pick out those patients whose alcohol consumption level is at risky levels or worse. Doctor or nurse then targets these people for a 'brief intervention'. However, in this instance, there is no intervention with people who are not yet drinking to excess, so the health promotion is focused on secondary rather than primary prevention.

THEORETICAL PERSPECTIVES UNDERPINNING HEALTH PROMOTION WORK IN PRACTICE

Work with individuals

One of the theoretical frameworks most commonly used in looking at effective health promotion is that of DiClemente and Prochaska (1982). This was originally developed in work with alcohol-dependent people. It rests on the idea that an individual will only change his behaviour when he is ready, having weighed up the pros and cons for him, and will only sustain change when he has reviewed the implications of change and found ways of managing them and making them acceptable. The behaviour – change cycle, as it is commonly known, identifies a series of stages (Box 3.2) through which the individual will pass on the way to a new way of behaving.

The theories which underpin the behaviour – change cycle include Becker's (1974) health belief model, which indicates some of the ways in which individuals may be moved from a pre-contemplative to a contemplative state, or from a contemplative to a planning stage, as well as indicating the factors which may help to sustain behaviour. Another important linked theory is Skinner's (1951) stimulus – response theory, which developed ideas about ways of reinforcing and extinguishing certain sorts of behaviour by offering rewards or punishments. In the context of the behaviour – change cycle this indicates the importance of looking for the rewards and 'punishments' delivered by different behaviours: the comfort of a familiar chair by the fire versus the run in the cold and rain.

BOX 3.2	*Stages of change (adapted from DiClemente & Prochaska 1982)*
Precontemplative	Not even thinking about making a change in this area
Contemplative	The idea of change has been triggered – perhaps by an event, a coincidence, a conversation or an advert – but the individual has no plan for its achievement
Motivated/ planning change	At this stage the individual has begun to plan how he can make a specific change, setting goals for doing more exercise, giving up smoking or eating more healthily. At this stage he will also be considering the factors which will either help or hinder in this, for example peer pressure, breaking routine
Putting change into action	Change goes into action – the plan begins
Keeping change going (or) Relapsing	The individual has to operate strategies to maintain the new behaviour, working to overcome adverse effects of change such as stiffness after exercise, or exacerbation of cough on giving up smoking. In many cases, the individual relapses back to previous patterns of behaviour. He requires reassurance that this is normal. Many people will need to go around the cycle perhaps three or four times before achieving successful change

Work with groups and organisations

Increasingly, policy development is moving towards the promotion of health within communities or across organisations and institutions. Theoretical development in this area has taken place in the study of urban regeneration and in organisational and community development. Much of the thinking has been located in other countries and cultures. The elements of theoretical development have predominantly been in two areas.

First, attention has been paid to the involvement of people within communities and organisations in decisions about change: The importance of public participation in the process of seeking to achieve and maintain health is a central tenet of the 1978 Alma-Ata Declaration on Health for All by the year 2000 (World Health Organization 1978). In the UK it was the Griffiths Report on NHS management in 1983 which first set out the policy shift towards consumerism. While this was seen as empowering people by increasing the choices open to them in a market model of health care, more recent policy shifts have also been motivated by notions of transparency, autonomy, equity and justice. It is now believed by those guiding policy that,

> 'Successful action to reduce inequalities and to promote health can only
> be taken with the active participation of the communities and
> individuals that have been excluded from the benefits available to more
> affluent members of society' (NHS Executive 1998).

The World Health Organization (1991) set out the overall benefits of community involvement and participation in health care as five-fold: Increased coverage of the population, increased efficiency through better coordination of resources, increased effectiveness – through more relevant goals – increased equity through greater recognition of need, and increased self-reliance as a result of increased opportunities for people to control their lives. As noted earlier, in the White Paper 'The New NHS, Modern, Dependable', the importance of including 'a strong public voice' has been emphasised (Department of Health 1997).

Secondly, the way in which organisations and systems operate to bring about change has been explored, and theories constructed about how and why to achieve successful change. For example, Nelson and Wright (1995) suggest that 'stakeholders' and 'transformation' are key concepts within this process. They indicate that these concepts are related to the introduction of ideas from North American organisational management, which view organisations as made up of free-floating actors (stakeholders) with interests which they pursue by a process of bargaining. Transformation is seen as the structural change which results from this.

Work at policy level

Health promotion work at the level of policy appears to be driven by theories on a different scale. Economic theory is perhaps influential in the slow pace of change in relation to advertisement of cigarettes, while it was used effectively in the move to seat-belt legislation. Ideas about potential economic benefit remain among the strongest drivers for health promotion policy: European health policy, in particular, seems to demonstrate concern for the economic benefits of health-promoting activity. In the UK, the Treasury led the move to pump-prime Sure Start initiatives to the tune of £540 million, when faced with massively rising costs of juvenile crime, mental illness and drug use in young people, a trend that the evidence suggested could be reduced or even reversed by early interventions focused upon the most disadvantaged 5% of the pre-school population (see Chapter 13).

EXAMPLES FROM PRACTICE

To conclude this section, a few examples of health promotion work in practice are described. These will be developed further in later chapters. First, at the individual level, a practice nurse working in a large primary care team in Gateshead noticed that many patients of the practice were experiencing difficulties with warfarin treatment. They highlighted two main problems. The first related to the outpatient clinic at which levels were monitored, which had long waiting times and very brief consultations. The second was that people remained uncertain, despite attendance at the clinic, about how they should adjust their dosage according to their day-to-day needs. The practice nurse read up on warfarin. She talked to the GPs and to the consultant haematologist running the outpatient clinic. Then she set up a pilot scheme to provide warfarin-monitoring sessions through the practice, within very strict protocols. The patients were keen to attend, and appreciated having a local service with clear appointments. They continued to ask questions about their dosages, many of which she could not initially answer. However, she found out the answers, and after a while produced a number of leaflets which addressed particular issues which recurred. Evaluation of the service showed that not only was this seen as more accessible and helpful in addressing individual questions – partly through longer consultations – it was also cheaper than the standard option.

An example which takes place at the level of a local school involved issues of both participation and of successful work to change an organisation's culture. Two school nurses in Newcastle worked together to identify the health needs of young adolescents through lunch-time health fairs, at which students were encouraged to put their questions into an anonymised box. Considerable concerns about sexual health and development, as well as mental health, were highlighted. However, offers of discussion with the nurses failed to generate many takers: consultation with young people suggested that sessions would be more effectively located off the school premises, after school hours. When sessions were set up at a local clinic after school hours, these proved to be well-used. Feedback from students enabled the school to reduce bullying and other threats to mental health.

Health-promoting policy has not always been recognised. The examples which exist are often those where an individual city or county has been influenced by relatively small-scale initiatives which challenge traditional ways of thinking. One such example arose out of the secondment of a health visitor and later a district nurse to the housing department in Newcastle. She was exploring housing patterns across the city and decided to visit all the sheltered-housing units. As a result, she discovered a number of issues ranging from training deficits for sheltered-housing wardens, to decision-making by housing officers. Sheltered wardens complained of the 'TWIT' syndrome – The Warden Is There. They were often cast in the role of semi-formal carer for an increasingly frail group of people, while in reality having a very limited knowledge base. This was addressed by collaborative sessions with local district nurses and social workers, and contributed to the development of a new organisational structure for wardens, including a 24-hour centralised control room, and greater use of a mobile service as back-up. Housing officers often made their decisions about housing in the virtual absence of health information. They were encouraged to make links with local health professionals to facilitate appropriate sharing of knowledge, and more timely and suitable placements.

CONCLUSION

This chapter began by setting out some definitions. In particular, it was asserted that health is not one, but a number of ideas, which operate differently in different people's minds at different times, as they consider how the health of the public can be promoted and maintained. The historical development of ideas about health and its promotion and maintenance have been outlined, and set in the context of political change. At various points along the way, public health work had to reinvent itself to respond to the mood of the day. The related notions of health promotion, health education and of primary health care have been explored, and different perspectives on these described.

Negotiation of perspectives within primary care groups or local health groups, in the construction of a Health Improvement Programme, has been outlined. Evidence on the relative effectiveness and feasibility of targeting individuals or population groups has been described. Theoretical frameworks have been set out in relation to individuals, groups and at policy level, linking ideas about participation and organisational change. These theories are illustrated in practice using some examples.

DISCUSSION QUESTIONS

- In considering how the health of the public may be promoted and maintained, what theories and models are most important to you?
- Wass (1994) and Kelly and colleagues (1993) have sought to describe health promotion activity as a range of levels. How far do their suggestions fit in with practice in your area?
- What is your view on the appropriateness of targeting health promotion interventions with individuals or population groups? Why?
- In your own context, can you identify examples of health-promoting activity at the individual, community and policy levels?

FURTHER READING

Naidoo J & Wills J 1998 Practising Health Promotion: Baillière Tindall, London
This book addresses health promotion practice. It is well presented with good use of case studies, activities and discussion points. It considers the policy context in which health promotion takes place, although is slightly dated due to the fast pace of change. One of its particular strengths is the 'challenges in practice' section. In this, the research base provided is helpful – for example in looking at the prevention of coronary heart disease and stroke – reference is made to reports of the OXCHECK study amongst others, though again, this material dates quickly.

Allott M & Robb M (eds) 1998 Understanding Health and Social Care: An Introductory Reader. Sage Publications, London
Although this book is a very broad reader, it is an excellent resource in thinking through the context of public health and health promotion, primarily from a sociological perspective. It is a collection of papers gathered from a range of sources. The two particularly relevant sections are Section 2 (Where Care Takes Place) and Section 5 (Contexts of Care: Policies and Politics), but there are also pieces exploring empowerment, professionalism, and social control among others.

Popay J & Williams G (eds) 1999 Researching the People's Health. Routledge, London
This book is particularly helpful in exploring ways in which researchers can help practitioners to identify the health needs of the people they work with. It includes sections on the theory and methods of health needs assessment and on ways of involving the public in this. It is well referenced and includes a number of practical examples.

REFERENCES

Acheson D 1998 Independent Inquiry into Inequalities in Health. The Stationery Office, London

Antonovsky A 1996 The salutogenic model as a theory to guide health promotion. Health Promotion International 11(1):11–18

Ashton J & Seymour H 1988 The New Public Health. Open University Press, Buckingham

Ashton J, Grey P & Barnard K 1986 Healthy Cities: WHO's new public health initiative. Health Promotion 1(3):319–323

Becker M H (ed) 1974 The Health Belief Model and Personal Health Behavior. Thorofare, New Jersey

Board of Education 1928 Handbook of Suggestions on Health Education. HMSO, London

Bhopal R 1995 Public health medicine and primary health care: convergent, divergent, or parallel paths? Journal of Epidemiology & Community Health 49(2):113–116

Blaxter M 1982 Mothers and Daughters: a three generational study of health attitudes and behaviour. Heinemann Educational Books, London

Brown V 1985 Towards an epidemiology of health: a basis for planning community health programs. Health Policy 4:331–340

Boyd M, Brummell K, Billingham K & Perkins E R 1993 The Public Health Post At Strelley: Nursing Development Unit, Nottingham. Community Health NHS Trust, Nottingham

Chadwick E 1965 Report on the Sanitary Condition of the Labour Population of

Great Britain (Reprint of Chadwick 1842). Edinburgh University Press, Edinburgh

Clark J 1986 A model for health visiting. In: Kershaw B & Salvage J (eds) Models for Nursing. John Wiley & Sons, Chichester

Collin C, Wade D, Davies S & Horn V 1988 The Barthel ADL Index: a reliability study. International Disability Studies 10:61–63

Cornwell J 1984 Hard-earned lives: accounts of health and illness from East London. Tavistock Publications, London.

Council for the Education and Training of Health Visitors 1977 An Investigation into the Principles and Practice of Health Visiting. Council for the Education and Training of Health Visitors, London

Cox J & Hill S 1993 Tackling language delay: a groupwork approach. Health Visitor 66(8):291–292

Department for Education and Employment 1999 Sure Start. DfEE, London

Department of Health 1992 The Health of the Nation: A Strategy for Health in England (Cmnd 1986). HMSO, London

Department of Health 1997 The New NHS: Modern, Dependable (Cmnd 3809). The Stationery Office, London

Department of Health 1999 Saving Lives: Our Healthier Nation (Cmnd 4386). The Stationery Office, London

DiClemente C C & Prochaska J O 1982 Self-change and therapy: change of smoking behavior: a comparison of processes of change in cessation and maintenance. Addictive Behaviors 7(2):133–142

Ewles L & Simnett I 1985 Promoting health: a practical guide to health education. John Wiley & Sons, Chichester

French S 1993 Disability, impairment or something in between? In: Swain J, Finkelstein V, French S & Oliver M (eds) Disabling Barriers – Enabling Environments. Sage, London

Home Office 1998 Supporting Families. Home Office, London

Kaner E, Heather N, McAvoy B, Lock C & Gilvarry E 1999 Intervention for excessive alcohol consumption in primary health care: attitudes and practices of English general practitioners. Alcohol and Alcoholism 34(4):559–566

Kelly M P, Charlton B G & Hanlon P, 1993 The four levels of health promotion: an integrated approach. Public Health 107: 319–326

Kerr S M, Jowett S A & Smith L N 1996 Preventing sleep problems in infants: a randomized controlled trial. Journal of Advanced Nursing 24(5):938–942

Leavell H R 1953 In: Leavell H R & Clark E G (eds) Textbook of Preventive Medicine. McGraw-Hill, New York

Luker K 1982 Evaluating Health Visiting Practice. Royal College of Nursing, London

Mayall B 1986 Keeping children healthy: the role of mothers and professionals. Allen & Unwin, London

McEwan R T, Davison N, Forster D P, Pearson P & Stirling E 1990 Screening elderly people in primary care: a randomised controlled trial. British Journal of General Practice 40:94–97

Nelson N & Wright S 1995 Participation and Power. In: Nelson N & Wright S (eds) Power and Participatory Development: Theory and Practice. Intermediate Technology Publications, London

NHS Executive 1998 In the Public Interest: Developing a Strategy for Public Participation in the NHS. Department of Health, Wetherby

Parsons T 1951 The Social System. Free Press, New York

Pearson P 1991 Clients' perceptions: the use of case studies in developing theory. Journal of Advanced Nursing 16:521–528

Pearson P, Mead P, Graney A & McRae G 2000 Evaluation of the Developing Specialist Practitioner Role in the Context of Public Health. University of Newcastle, Newcastle upon Tyne

Rodgers H, Soutter J, Kaiser W, Pearson P, Dobson R, Skilbeck C & Bond J 1997 Early supported hospital discharge following acute stroke: length of stay and three month outcomes. Clinical Rehabilitation 11:280–287

Skinner B F 1953 Science and human behavior. Macmillan, New York

Tannahill A 1985 What is health promotion? Health Education Journal 49:10–12

Titmuss R 1970 The Gift Relationship: from human blood to social policy. Allen & Unwin, London

Wass A 1999 Promoting Health: the primary health care approach, 2nd edn Harcourt Australia, Marrickville

Watkins S J 1994 Stockport Health Promise. Stockport Health Authority, Stockport Metropolitan Borough Council

Watkins S J 1996 Health 2000: four years to go. 8th Annual Public Health Report for Stockport. Stockport Health Authority, Stockport

Whyte W F 1993 Street Corner Society, 4th edn. University of Chicago Press, Chicago

World Health Organization 1946 Constitution. World Health Organization, Geneva

World Health Organization 1978 The Declaration of Alma-Ata. International Conference on Primary Health Care, Alma-Ata, Kazakhstan

World Health Organization 1984 Health Promotion: A Discussion Document on the Concept and Principles. World Health Organization, Copenhagen

World Health Organization 1986 Ottawa Charter for Health Promotion. World Health Organization, Ottawa

World Health Organization 1991 Community Involvement in Health Development: Challenging Health Services. World Health Organization, Geneva

Zola I K 1973 Pathways to the doctor – from person to patient. Social Science and Medicine 7:677–689

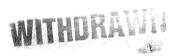

THE POLICY AGENDA IN PUBLIC HEALTH PRACTICE

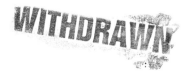

INTRODUCTION TO SECTION 2

Sarah Cowley

Nationally, some priority has been given to the needs of public health specialists in order to develop the capacity for public health. Hitherto, all such specialists were from a medical background, but it is no longer considered necessary for them to be doctors (Department of Health 1999). Following discussion and a small scoping study, however, it has been widely agreed that, in future, public health specialists from all backgrounds will be expected to achieve certain national standards (Lessof et al 1999). Initial proposals include ability in the following key areas:

- Understanding health and disease; measuring disease status
- Disease surveillance and control
- Promoting health and well-being
- Evaluating and improving the effectiveness and efficiency of health care
- Evidence based decisions, information management and research
- Advocacy
- Communications and coordination
- Intersectoral and collaborative working
- Management and leadership
- Modelling the future of public health.

It is proposed that, in future, educational programmes should include these standards at least to diploma level, leaving the final year of a degree to be completed in the particular field of choice, such as health promotion or environmental health. This would mean that such graduate practitioners would be well placed to undertake Masters preparation in which they further develop these skills, should they wish to develop their careers as public health specialists. There are no plans, at present, for changes to the preparation of health visitors or public health nurses to take account of these standards before they qualify.

The extent to which hands-on practitioners, working at a grass roots level, need to be skilled in all of these is not clear and has been little discussed. This section of the book is not intended to inform the development of all these specialist public health skills. It has been planned, instead, to help practitioners understand how they can contribute to the wider public health agenda whilst continuing to maintain a base at the grass roots.

In Chapter 4, Rowe sets the scene for the rest of the section by providing a broad overview of how health strategies are developed at different levels, from national policy to a local plan. Not every nurse working in primary care or a local community will be operating as a public health specialist, but changes in the structure of the health service mean there are now more opportunities to influence the type of service provision than ever in the past. This chapter is complemented by the next, which explains why primary care has risen so high on the agenda for achieving public health outcomes. The changes in primary care are as extensive as those in public health and could be the subject of a whole book in themselves, so this chapter has not attempted to encompass the range of variations and innovative service developments in this field. Instead, Walters draws on her experience of operating as a primary care group board nurse to emphasise the importance of organisational development, management and leadership. The chapter highlights the huge agenda for the small number of nurses serving on boards, so all practitioners need to support their representatives and become involved in developing local service plans.

A key reason for promoting primary care as the lead sector in developing services is that the primary care team, between them, have contact with the whole local population and are therefore best placed to identify the health needs of those people and to know which services are most needed. This contributes to both the prioritising and advocacy aspects of public health, which requires a clear statement about what the health needs are in an area. In Chapter 6, Billings demystifies the process of needs assessment, giving clear examples and a range of options to show how this process can be achieved.

Having identified the needs in an area, the next step is to see whether services are meeting the needs, or if they might have to be developed or changed. Services cannot be planned sensibly unless it is known which approaches work and which do not. In Chapter 7, Griffiths explains how to tell whether or not an intervention will do what it is expected to do, using standard approaches to determining the extent of its effectiveness. Critical appraisal skills have traditionally been associated with public health and service commissioning, but are no longer confined to that field. Understanding these issues is increasingly part of everyday practice, as all practitioners are expected to contribute through their own personal development to clinical governance and the implementation of official guidelines or national service plans.

However, there is a great deal of grass roots public health work that involves whole communities and multiple interventions applied in a deliberately unstructured and often informal or unpredictable way. Empowerment practice, whether directed at whole communities, groups, families or even individuals, needs to start with the client and their view of what is needed; not with a preplanned intervention. In the final chapter of this section, Graney explains why these approaches create such difficulties for standard approaches to assessing the effectiveness of interventions and offers some alternative ideas and solutions to evaluation.

REFERENCES

Department of Health 1999 Saving Lives: Our Healthier Nation (Cmnd 4386). The Stationery Office, London

Lessof S, Dumelow C, McPherson K 1999 Feasibility study of the case for national standards for specialist practice in public health. Cancer and Public Health Unit, London School of Hygiene and Tropical Medicine, London

4 Planning Public Health Strategies

Jean Rowe

KEY ISSUES

- National policy requirements.
- Public health strategies.
- User involvement.
- Clinical effectiveness, research and development, evidence and outcomes.
- Public health roles in primary care.

INTRODUCTION

The National Health Service (NHS) is a huge and complex organisation and employs large numbers of people, many of whom are from professional groups, in particular nursing. Nurses are the largest professional workforce in the NHS and are responsible for the majority of care delivered within the NHS (Standing Nursing and Midwifery Advisory Committee 1995). Health care is also administered through the independent and voluntary sectors, members of whom may have contracts with the NHS or work at the interface between their respective organisations in order to care for people who have health needs. Community nurses therefore play a major role in delivering care and liaising with nurse colleagues and many other organisations for and on behalf of their clients and patients. Whichever organisation delivers care, it does so within a structural framework through an overall health care plan. The difference between institutional care and community care is the mode or plan of delivery. For community nursing, access to other parts of the health care system entails knowledge of the local systems, good communication and liaison and negotiating care with other providers, as well as an intimate knowledge of the individual needs concerned.

HEALTH STRATEGY

A strategy is a grand plan, an approach, a programme or a scheme. A strategic policy and plan is a key framework for a service. In public health, modern practice involves needs assessment, which includes social indicators of health, clinical effectiveness and practice, informing commissioning processes and working with the inter-agency networks.

The broad-based NHS strategies are set by government and will be based on the party ideologies and what the electorate has mandated. Hence, the most recent changes for the NHS have been the removal of the 'internal market' and

GP Fundholding schemes to form a less-fragmented system of a partnership approach to care through a primary care-led NHS and the development of the primary care groups and trusts. This indicated major changes for both the GP practices and community trusts (Department of Health 1999c). It has meant that community nurses can now take a more strategic and commissioning role.

HEALTH IMPROVEMENT PROGRAMMES

Most of the health care priorities and improvements in health will be carried out through the Health Improvement Programmes (HImPs) based on the 'Our Healthier Nation' objectives (Department of Health 1998a).

The core objectives of the Health Improvement Programmes are:

■ Needs assessment
■ Resource mapping
■ Identification of priorities for action
■ Strategies for change
■ A Service and Financial Framework for the NHS.

Inclusiveness will be sought through the widest possible involvement from the outset, rather than consultation on a near-final product

What have been recently stressed (Department of Health 1997a, Secretary of State for Health 1999, Department of Health 1997c) are the user-involvement aspects of health. This area has been less well-developed in the NHS, but there is now an expectation that more work should be done to include local people's thoughts about health and health services. The role of users of health services is now a priority in the NHS reforms within the NHS Plan (Secretary of State for Health 2000).

Health care organisations have to work within a grand plan, otherwise health planning and care delivery would be chaos. Each part of the organisation works within the overall strategy, but all levels have their own local strategy for delivery of a service. A public health strategy would be based on the local demography, the deaths by age and cause, and incidence and prevalence of disease. The strategy would identify the potential to improve health and quality of life, and through coordinated health programmes aim to reduce the impact of disease and disability for the population. It should identify gaps in the services so that either a new service, or a plan to organise delivery of services in a different way, can be developed.

The NHS Executive regional offices have responsibility for giving guidance to the local district health authorities on the national plan for the NHS (Secretary of State for Health 2000). This has explicit objectives to be met by health authorities, and trusts are monitored on their performance against those objectives in terms of both the national plan for the NHS and the Health Improvement Programmes. In the hierarchy of responsibilities, each unit of an organisation will adjust their focus to meet the national priorities, whether it is to reduce the waiting-list times or reduce the number of under-age pregnancies. All these priorities have to be translated into local action. It is the health authorities who will ask the trusts, including primary care groups and trusts and health promotion departments, how they intend to do it. Some of the issues will be of national concern, such as the care of people with enduring mental illness or how employers might put in place mechanisms to reduce the level of nurses' back injuries. Some of the health improvement priorities will be locally sensitive to the ethnic mix and/or areas of high deprivation.

SETTING THE CONTEXT: PUBLIC HEALTH

Public health is about the health of the population (see Box 4.1). Its origins lie in economic, social, environmental and ecological aspects of health and disease. Public health is both a collective and an individual issue. What affects population health includes health-sustaining policies of the other government departments who have responsibility for agriculture and food production, the fiscal system and transport. Inequalities and health outcomes have as much to do with community and individual resources, as with an individual's genetic blueprint, and it is the reduction of health hazard which can help reduce the burden of disease.

In order to decide that any health issue is a priority, information must be collected nationally and locally. It is information that informs the agenda for action. However, data collection is complex. Huge amounts of information are collected from many differing sources including the Public Health Common Data set, Office of National Statistics, General Household Survey, local authorities, acute and community trusts, primary care, and from studies carried out on local populations. Other sources of information and 'grey literature' used will be from university research. The collection mechanisms themselves are a problem, as data that meets the need of one organisation may not be presented in a useable way for another organisation. So health intelligence and information departments have the crucial task of analysing information and presenting it in such a way that health services can use it.

BOX 4.1	Concepts that underpin public health work (Standing Nursing and Midwifery Advisory Committee 1995)

Public health approaches feature:

- Identification of health needs and desired outcomes
- Agreement on the most effective and acceptable action
- Evaluation
- User perspectives
- Knowledge of population health needs even when caring for individuals
  - identified client groups
  - whole communities
  - geographical areas
- Emphasis on collective and collaborative action
- Recognition of people as members of groups, not only individuals
- A public health perspective that anchors clinical and non-clinical care in the social, organisational and policy aspects of health development
- A focus on health promotion enabling people to increase control over and improve their health, combined with preventing disease

Public health departments are required to produce an annual Public Health Report, which will focus on health priorities and local epidemiology. This will include comparative national and local district data and information on the health services' performance in relation to health targets set. Data from the communicable disease control sections of public health are also included in the report. It is a public document and therefore open for scrutiny by the public. Public health departments take a population approach and measure health at different levels by age-group, condition-specific groups and disease prevalence. Primary care groups and trusts now have the responsibility for assessing health needs locally and therefore need support to take on this wider role. The assessment of need might include participative techniques such as rapid appraisal through key informants and may commission other *ad hoc* studies. Each information source gives a different standpoint, but probably what is less developed is the user perspective. The Public Health Report has the purpose of ensuring the longer-term health planning, and identification of unmet health needs. Health intelligence therefore involves the bigger picture of health, which is not just about how resources are used for health services but how the total community impacts on health (Pearson 1998).

PUBLIC HEALTH AND ITS RESPONSIBILITY FOR HEALTH IMPROVEMENT

The Health Act 1999 gave health authorities responsibility for the Health Improvement Programmes with an emphasis on promoting health, reducing inequalities and social exclusion, working in partnership and involving communities. 'Saving Lives: Our Healthier Nation' (Secretary of State for Health 1999) and 'Reducing Health Inequalities' (Department of Health 1999a) build on the previous requirements under 'The Health of the Nation' (Department of Health 1992) targets. Providers are expected to take action on health targets at all levels, including the primary care groups and trusts (Table 4.1) (Department of Health 1997a, 1998a). What has been recognised is that, in order to reduce the burden of ill-health and narrow the health gap, all the major government departments must play a part.

TABLE 4.1	Roles and responsibilities of health authorities and primary care groups/trusts (Secretary of State for Health 1999 p 122)	
	Health authorities	*Primary care groups/trusts*
	Enabling	Doing
	Gaining multisectoral commitment and coordination	Forging local partnerships
	Setting strategy (jointly with others)	Planning action
	Prioritising and investing in public health programmes	Resourcing action plans
	Developing public health organisational and people capability	Building workforce capacity and public health infrastructures
	Monitoring progress	Meeting objectives

The Health Improvement Programmes will encompass:

- Needs assessment and how partnership can broaden the action on public health
- How local services can be developed to meet needs directly through the NHS and jointly with other agencies
- The range, location and investment required in the local health services to meet the needs of local people.

The national priorities are heart disease and stroke, accidents, cancers and mental health. These were priorities in the previous 'Health of the Nation' targets (Department of Health 1992). What is different now is that the environments in which health promotion may be delivered are specified through identified settings – healthy schools, workplaces and neighbourhoods – emphasising a partnership approach. Health authorities must also focus on social exclusion and tackle the inequalities in relation to poverty, poor housing, low educational attainment and joblessness. This is where they must work in partnership with their local authorities (Department of Health 1998a).

IDENTIFYING NEED

The definition of need according to Bradshaw (1972) is that 'need' could be categorised into four areas: normative, felt, expressed and comparative. Normative need is defined as a desirable standard set down by a professional or expert, felt need is limited to the perception of individuals who may express a desire for a service without needing it, expressed need is turning it into action. Comparative need is when individuals or communities who experience the same problem may or may not be receiving the same services. Some areas might have an inequitable distribution of services, for example concerning continence promotion, where some community trusts may have to put a financial limit on access to supplies.

Methods for assessing need described by Jolly and George (1996) are:

- Comparison – by seeing what is provided elsewhere
- Consensus – by asking different groups of people (purchasers, providers and patients) what they want and coming to an agreement
- Epidemiology – by assessing scientifically the burden of disease and the cost-effectiveness of interventions to control it.

Needs assessment methods then use data and information to present a case for health improvement, service change or investment in a health programme. Much of the information currently gathered is used for the purpose of estimating total activity and total cost of services, which is an inefficient method of contracting services. The health authority needs to consult with any stakeholders who may be affected by any change. GP Fundholding was a major policy change for primary care. Now, the NHS Primary Care Act 1997 Personal Medical Service pilots (Department of Health 1997b) has given primary care an opportunity to make services more sensitive to local needs and has spawned new innovations in practice. (Lewis et al 1999). Policy changes such as the primary care-led NHS will need major shifts of culture and with that, the development of mechanisms by which primary care practitioners can influence the commissioning of services needed by the local population (Department of Health 1997a)

COMMUNITY-BASED NEEDS ASSESSMENT

Community-based needs assessment has three main approaches: sociology, epidemiology and health economics (Billings & Cowley 1995). Biomedical models of health have been the most prominent features of medical and nursing education, but it was the inclusion of social aspects of health and disease figured in health visiting and school nurse education that gave them the specialised knowledge and skills of public health in a wider context. Poverty and deprivation in childhood have had a major impact on the health of adults. This has been illustrated in the study of a cohort of children in Newcastle in 1948, where repeated infections in childhood greatly increased the risk of chronic respiratory disease by the age of 15 years. Class differences accounted for heavier and taller children in the professional and managerial families (Lamont et al 1998).

Careful consideration of community-based needs assessment is essential, and should be carried out for an identified reason. According to research by the London Health Economics Consortium (1995) needs assessment has not yet had any major impact on purchasing decisions. The study found that purchasers and staff in primary and community services made a fairly accurate assessment of need in their local communities. But it did suggest that it may not be worthwhile going into detailed community enquiries, as needs may have already been identified by the local agencies. Local community nurses, in particular health visitors and school nurses, have been required to produce community profiles, which have included a needs-based approach to their caseloads. What appears to be important in the process is staff with good local knowledge of the area, good lines of communication and stable management structures within the organisation (London Health Economics Consortion 1995).

DIFFERENCE BETWEEN NEED AND WANT

To take a pragmatic view, need is about those things that are life-sustaining, e.g. food, water, heat, shelter and health care. 'Want' may be a demand to have health and social care which is felt to be a right in a modern society, and which many older people may feel that they have invested in during their working lives. It may be more meaningful to ask what people require. Requirement lies somewhere between need and want, and may be about quality. It is about balancing competing demands and expectations. In the health services it is usually in the basics of communication and response to human dignity that users make value judgements in terms of satisfaction or dissatisfaction. These are often related not so much to clinical interventions but the way people are treated on a personal level (Stewart & Turner 1998 p 142). Quality in the new NHS becomes a statutory duty for health service providers, since their performance will be measured in terms of 'prompt access, good relationships and efficient administration' (Department of Health 1998a).

A STRATEGIC PLAN FOR HEALTH

What does a strategic plan involve? It is usually a corporate plan either at a health authority or trust level. At health authority level, it may be an overall health strategy or a service specification that includes all the elements required to meet a particular health need. A local community nursing strategy can be developed as an agreed plan with a statement of intent, health outcomes and what will be delivered for the population for whom they have the responsibility to care. It could be a case for change, a new service or a further development of an existing service. The strategy can involve major changes or relatively minor changes but with any change, certain elements need to be in place.

A useful model for thinking about a strategy is the 'Seven Ss' model (Pascale 1990). Included in the model are hard Ss – structure, strategy and systems, and soft Ss – staff, skills, style and shared values (Figure 4.1). Marsh and McAlpine

---

FIGURE 4.1   *A community health strategy framework.*

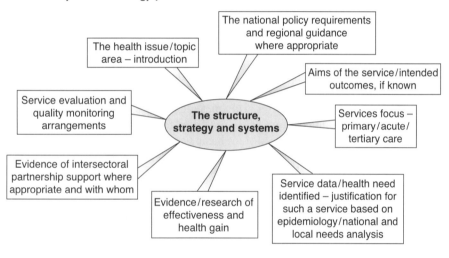

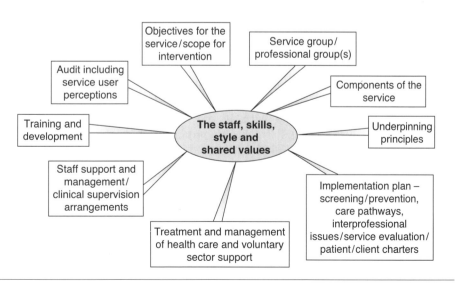

(1995) found that nurses tend to focus more on the soft Ss, but need to develop their skills to include the hard Ss.

VALUES IN PUBLIC HEALTH

Health authorities must have a value system, since they are accountable for which services are purchased on behalf of the local population. Central values are openness, fairness, equity, effectiveness, value for money and responsiveness (Ham & Appleby 1993). Decisions have to be made on what the NHS will offer in terms of health care, since resources are limited. These decisions made may be on the basis of clinical efficacy. New drugs and technology have greatly increased health opportunities, which brings dilemmas in decision-making, since patients are much better informed of the possibilities and will wish to have any life-saving treatments available. Decisions must therefore be considered on the balance of clinical possibilities, outcome probabilities and quality of life issues. Sometimes these decisions are reasonable, but may be unpalatable for patients. Therefore, the National Institute of Clinical Effectiveness (NICE) was set up in the UK in 1999, to give guidance to clinicians on the most effective treatments. NICE has three broad functions including appraisal of existing and new technologies, development of clinical guidelines and promoting clinical audit and confidential inquiries (Department of Health 1998c).

International principles identified by the World Health Organization in 1985 included peace, freedom from fear of war, equal opportunity and social justice for all, satisfaction of basic needs, public commitment and public support. In an address to the American Public Health Association in 1997, the president recognised values that are general: human dignity, health and well-being, quality of life, social justice and community responsibility. Skills necessary for public health practice were values, vision and leadership. Public health professionals need the skills to listen, educate and inform, advocate, and develop partnerships (Levy 1998).

HEALTH PROMOTION AND PUBLIC HEALTH

Health promotion departments in some areas are part of the public health and commissioning role in health authorities. They will be instrumental to the health strategy and planning for health gain. Their role involves a broader influence, working with all other sectors that have a health remit and mutual interests. Skills of health promotion specialists at strategic level can help to forge closer links within and outside health organisations. Many inner city areas have large populations from minority and ethnic groups and there are health needs and health promotion concerns, especially regarding uptake of services and cultural sensitivities. All areas have access to departments where there are resources and health information. Even if departments do not have all the specific information they will be in touch with organisations that represent the public health concerns.

USER INVOLVEMENT

All through 'The New NHS' (Department of Health 1997a) and 'Saving Lives: Our Healthier Nation' (Secretary of State for Health 1999) is the concept of user involvement. Most people use the health services for both preventive and diagnostic services, or for a diagnosed medical condition. The NHS Plan (Secretary of State for Health 2000) now requires trusts to take more account of the views of the users and of the local population, through representation on the boards of trusts including the primary care trusts. The NHS Plan acknowledges the role of the patient organisations that do much to support people with medical and disabling conditions. Alongside the reforms each trust will have patient advocacy services that will help and guide people using the NHS.

Many user groups have lobbied for more involvement in the health agenda, but live a hand-to-mouth existence, with constant worries about income and use of volunteers to get their needs met. The rise in the number of organisations over the past twenty years or so might reflect the minimal power people felt they had within the health care system – that decisions were made on their behalf without consultation. This can happen at an individual or community level. It is similar to constructing a building, not asking the buyers what fittings they would like, but then expecting them to pay for them.

How can the users of the services become engaged with designing the services and who knows best about their needs? Was the practitioner being set up as the proxy for the user and is there real consultation? Interestingly, the user views on maternity services have, for many years, been represented on the Maternity Services Liaison Committees that operate in each maternity unit. Now, through the establishment of the Patient Advocacy and Liaison Service (PALS), the new patient advocate team will be the independent facilitator handling personal and family concerns (Secretary of State for Health 2000 p. 91). This service will take on the role of the Community Health Council of supporting complainants. At a strategic level the user perspective will be built into Citizens' Council to advise the National Institute for Clinical Effectiveness (NICE) and support the work of the NICE Partners Council (Secretary of State for Health 2000 p 95).

Models of user involvement

Models of user involvement indicate that there is a continuum of involvement, which was developed by Arnstein as described in Leonard et al (1997), which uses the concept of a ladder of participation. Each rung corresponds to a position of citizen power (Figure 4.2).

While citizen control might be difficult to manage in terms of accountability for delegated resources, the primary care trusts will have more user, non-executive, representation on their boards.

Research carried out by the Long Term Medical Conditions Alliance (Lewthwaite 1997) to promote the needs of patients, estimates that 32% of the population have some medical condition. It identified issues where patients

FIGURE 4.2 *The 'ladder of participation' of user involvement (Adapted from Leonard et al 1997).*

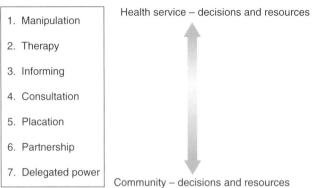

1. Manipulation

2. Therapy

3. Informing

4. Consultation

5. Placation

6. Partnership

7. Delegated power

Health service – decisions and resources

Community – decisions and resources

could influence commissioning. Common themes emerging from their research on customer feedback were about basic quality of the services. The facilitator role of the health authority was absolutely crucial, and helped to empower doctors and nurses to engage and say what they felt about the issues.

The Chief Medical Officer set up a taskforce to design a new programme for expert patients (Department of Health 1999a). This intended to address the needs of people with chronic disease or disabilities. What was apparent from observing changes that have taken place within the groups of people who have long-term chronic disease is the amount of self-management that happens. Children with diabetes, for example, are now taught to administer their own insulin, and school children their asthma drugs. Many cancer patients cope with quite devastating conditions but do so because they have more control over their lives and have been enabled to do so by the professionals and by organisations such as Cancerlink and BACUP. Many of these organisations have a research arm and will keep research information in their libraries and archives.

METHODS OF OBTAINING THE VIEWS OF LOCAL PEOPLE

Differing methods can be used according to the type, quantity and quality of the information needed to inform the delivery of health services.

Patient's Charter

Probably most well-known of the methods used in the past was the Patient's Charter, introduced in 1991 (Department of Health 1991), which will now be replaced by the NHS Plan (Secretary of State for Health 2000). Users' and patients' standards have been set nationally and performance will be monitored on a regular basis.

Although many professionals found problems arising from the Patient's Charter, with higher expectations of the users, it did encourage the reporting of performance in relation to standards and had to be taken seriously by the providers of services.

Public meetings

Health authorities, primary care groups/trusts and local authorities have public meetings on a regular basis, so that information about local services can be disseminated through the local networks and media.

Users' forums

Forums can be useful when trying to look at the aspects quality of service, and in particular a specific service.

Much of the work of hospices and treatment centres, for example for people with HIV/AIDS, have made a huge impact on the emotional, social and spiritual care of people with terminal illnesses. Hospices now have homely environments and people do not have 'routines' imposed on them.

Focus groups

Many organisations use focus-group meetings to canvass the views of both service users and the practitioners involved. This usually involves setting up a group of people who use certain services and gathering views and opinions about a specific issue or service. It is a skilled activity because the facilitator must be careful not to lead the discussion but to listen.

Citizens' jury

Another type of public consultation, which is now being used more extensively, is the 'Citizens' Jury'. An experiment was tried out in Oregon USA. The plan was to involve the public in health decisions and to establish what values were important to the people. The Oregon Health Plan was the first attempt to ration health care on the basis of clinical effectiveness and values held by the public (Rutt 1995).

Questionnaires

Questionnaires are a useful method of assessing views but can be complex to devise, as they may not ask the questions for which answers are needed. Questionnaires have a tendency to generalisation. Help when drawing up a questionnaire may be necessary and in some cases ethical approval may be required if people are to be asked personal or sensitive questions

Individual interviews

Interviews will capture very rich data but will only represent single views. They are very useful in ascertaining what health issues affect, for example, people with disabilities or a particular health problem, where access to information and help may be limited. This method is often used where there may be sensitive issues or when complaints are being handled by the services.

Using 'layperson'/peer education

Schemes that increase health knowledge and personal self-esteem have been shown to be highly beneficial, particularly where access to services was difficult because of cultural or language difficulties.

Use of health advocates in the East End of London resulted in reductions in caesarean sections and women spent less time in hospital during the antenatal period (Parsons & Day 1992). First Parent Visitors and Community Mothers programmes have also demonstrated good outcomes in positive parenting for socially disadvantaged families (Barker 1984).

Community Health Council and formal consultations

Any changes to the way in which health services are delivered have to be notified to the Community Health Councils, including any shifts in contracts from one provider to another. The consultation process may need to involve local users and professionals concerned, especially the general practitioners. The consultation periods or notification of changes must be carefully considered since setting up focus groups or putting information in the local press takes time.

As part of a King's Fund Initiative, the local health authority decided to look at the issues and problems of primary care services in a disadvantaged area of Sunderland (Alderman 1997). There was a problem of recruitment of GPs in Sunderland. The jury panel of sixteen people from a range of backgrounds was asked whether they would accept services from a nurse practitioner, a pharmacist or another doctor. Instead of deciding on any of the options, the jury recommended that the nurse practitioner role should be developed and piloted. They felt that the nurse practitioner should be accountable to the general practitioner and nationally agreed standards developed. They felt the health authority should provide incentives for general practitioners to work in the area. This whole process would be very expensive and time-consuming and could not be a panacea for all the problems and issues within health services.

The NHS Plan (Secretary of State for Health 2000 p 94) now requires local government to be involved as scrutinisers of the NHS and any changes to local services to be discussed in the council's scrutiny committees.

COMMISSIONING AND NEEDS ASSESSMENT

Commissioning entails:

- Assessing health needs of the relevant population
- Developing strategies to meet that need
- Negotiating with providers to deliver services, which would include both the NHS and other health care providers
- Monitoring performance of that service, including the quality.

BOX 4.2	*Options for change in commissioning services (Jones 1997)*

- Medium-term strategic components
- Emphasis on performance and contributions to health
- Greater precision in service specifications
- Longer timescales for service provision
- More appropriate contract currencies for community and primary care
- Reimbursement for strategic achievement

Health authorities will have to support commissioning for the primary care groups with a population of 100 000, which may increase fragmentation, although primary care trusts will serve larger populations and develop their public health infrastructure, which could include partnership with local authorities. Working through a partnership approach with the local authority and community networks is where the community nursing intelligence and perspectives will be invaluable. Primary care groups/trusts will be accountable to the health authority and local population for the Health Improvement Programmes.

Commissioning is an elaborate process that consumes many resources in terms of people and time. Information on existing levels of investment in services and the future funding allocation must be considered in the light of necessity. Public health personnel have to produce data or carry out needs assessments. This gives planners a picture of the present situation in order to produce options for change (Box 4.2), which can be considered as part of the contracting process.

Local level

Community nurses hold both quantitative and qualitative information that is very live. Caseload analysis presents a picture of local need and outcomes of services accessed by clients or patients. It can have the advantage of informing the local practice but how does this fit with locality need? The aggregation of data and profiles of the practices in a locality or for the primary care group has a local intelligence function, so that community nursing resources can be estimated (Figure 4.3). Equally, by gathering information, levels of unmet need can be ascertained.

Stages to public health action

Is there a need and what is the question (CPHVA 1997)?

1. What is the social context of this health need?
2. What does the health data tell you about this need?
3. Are there any other sources of information, e.g. health or local authority?

FIGURE 4.3   *Community health aggregated data and community profile.*

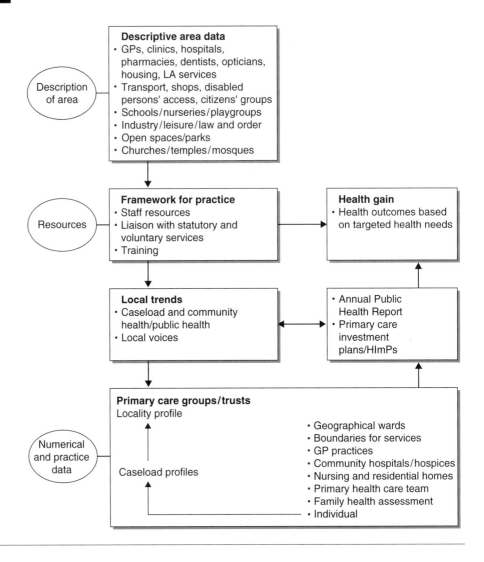

4. Is the health need important enough to do something about?
5. What are people doing already?
6. What does and does not work?
7. What do local people think and want to see happen?
8. Who else should be involved – from health, other agencies, and voluntary sectors?
9. How will we know if we have made a difference?

Having addressed these questions, providers then need to develop a proposal for commissioning that must include an estimate of costs (Figure 4.4).

FIGURE 4.4	*Preposal for a service development, including costings.*

PROPOSAL FOR A SERVICE DEVELOPMENT

❏ Name of provider ....

❏ Funding proposal to ....

❏ Total amount sought ....

❏ Period of project ....

❏ Health needs to be targeted ....

❏ Significance of health need ....

❏ Proposed service to meet health need ....

❏ New service ....

❏ Changes to present service ....

❏ Who else has been consulted/what other partners involved in the service
      changes? ....

❏ What health benefits are anticipated from proposed service/changes? ....

      ....

❏ How will the service be evaluated? ....

❏ Explanation/justification for funding sought ....

❏ Key references ....

Financial profile

Staff costs

Posts	Grade	WTEs	Starting salary	Weighting	On-costs	Total costs Year 1	Total costs Year 2

Total funds required

Non-recurring costs – equipment etc.	
Other recurring costs – specify	
Total for staff costs year 1	
Total staff costs year 2	
Grand total	

Health outcomes

There would be no point in carrying out a needs assessment if it had no end function, and that must be to produce health gain. How do community nurses know that what they are doing will make any difference? Evaluation processes should always be part of any service offered to the clientele, and that includes assessing the value that the local population places on the services. From a public health perspective, the measurements may be longer term – to reduce the numbers of deaths in the population or to assess the health risk through prevalence studies or incidence of infectious disease occurring in the community. Public health measures, however, can be much more to do with air quality, accidents or teenage pregnancies. Any public health intervention, when used in practice, needs to incorporate an outcome-measuring process.

Many community nurses find it difficult to think about measurement of outcomes especially when the outcomes are very long-term, for example, prevention programmes in childhood that may have an impact in adult life.

Constant restructuring can bring insecurity and changes in the configuration of the services and policies where practice is not embedded. Job insecurity and changes to job roles may inhibit new ideas. It is a rare event for good practice to be mainstreamed. Often good practice is ignored and much time is spent on trying to find out why things have gone wrong.

Primary health care teams and primary care groups

GP fundholders and the total purchasing pilots have been at the forefront of commissioning processes, but nurses have not been included. 'The New NHS' (Department of Health 1997a) has sought to remedy this situation, by making sure that they are included on the boards of primary care groups. However, community nurses will need to develop skills in commissioning, including public health skills, needs assessment, strategic planning and influencing and measurement of outcomes. Primary care needs to justify what it does by measuring the outcomes of that care. Professionals, including community nurses, must learn the skills necessary to be able to prioritise and plan rigorous research to identify effective and ineffective practice (Vanclay 1998).

TEAMWORK

With the creation of the primary care groups and trusts, some of the public health functions are being devolved to locality level and with this will come the need for good networking and teamwork. Critical to this will be accountability and equitable accessibility and effectiveness of the services, not only for the registered population but also the unregistered groups who live in communities. This is where community nurses will play an important role. Many of the homeless and refugee populations may be known to the services but through differing access routes via the communities: accident and emergency departments, mental health, local authority housing and social services or through the voluntary sector. General practice tends to be demand-driven and will have to engage with the local population of unregistered people through the primary care groups (Peckham 1994, Department of Health 1997a). Poverty profiling should be part of the overall process of community profiling. In the case of the people that are socially excluded, community nurses will need to recognise that the effects of poverty on health are considerable and that inequalities can exist in any age-group and for almost any disease-group. So poverty profiling can help community nurses to identify equity issues in service provision and therefore to argue for more resources (Royal College of Nursing 1996).

Team approaches to care and integrated nursing teams

In many areas primary health care teams have set up integrated nursing teams. This was the vision of the Cumberlege Team, where neighbourhood nursing services would be established with the primary health care teams within that neighbourhood (Department of Health and Social Security 1986). Where an integrated nursing team has been properly planned and negotiated it has worked well (Bull 1998). However, there is a notion that community nurses are there to do anything that is asked of them and that their skills are interchangeable. Not only is this unrealistic, but it also puts community nurses and their clients and patients at risk. The Health Visitors' Association (1996) definition of the integrated nursing team is:

> 'A team of community-based nurses from differing disciplines, working together within a primary care setting, pooling their skills, knowledge and ability, to provide the most effective care for the patients within a practice and the community it covers.'

It has been through the United Kingdom Central Council (1992) 'Scope of Professional Practice' that community nurses have been able to have their skills recognised, but also to realise when they must have training and updating of these skills. It is not about territorial concerns, but about who has the most appropriate skills to care for the patient or client. If the patient becomes central, then the type of care need will flow from a care plan. Care may need to be offered by other agencies including social services.

The reality of teamwork is that it is not easy and involves complex relationships. Although it is thought to be a panacea for good practice, it involves a great deal of commitment to make it work and this takes time. The team must have shared goals, vision, values and aspirations. The roles of all the nurses in the team should be complementary, and respected by all the team members. Work will be needed to plan procedures and protocols. Regular team meetings and effective communication will aid the support and recognition of each others contributions. Audit and reflection time must be built-in to review the whole team performance (Vanclay 1998). Bull (1998) feels that the integrated nursing teams are extremely well placed to advise on the involvement of primary care in the public health role.

Public health teamwork

Where there is a health issue or problem for a specific condition or population-group, then the public health expertise will be concentrated around this problem. It depends on the health issue and therefore brings together the most appropriate team-skills (Table 4.2). The members will come from very different agencies

TABLE 4.2	*Examples of public health teamwork*

Community health problem	Public health team	Possible strategy for action
Outbreak of diarrhoea in a local nursing home	Director of Public Health PCT Public Health Team Nursing Team Communicable Disease Control Team Registration and Inspection Team Environmental Health Infection Control Nurse	Notify Public Health Department of Health Authority Collect stool samples Isolate patients if possible Alert any visitors Advise on infection control Teach and advise Care Assistants Monitor any new cases
Large numbers of children in school with diagnosed asthma A decision made to look at best practice with possible outcome so that children can have their medication with them in school	Primary care group/Community health services Form Teacher Head Teacher Parent Group School Secretary School Nurse Community Paediatrician Director of Education/Policy Special Needs Teacher Health Promotion Advisor	GPs, school nurses, community paediatrician, health promotion and Director of Education meet up and discuss possible strategy Head teachers and staff meet to discuss their needs School Governors, staff and parents meet to discuss how children can safely maintain their own care by having their medication with them in school Health and school staff develop an agreed protocol including what to do in an emergency situation. Group to agree review date
District nurses wish to set up a leg-ulcer clinic in the community Evidence from other areas suggest that community clinics have been very successful in improving healing rates	Lead Nurse – professional development District nursing teams Research link with university Director of Nursing Consultant in Vascular Surgery Community Podiatrist Local patient transport service Locality Manager Administrator Community Pharmacists GP Advisor PCG Commissioning Manager	Assess need through patient caseload profiles Identify the research evidence on venous leg-ulcer management Discuss plan with Trust/ commissioning manager and draft proposal to include accommodation, equipment, patient access Draft patient protocols and patient information sheets – send out for comments as appropriate Identify budget for treatment and dressings Set up appointment systems and GP communications Service promotion leaflets Teaching programme for nurses Audit outcomes, and patient satisfaction and review service

TABLE 4.2	Cont'd

The local hospital gynaecological ward sister has asked patients if they would like some support following a miscarriage. They agree that they do, but not in the hospital setting	Ward Sister Liaison Health Visitor Consultant National Miscarriage Support Group Health Centre manager Locality Manager Health Promotion Manager	Results of patient survey shared with immediate team in ward Information gained from national support groups Discussion with health centre manager re: evening accommodation and security Invitation flyer developed with health promotion support Plan for first evening meeting and facilitation Identify with parents what support they would like Discuss short pilot programme and review with group Identify materials and training needs for group to continue
The local GP has many patients who come from the Punjab area in India There is a high level of diabetes and coronary heart disease Many of the older members of the community do not speak English Literature suggests that other similar programmes have been successful but not yet tried with Ethnic groups	PCT Public Health Team GP Practice Practice Manager Practice Nurse Health Visitor (speaks Punjabi or accesses interpreter) Health Promotion Manager Diabetes Sister Consultant Cardiologist Coronary Rehabilitation Sister Public Health Specialist PCG Commissioning Manager	Review progress, budgets and future funding Identify numbers of patients who have had coronary event Arrange practice meeting with public health specialist Set up liaison with local cardiac rehabilitation nurses to refer patients for follow-up at surgery Plan with practice manager to tag those patients who have had a coronary event in the past year Set up appointments and protocols Plan lifestyle programme with health visitor Pilot some clinics and record outcomes including patient satisfaction Write-up results, share with practice staff and colleagues and commissioning manager Plan training for other practice nurses

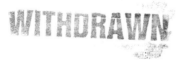

and will either advise or become the 'hands on' practitioners. This multidisciplinary team must work to a strategic plan that has a common aim and focus. The team must evaluate and review the outcomes, especially if an infection needs to be controlled or if it is a new service that might be commissioned if successful.

CLINICAL EFFECTIVENESS

The opportunity to bring practitioners together with academic centres may arise through clinical effectiveness and clinical governance in all the health care settings. Clinical governance has become a major feature of the new policy changes within the NHS and will include evidence-based practice, research, protocols and guidelines as a feature of service delivery. For practitioners, there needs to be continual evaluation and reflection on practice through peer-review (Department of Health 1998c).

Evidence of clinical effectiveness is difficult in some cases, and there is a possibility that because the evidence of effectiveness is not available, or the area has not been researched, that services may be cut on that basis. The Royal College of Paediatrics and Child Health (1997) has produced a useful document for the commissioners of services in child health and has graded the evidence as follows:

■ Statutory/legal requirements
■ Clear evidence for value
■ Of likely benefit in spite of lack of overwhelming evidence of effectiveness
■ Of common-sense benefit only
■ Of doubtful value.

This is particularly useful as some clinical practices might be deemed as unnecessary. In many cases, research in a clinical area may have already been carried out and practice developments or changes may have been proposed on the basis of that evidence. It is important, therefore, to check whether this has been done, so that community nurses are not reinventing the wheel. Literature searches through the professional organisations, academic libraries or through the national centres for the dissemination of evidence may be carried out, and will produce a wealth of material. However, there can also be a dearth of research in community nursing and so research on some topic areas may be breaking new ground.

A strategy for researching clinical effectiveness in practice should include:

■ Management structures
■ Staffing
■ Access to clients
■ Applied research and development
■ Training and support
■ Quality control systems including information technology
■ Resources
■ Facilities
■ Accommodation
■ Audit and outcomes measures
■ Health and safety concerns and ethical practices.

Critical appraisal training

This is now open to many community nurses through academic departments, library information technology training and professional organisations. It offers people the skills to look at the clinical research and evidence of good practice.

Internet access to databases is now available to more practitioners though the workplace and the colleges.

AUDIT

Clinical audit has now become a common feature in the health service and part of the clinical-effectiveness process. It is about monitoring what you are doing in the services against quality standards, clinical guidelines or protocols. Trusts have audit departments and help in understanding and carrying out audits can be provided. Practitioners may need help with the audit tools and setting up the collection of the information. A central fund of audit money is available through the health services and systems are usually in place for applying for the funding through Clinical Audit Committees. The contact for this may be through the health authority. The committee will consider all the submissions for topic areas for central funding, but each trust usually has its own clinical audit funds for local use.

At practice level, audit must be pertinent to the area of work. It is naturalistic, in that it will be from patients or clients themselves or from recording in clinical notes. It need not involve complicated statistics as in much research but can employ percentages, means, averages and ratios. It is internally-led but can be multiagency. Audit should feed into a cycle of change and into a practice-development programme for staff. Another type of audit could involve an understanding of why people do not comply with medication or why people have not turned up for appointments. This can indicate whether it was about the service administration or the patient's perceptions of the clinical care received. Many people do not like to complain but may vote with their feet, therefore it is important to find out the issues so that services may be made more accessible.

OUTCOMES – MEASURING

Why measure outcomes? For practitioners, outcomes can demonstrate accountability, improve quality of services and identify what is good or not about community practice. It can also aid risk-management and justify the use of resources, but equally it can generate better morale in cases where outcomes have never been demonstrated. Measuring outcomes is a broad concept. A traditional way of measuring outcomes has been through death rates associated with intervention or non-intervention. Health status can be measured via programmes of care. Examples could include immunisation levels for children and the elderly, smoking cessation in pregnant mothers or teenagers at school as a result of health-promotion input, or healing rates of venous leg ulcers as a result of a clinically-effective intervention.

Measuring outcomes for health has been a thorny issue for community nursing, and in particular for the groups of nurses such as school nurses and health visitors who have public health, prevention and health promotion as the major focus of their practice. Their work may have much longer-term outcomes for health gain. The Korner (Department of Health and Social Security 1987) requirements were a method of counting patient contacts within the NHS, and was incorporated into many of the hospital and community-based computer systems. The system was used as the origin of contract currencies, e.g. initial contacts and subsequent visits by health visitors to families, but was a very crude numerical estimation and may have hampered the development of much better performance indicators.

RESEARCH

Many more community nurses are involved in research, either on their own or as part of a multidisciplinary research programme. Research involves a more rigorous process that must produce results that are generalisable. There is a process in research design that involves:

- An explicit and defined question/topic area
- Ethical approval
- Writing proposals
- Systematic review of the literature
- Choice of research design
- Sample size/type
- Choice of tool – valid or standardised
- Knowledge and understanding of statistics
- Analysis of results and use of computer packages
- Interpretation of results
- Dissemination and publication of results.

Research aims to create new information about care, and possibly new ways in which care can be delivered. The health service is a rich source of both primary and secondary data and information. However, care needs to be taken that patients, staff and services are not exploited. Practitioners need education in research to help them understand research methods and the issues of ethics and confidentiality.

Research funding

Changes have occurred in terms of research and development funding since the Culyer report (Department of Health 1994) supported the move of more research funding into primary care. This does mean that both primary care and the community trusts can build their research profiles and apply for Culyer funding to support research and developments. Rather, it supports the idea that better quality research should be promoted in the community. There is a require-ment for better information on clinical effectiveness and efficiency of treatments for community services. The development of clinical guidelines and protocols is important to reduce the variations in clinical practice, and in particular to protect clients and patients from unacceptably poor practice (Royal College of Nursing 1998). Reforms in research and development funding to fit the NHS modernisation and clinical governance agenda will now allow that not only will the research and development costs be funded but also the service support costs supported by external funders (Department of Health 2000).

For community nurses, academic support may be required to carry out research. Many universities cover research awareness and methodologies as part of an academic course. Community nurses may well wish to carry out some local studies to inform practice. Support for the study or development can be offered through the research networks.

Research funding is important if the study or project could be in jeopardy of failing due to lack of skills, time and support, and for national or local recognition. Funding is available through many sources, and the proposal for funding should be as explicit and well-developed as possible. Each funding body will issue instructions and criteria which have to be met, and it is that refining process that is very time-consuming and difficult. The local research and development officer, who may be based at the health authority, is there for advice and guidance on research possibilities and funding.

There are several levels of evidence that practitioners may wish to explore, and knowing the difference between them is important in terms of resources. Does the area of study come into the category of research, audit or development? It depends very much for what kind of project or research community nurses need funding. Community health rarely attracts funding. This may be due to lack of acknowledgement that this area of the health services needs researching, or that the funding bodies may not have thought about community or primary care. Each year a set of priorities for funding is advertised through the research networks and the press. The local research and development officer can offer help to explore the range of possibilities. There are small grants or funds that may help an innovative project or even to set up a learning set to raise the level and awareness of research and project management. Many areas will have a journal club or a research society, but again these are not so common in the community. It may be possible to join a journal club locally to explore the most recent nursing research.

DEVELOPMENT

This will be more to do with application of the research, which has been critically examined, to an area of practice. Examples of this would be the research into treatment and care of pressure sores in the community, or into the identification of postnatal depression and the therapeutic interventions available. It is not about increasing the level of resourcing of existing services, although as a result of pilot programmes the developments may inform the commissioning of changes within the service provision.

PREPARING A PROPOSAL OR A BID FOR A RESEARCH PROJECT

One of the first things to do is to formulate an action plan and if possible discuss it with the research and development officer. Box 4.3 sets out the main steps in the process.

BOX 4.3	*The process of preparing for a research project*

- Discuss ideas with other people concerned
- Draw up a skeleton of the idea
- Identify support for the project
- Determine approximate resources required for the project
- Identify possible funding routes
- Submit project proposal to funding bodies
- Network with possible alliances
- Form a steering group or project committee
- Allocate responsibilities to members
- Plan start date
- Pilot idea
- Evaluate pilot
- Consider any changes as a result of pilot experience
- Consider exit strategies where appropriate, e.g. future resourcing of project or service development: will health authority consider?
- Plan dissemination strategy, including articles and possible workshops and conferences

Fitting the brief in terms of funding

Many community practitioners identify phenomena that they experience in the everyday course of their work. If these observations are made on a regular basis, there is the possibility that they are worthy of research. It is always advisable to discuss any idea with someone else, as it is at this point that the decision to seek answers or otherwise needs to be made, before investing time and energy.

Questions that may need to be asked are:

- Is there evidence of a need for change or improvement?
- What strategic direction or policy initiatives would be the focus (national or local health authority)?
- Has a literature search on the evidence been carried out?

There are now multiple sources of information available through professional libraries, academic departments, and centres for clinical trials, but it does take time and energy to complete a search enquiry.

Commissioning priorities

Does the project or research fit with the 'Our Healthier Nation' target areas (Department of Health 1998a), the National Service frameworks or commissioning priorities of the health authority or primary care group? If it does, then your chances of having a successful bid will be greater. To access this information, practitioners can ask their provider unit business manager or ask the health authority directly.

Steering groups

The steering group is a group of people who will monitor the progress of the project. The group needs to have representation with people who have appropriate clinical backgrounds and senior people in the organisation, in order to get support.

Informing people

In order to get the plan accepted and owned by all members, it is necessary to inform the organisation and the people who may be affected by your project or research. If people are not well-informed, they are less likely to participate in its achievement. However, in some cases, information may need to be restricted as part of the research process.

Outline plan

Once the outline plan is in place, ask the research and development officer, other practitioners and supervisors to critique the plan. Often this is very helpful in preventing pitfalls in the early stages, especially if it is your first project. Other people can see things from different perspectives and the practitioner may not have thought about some fundamental and pragmatic issues. Once it has been critiqued, refinement of the protocol may be necessary. Other people may need to be included as stakeholders.

Resources needed

Time is a major resource for people working in the health services and is often at a premium. When undertaking *any* developments or research, more time than is envisaged will be needed. As a general rule, researchers need to spend a third of the time available on literature reviews, a third of the time collecting and analysing data and another third writing it up. If the research needs funding, it may take many months to develop, write and submit a funding proposal; and it may not be accepted. However, even if one funding body does not accept it another may, so that the work invested may be worthwhile. Funding sources include European funding through partnerships with other European countries, Department of Health funding for research, nationally via centrally commissioned research and development, jointly commissioned national research, the Medical Research Council, the NHS Ethnic Health Unit, the Sports Council, the National Lottery and locally through regional project grants schemes and trustees schemes. For specific topic areas, grants may be available through professional organisations, charities and private companies.

Ethics, trust and health authority approval

It is most important before going ahead to think about whether ethics approval is needed. If there is any doubt, it is wiser to assume that it will. Ethics approval always takes time and the committees concerned only meet at certain times. Research protocols, consent forms and explanatory letters have to be drafted to accompany the application forms. Even if the study is approved, the committee will expect feedback at certain points and notification of any changes made to the protocol.

PUBLIC HEALTH PROFESSIONALS

There is a growing recognition that many other professionals work in the area of public health, not just the doctors working in public health medicine (Department of Health 1998d). The Standing Nursing and Midwifery Advisory Committee (1995) report identified the public health roles of nurses in communicable disease control, but also that health visitors, school nurses and occupational health nurses have had a long tradition of public health practice. The Chief Medical Officer's (Department of Health 1998b) project recognised the diversity in public practice. It identified the 'hands on' public health practitioners, including public health nurses, health promotion specialists, health visitors, community development workers and environmental health officers, who will need more specialised knowledge and expertise in their respective fields. The role of health visitors as public health professionals is recognised in the modernisation agenda and 'health visitors will lead public health practice and agree local health plans' (Department of Health 1999b para 11.17).

CONCLUSION

Developing public health strategies is a complex process. It must involve more population-based approaches at primary care level, so that services are maintained on an efficient, accessible and equitable basis for the total population. Health improvement programmes will have to be developed to bring health gain. Health Action Zones (Department of Health 1997c) will increase resources for certain priority health programmes. The nursing strategy in 'Making a Difference' (Department of Health 1999b pp 60–62) identifies health visitors, school nurses and midwives as having a major role in the public health function:

> 'Health visitors will lead public health practice and agree local health plans, school nursing teams will provide a range of health improvement activities, midwives are uniquely placed to improve health and tackle inequality through services to women and their babies.'

Community nurses are very well placed to identify needs and resources and can use innovative approaches for people in local communities. They know about the local health problems within their communities and can identify the priorities in terms of health and social care.

Trusts and education providers need to work in partnership to enable nurses to gain knowledge and competencies in public health for the 'New NHS' if it is to become modern and dependable. Commissioning health services and working with the primary care groups and trusts will be a challenge. Community nurses are vital to the public health function at local level, so health and appropriate health care can be the aim and philosophy of primary care services.

DISCUSSION QUESTIONS

- What are the dilemmas that community nurses face when commissioning healthcare alongside GPs and social services?
- Primary care groups/trusts have community nurses on the boards but what and whom do they represent?
- How can community nurses make sure that community profiling is part of the public health role and, if needs are identified, how can they change the strategic direction?
- What do community nurses feel about the the advantages or otherwise of involvement of the user perspectives as described within 'The NHS Plan'?
- What access do community nurses need for the development of research bases in practice?

FURTHER READING

Arora S, Davis A & Thompson S 1999 Developing Health Improvement Programmes: Lessons from the first year. Kings' Fund Publishing, London

Department of Health 1998 Our Healthier Nation: a contract for health (Cmnd 3852). The Stationery Office, London

Department of Health 1998 Partnership in Action: new opportunities for joint working between health and social services. Department of Health, London
Possibilities of 'pooling budgets' – health and social services. Lead commissioning (e.g. elderly) – transfer of funds from one agency to another under delegated authority of Section 28a of the NHS Act 1997 and vice versa to support objectives under the HImP. Integrated provision that allows providers to deliver services beyond the level possible under current powers

Harris A 1997 Needs to know: a guide to needs assessment for primary care. Churchill Livingstone, London
A useful guide to needs assessment with models and frameworks for assessing health needs from a general practice and public health perspective.

Koch H 1994 Towards Total Quality in Community Nursing Services. Longman Health Management, Harlow
A textbook full of examples of quality assurance in community nursing, as well as information on how information can be presented.

Naidoo J & Wills J 1994 Health Promotion: Foundations for Practice. Baillière Tindall, London
This book looks at health promotion in a very wide setting and includes needs – assessment planning and evaluation. Both national and international concepts of health and health promotion are discussed with examples used in practice.

NHS Centre for Reviews and Dissemination 2000 Evidence from systematic reviews of research relevant to the 'wider public health agenda'. University of York, York Electronic version available from http://www.york.ac.uk/inst/crd/wph.htm
Wide-ranging review of evidence collated under headings like 'mental health', 'social and economic interventions' or 'service interventions'. Very useful and user friendly basis for developing specific health strategies.

NHS Executive 1996 Clinical Effectiveness Reference Pack. NHS Executive, Leeds
The pack contains information on how to get hold of the bulletins, clinical guidelines, protocols and systematic reviews plus a list of academic centres.

Office for Public Management 1997 Achieving Health Gain through Health Promotion in a Primary Care-Led NHS. Health Education Authority, London
This is an account of a simulation exercise for shaping commissioning and achieving health gain. It explores the capacity within primary care to manage the future.

REFERENCES

Alderman C 1997 Citizens of Sunderland. Nursing Standard 1(32):22–23

Barker W 1984 Child Development Programme. Early Childhood Development Unit, University of Bristol, Bristol

Billings JR & Cowley S 1995 Approaches to community needs assessment: a literature review. Journal of Advanced Nursing 22:721–730

Bradshaw J 1972 A taxonomy of social need problems and progress in medical care. Seventh Series. Nuffield Provincial Hospitals Trust. Oxford University Press, Oxford

Bull J 1998 Integrated nursing: a review of the literature, B. Journal of Community Nursing 3(3):124–128

Community Education Development Centre 1995 User Involvement in Health Services for Children and Young People: A CEDC Project. Community Education Development Centre, Coventry

Community Practitioners' and Health Visitors' Association 1997 Public health: the role of nurses and health visitors. Community Practitioners' and Health Visitors' Association, London

Department of Health 1991 The patient's charter – a summary. HMSO, London

Department of Health 1992 The Health of the Nation (Cmnd 1986). HMSO, London

Department of Health 1994 Supporting Research and Development in the NHS. EL(94)79. HMSO, London

Department of Health 1996 Primary care: delivering the future. The Stationery Office, London

Department of Health 1997a The New NHS – modern, dependable (Cmnd 3807). Department of Health, London

Department of Health 1997b Personal Medical Services Pilots under the NHS (Primary Care) Act 1997: a guide to the application and approval process. NHS Executive, Leeds

Department of Health 1997c Health Action Zones: Invitation to bid. EL(97)65. Department of Health, London

Department of Health 1998a Our Healthier Nation: A Contract for Health (Cmnd 3852). Department of Health, London

Department of Health 1998b Chief Medical Officer's Project to Strengthen the Public

Health Function in England. Department of Health, London

Department of Health 1998c A First Class Service: Quality in the new NHS. Department of Health, Leeds

Department of Health 1998d Shared Contributions, Shared Benefits: The Report of the Working Group on Public Health and Primary Care. Department of Health, Leeds

Department of Health 1999a Reducing Health Inequalities: An Action Report. Our Healthier Nation. The Stationery Office, London

Department of Health 1999b Making a Difference: Strengthening the nursing, midwifery and health visiting contribution to health and healthcare. Department of Health, London

Department of Health 1999c Primary care trusts establishment, the preparatory period and their functions. Department of Health, Leeds

Department of Health 2000 Research and Development for a First Class Service: R&D funding in the new NHS. Department of Health, Leeds

Department of Health and Social Security 1986 Neighbourhood Nursing – A Focus of Care (Chair J Cumberlege). HMSO, London

Department of Health and Social Security 1987 Körner Implementation: Statement of Central Requirements for Aggregated Returns on Community Health Services Ref. No. B6. HMSO, London

Dixon M, Murray T & Jenner D 1998 The Locality Commissioning Handbook: from vision to reality. Radcliffe Medical, Oxford

Gastrell P & Edwards J 1996 Community Health Nursing: Frameworks for Practice. Baillière Tindall/RCN, London

Ham C & Appleby J 1993 The Future of the NHS. National Association of Health Authorities and Trusts, Birmingham

Health Visitors' Association 1996 Integrated Nursing Team – Initial Information. Professional Briefing 1. Health Visitors' Association, London

Jolly K & George S 1996 Demographic Changes. In: Gastrell P & Edwards J (eds) Community Health Nursing: Frameworks for Practice. Baillière Tindall/RCN, London pp 18–27

Jones T 1997 Strategic planning for purchasers B. Journal of Health Care Management 3(8):441–443

Leonard O, Allsop J, Taket A & Wiles R 1997 User involvement in two primary health care projects in London. Social Science Research Papers No. 5. South Bank University/College of Health, London

Levy B S 1998 Creating the future of public health: values, vision and leadership. 1997 Presidential Address. American Journal of Public Health 88:188–192

Lewis R, Jenkins C & Gillam S 1999 Personal medical services pilots in London: re-writing the Red Book. King's Fund, London

Lewthwaite J & Haffenden S 1997 Patients Influencing Purchasers: report of an action research project sponsored by Long Term Medical Conditions Alliance. NHS Confederation Research Paper No 3. NHS Confederation, Birmingham

Liddell A 1998 Guidance Notes for GP Commissioning Group Pilots. Department of Health, Leeds

London Health Economics Consortium 1995 Community based needs assessment. Test bed sites study: overview paper and summary of findings. Report to the Steering Group. London School of Tropical Hygiene and Medicine, London

Marsh S & Macalpine M 1995 Our Own Capabilities: clinical nurse managers making a strategic approach to service improvement. King's Fund/Nursing Development Units, London

NHSME 1992 Local Voices: The Views of Local People in Purchasing for Health. Department of Health, Leeds

Peckham S 1994 Local voices and primary health care. Critical Public Health 5(2):36–40

Parsons L & Day S 1992 Improving obstetric outcomes in ethnic minorities: an evaluation of health advocacy in Hackney. Journal of Public Health Medicine 14(2):183–191

Pascale R 1990 Managing on the edge: how successful companies use conflict to stay ahead. Penguin, Middlesex p 40

Pearson V 1998 Who needs needs assessment? Assessing health needs and integrating public health into locality commissioning. In: Dixon M et al (eds) The locality Commissioning Handbook. 60–68. Radcliffe Medical Press, Oxford

Royal College of Nursing 1996 Profiling Poverty: A Guide for Nurses in the Community. Issues in nursing and health 40. Royal College of Nursing, London

Royal College of Nursing 1998 Clinical Guidelines: What you need to know. Royal College of Nursing, London

Royal College of Paediatrics and Child Health 1997 The Essentials of Effective Community Health Services for Children and Young People: Report of a Working Party. Royal College of Paediatrics and Child Health, London

Rutt H M 1995 Listening to local voices in Oregon. British Journal of Health Care Management 1(11):556–560

Secretary of State for Health 1999 Saving Lives: Our Healthier Nation (Cmnd. 4386). The Stationery Office, London

Secretary of State for Health 2000 The NHS Plan: A plan for investment; a plan for reform (Cmnd 4818-I). The Stationery Office, London

Standing Nursing and Midwifery Advisory Committee 1995 Making it happen. Public health – the contribution, role and development of nurses, midwives and health visitors. Department of Health, London

Stewart R & Turner I 1998 Achieving quality in residential care and nursing homes. In: Mason C (ed) Achieving Quality in Community Health Care Nursing. Macmillan, Basingstoke pp 138–159

United Kingdom Central Council, 1992 Scope of Professional Practice. United Kingdom Central Council, London

Vancay L 1998 Teamworking in primary care. Nursing Standard 12(20):37–38

5 Public health and primary care

Susan Walters & Sarah Cowley

KEY ISSUES

- Primary healthcare is viewed internationally as the mechanism through which public health can be achieved.
- Primary care services may be selective, when they focus only on providing medical services, or comprehensive when they integrate hospital and community health services and incorporate other sectors relevant to health, like housing, voluntary services and social care.
- The Health Act 1999 has shifted towards a comprehensive model of primary healthcare, providing a mechanism by which general practitioners and community nurses lead strategic decisions that feed into the Health Improvement Programmes (HImPs) across an area.
- The role of community nurses serving on primary care groups and trusts is of central importance in identifying and prioritising the needs in an area and deciding the best way of delivering services to meet them.
- The position of primary care group board nurses gives increased legitimacy and power to practice-level knowledge, creating a need for leadership, executive level skills and organisational development.
- Varied understandings of how 'public health' can be implemented through 'primary healthcare' can be a barrier to effectiveness, especially given the diversity encompassed within nursing and the lack of additional time for practitioners to contribute at the strategic level implied in the new organisational structures.

INTRODUCTION

Since the last quarter of the twentieth century, primary health care has been increasingly hailed as the best way to achieve public health. This view has sometimes been greeted with confusion in the UK where, traditionally, the medical profession has seen public health as one speciality, while general practice, another distinct specialism, has claimed a near-monopoly on primary health care. This chapter will begin by outlining the different meanings and ideas linked with the term 'primary health care' to explain both the attraction of using it as a strategy for delivering 'public health' and the similarities in practice between the two terms. This introduction will be used as the basis from which to explain and critique the emerging English system of primary care groups (PCGs) and trusts, which are directed toward improving the public health. In the second half of the chapter, the challenges and responsibilities faced by PCG Board Nurses in trying to achieve this will be detailed.

WHAT IS PRIMARY HEALTH CARE?

In 1978, the World Health Organization (WHO) held an international conference in the Russian town of Alma-Ata, to begin planning a global strategy for improving health. It culminated in a declaration expressing the need for a concerted effort by governments and communities to protect and promote the health of all people of the world. This was clearly a public health strategy on a grand scale. Primary health care was viewed, then, as the mechanism by which this vision could be achieved, and it remains a key target for health for the twenty-first century (WHO 1999). A comprehensive definition of 'primary health care' was included as part of the Alma-Ata declaration; excerpts are shown in Box 5.1.

The Alma-Ata declaration was much discussed in developing countries when it was first made. However, since the start of the NHS, all residents have been entitled to register with a local general practitioner and, from thence, to access other members of the primary health care team. International expectations seemed less important in the UK, therefore, and discussion has focused on service definitions and responsibilities rather than on how services could or should be reorientated. Even so, primary health care teams became generally wider and practices larger throughout the 1980s, setting the scene for an increasing and rapidly escalating legislative and policy emphasis on primary health care in the UK in the final decade of the twentieth century.

In 1990, the NHS and Community Care Act empowered general practitioners (GPs) to apply for fundholding status and to engage in purchasing health services for patients on their lists. This function was, for the rest of the population, undertaken by health authorities under the auspices and guidance of the Directors of Public Health, who were expected to draw up epidemiological assessments of need in their areas and ensure that appropriate services were available, within the resource base, to meet those needs. The phrase 'primary care-led NHS' was introduced to promote the diversity of structures and purchasing models available to GP fundholders and other NHS purchasing authorities (NHSE 1994). There have been numerous changes since that time, but the focus on commissioning of services continues to be a key aspect of the public health function undertaken within the primary care sector.

Service arrangements that focus heavily on selected health services and that are driven by professionals trained in medical interventions have been heavily criticised for 'medicalising primary health care' (Macdonald 1992). This is considered unhelpful because such a narrow focus goes against the philosophy and potential of comprehensive primary health care envisaged at Alma-Ata, which rests on the 'three pillars' of participation, intersectoral collaboration and equity (Macdonald 1992). In addition to the debate about whether primary health care is best delivered through a selective or comprehensive system, are concerns about the extent to which it is integrated into the whole of the health system. Achieving an integrated health sector is a key target in the WHO's updated plans to achieve health for all in the twenty-first century:

'Target 15: An integrated health sector. By the year 2010, people in the [European] Region should have much better access to family- and community-oriented primary health care, supported by a flexible and responsive hospital system.' (WHO 1999 p 119)

| BOX 5.1 | *Primary health care: excerpts from the declaration of Alma-Ata (WHO 1978 p 2–5)* |

Primary health care is essential care based on practical, scientifically sound and socially acceptable methods and technology made universally accessible to individuals and families in the community by means acceptable to them, through their full participation and at a cost that the community and country can afford. It forms an integral part of both the country's health system of which it is the nucleus and of the overall social and economic development of the community. It is the first level of contact for individuals, the family and community with the national health system, bringing health care as close as possible to where people live and work, and constitutes the first element of a continuing health care process.

Primary health care:

- Reflects and evolves from the economic conditions and socio-cultural and political characteristics of the country and its communities and is based on the application of the relevant results of social, biomedical and health services research and public health experience

- Addresses the main health problems in the community, providing promotive, preventive, curative and rehabilitative services accordingly

- Includes at least: education concerning prevailing health problems and the methods of preventing and controlling them; an adequate supply of safe water and sanitation; maternal and child health care, including family planning; immunisation against the major infectious diseases; prevention and control of locally endemic diseases; appropriate treatment of common diseases and injuries and provision of essential drugs

- Involves, in addition to the health sector, all related sectors and aspects of national and community development, in particular, agriculture, animal husbandry, food, industry, education, housing, public works, communications and other sectors; and demands the coordinated efforts of all those sectors

- Requires and promotes maximum community and individual self-reliance and participation in the planning, organisation, operation and control of primary health care, making fullest use of local, national and other available resources; and to this end develops through appropriate education the ability of communities to participate

- Should be sustained by integrated, functional and mutually supportive referral systems, leading to progressive improvements of comprehensive health care for all, and giving priority to those most in need

- Relies, at local and referral levels, on health workers, including physicians, nurses, midwives, auxiliaries and community workers as applicable, as well as traditional practitioners as needed, suitably trained socially and technically to work as a health team and to respond to the expressed health needs of the community.

The NHS and Community Care Act 1990 did help to move the NHS towards an integrated sector in which hospital services support those in primary care, by giving some GPs the power to purchase a wide range of services in their local area, through total purchasing pilots and consortium-based multifunds. However, the division between health and social needs continued to be emphasised, and the whole system was based on the ethos of competition rather than collaboration. The changes continued the earlier emphasis on primary care as a first level of contact and universal access to essential health care through a GP who could refer to secondary services; but primary care remained selective, narrowly focused on the health sector and professionally led.

A major shift in policies after 1997 was developed by the incoming Labour government to focus on those 'three pillars' of equity, participation and inter-sectoral collaboration. This was not only to develop a more comprehensive and integrated system of primary health care, but was seen as a way of improving both the public health and health services across the board.

REORIENTATING HEALTH SERVICES

The Health Act 1999 brought in new responsibilities and structures for the health service, that had been set out in the White Papers the 'New NHS' (Department of Health 1997) and 'Saving Lives: Our Healthier Nation' (Department of Health 1999a). The overall plan was to develop a comprehensive primary health care sector that would be fully integrated into the wider health service, that would reorientate hospital services so that they met the needs of the local population and that would begin to break down the barriers between health and social care. These would be achieved by bringing together representative primary health care workers (doctors and nurses) from a local area, along with someone from social services and a lay person, and giving them new powers and responsibilities to determine the shape of health services.

This was the basis for the primary care group (PCG) in England. There were variations across the UK with different terminology (that is, health cooperatives and local health groups) and details of working practice in Scotland, Wales and Northern Ireland. However, the underlying principles were all similar, with a clear intention that primary care would have a major say in the way services developed in future. Furthermore, PCGs were not only about commissioning services, but about improving health. PCGs were to fulfil three main functions:

- Improving the health of, and addressing health inequalities in, their communities
- Developing primary care and community services across the PCG
- Advising on, or commissioning directly, a range of hospital services for patients within their area which appropriately meets patients needs.

From the start, therefore, PCGs were expected to tackle health inequalities, as well as improving the quality and efficiency of services. The ideals of primary health care could be seen in the plan that decisions about priorities and health service commissioning would be made at a local level, involving local people. Decisions are to be based on clinical need as assessed and perceived by local professionals whose everyday work involves caring for local people in some way; this marked a reorientation of former structures to a more bottom-up approach. The explicit requirement for leadership from the practice level was a radical change from the former system, in which commissioning was seen as a senior managerial responsibility, undertaken within large health authorities that could seem remote from the population and local practices.

Another major change was the requirement to have both social services and lay representation on PCG boards, working as equal partners with the doctors and nurses to help shape local services. From the start, a typical PCG board would consist of up to seven GPs and one or two community nurses, who would all be in practice locally, undertaking PCG duties as an additional responsibility alongside their everyday work. PCG boards also have a single social services representative, one lay member and a non-executive director from the relevant health authority. The chair of the board is selected by the members; this must be a GP unless those on the PCG board agree to waive this right. Finally, each PCG has an appointed chief executive who will additionally serve as a member of the board.

Such a radical overhaul to the system needed to be implemented gradually, although it should be said that the pace of change felt very frantic at the time. Initially, four different levels of responsibility were set out (Department of Health 1997). The levels were:

- **Level 1** – at a minimum, act in support of the health authority in commissioning care for its population, acting in an advisory capacity
- **Level 2** – take devolved responsibility for managing the budget for health care in their area, acting as part of the health authority
- **Level 3** – become established as free-standing bodies accountable to the health authority for commissioning care
- **Level 4** – become established as free-standing bodies accountable to the health authority for commissioning care, and with added responsibility for the provision of community services for their population.

When they first started in 1999, PCGs could choose to operate at Levels 1 or 2; some 87% immediately moved to the second level. At levels 3 or 4, PCGs change in status as well as scope, becoming 'primary care trusts' (PCTs) that have a higher level of responsibility and accountability. By the end of 2000, there were 40 PCTs in England. This number is expected to rise rapidly with 130 PCGs actively seeking trust status by April 2001 and the remaining 300 expected to follow suit soon after. The transition is expected to be complete by 2004 (Department of Health 2000).

Further developments have been proposed in the NHS Plan (Department of Health 2000), which sets out an even broader level of 'care trusts'. These will build on the joint commissioning powers established under the Health Act 1999; they will be able to commission and deliver primary and community health care, as well as social care for older people and other client groups. Care trusts may be established where there is a joint agreement locally that this model offers the best way to deliver fully integrated services.

Alternatively, the government proposes taking powers to establish care trusts where there is a failure to establish effective joint partnerships or where inspected services are deemed to be failing. Full details of how care trusts will be established had not been published by the time this chapter was being prepared. However, the NHS Plan suggests that some may be in place as early as 2001, with a wider roll-out depending on implementation of Level 3 and 4 PCTs across the country.

As primary care trusts take over more of the day-to-day commissioning of services, so health authorities will be able to concentrate more of their time and expertise on the essential, wider public health functions. They are expected to develop an over-arching, strategic and enabling approach to improving health across a wider area, not only through commissioning health services, but by working in partnership with a range of other sectors and services and developing Health Improvement Programmes (HImPs). The key features of core roles of health authorities compared with primary care groups and primary care trusts were set out in the white paper 'Saving Lives' (Department of Health 1999a) as shown in Table 5.1.

The new policies have brought together all the necessary ingredients for a fully comprehensive and integrated service, based on the three primary health care pillars of equity, participation and intersectoral collaboration. This does not mean the recipe is complete! Despite the stated intention that the changes should be evolutionary, implementation of the new policies seemed to progress at a hectic pace. Given the right environment for change and learning, there is an enormous potential for community nurses and health visitors to participate in PCGs and PCTs. Yet, despite the changed agenda and new ways of working being recognised in policy (Department of Health 1999b), we continue to debate our potential (Community Practitioners' and Health Visitors' Association 1999). This is significant in itself and indicative of the underlying tensions within a rapidly changing health care environment; it suggests there is a need to focus on the development of both leadership skills and empowerment of staff within organisations. The second half of this chapter will focus on these developmental needs, along with the potential and practicalities of implementing the new agenda from a nursing perspective. It will draw on Sue Walter's personal experience of being a health visitor and board nurse from the time the PCGs were first set up in shadow form at the end of 1998.

PRIMARY CARE: POTENTIAL FOR NURSING?

When the 'New NHS' white paper (Department of Health 1997) first introduced the concept of PCGs in England, there was general excitement among nursing groups that at last their voice could be heard on a governing body. Soon after, there was a sense of trepidation as detailed working papers set out the

TABLE 5.1	Key features and core roles (from Department of Health 1999a)	
Health authorities	**PCGs and PCTs**
Enabling	Doing
Gaining multisectoral commitment and coordination	Forging local partnerships
Setting strategy (jointly with others)	Planning action
Prioritising and investing in public health programmes	Resourcing action plans
Developing public health organisational and people capacity	Building workforce capacity and public health infrastructure
Monitoring progress	Meeting objectives

extent of imbalance between the numbers of nurses and GPs on the PCG boards. As members of the PCGs, nurses were to work in partnership with other members to develop primary care and other services in their areas. It soon seemed apparent that whenever this partnership arrangement was mentioned it was in terms of 'the GP and others', always giving greater status to the one group. In practical terms, the workload created by the need for board members to sit on the various sub-committees and groups was relatively greater for nurses, who had only two members to share the load, than for GPs who could divide the duties between seven colleagues.

Even so, awareness of the importance of multiagency working grew, and of the greater contribution of other agencies such as housing, in improving health. The government's challenge to address health and social inequalities by this new way of working was appealing, because it seemed that at last positive changes could be made within communities. This was a clear public health remit, articulated in 'Saving Lives' (Department of Health 1999a). Here, in theory at least, was a bottom-up approach to the development of health. It held promise of great potential for the nurses, midwives and health visitors to contribute to Health Improvement Programmes, sharing power in the interests of improving services.

HEALTH IMPROVEMENT PROGRAMMES

As explained above and in Chapter 4, Health Improvement Programmes (HImPs) are a key part in the government's health policy, and are crucial in its strategy to modernise and change. The programmes are designed to introduce a more strategic and longer-term planning process into the NHS, with the introduction of 3-year rolling contracts. However, they are supposed to be formed from the 'bottom up', taking account of input from local government and local communities; information that may be submitted directly to committies formed by the health authority or through the PCG. Local government colleagues are key allies for nurses who want to influence the formation of policy. Local elected officials are also an important lobbying force, and many are represented on PCGs. Health visitors in particular, with their extensive knowledge of the impact of housing on health, and knowledge of local families, needs, can use these links to further influence the Health Improvement Programme, and its local priorities.

The HImP is an umbrella strategy for all the local health policy with its aim to reduce inequalities in terms of access as well as to improve health. Thus, it is through the HImP that the government intends to achieve and move forward its modernising agenda. National targets will have to be delivered in each health authority area through long-term service agreements. Underpinning the above are new duties of partnership with the NHS and local authorities, who take their roles extremely seriously in terms of health outcomes. This is another major area of influence, as nurses and health visitors are able to take advantage of new joint roles. Often these roles are only at a strategic level, but there is much scope and potential for, for example, health visiting roles to be placed in housing departments – these would then be ideally placed to influence the health agenda.

It is surely within the development of the HImP that practitioners can have the most influence. Key stakeholders in the process are people within the PCG/PCT area who can accurately reflect the views of the local community. It is not only the lay member who is close to the community, but also the local nurses, midwives and health visitors who see the day-to-day hardships of people on their caseloads. Here is an opportunity to translate public health knowledge into action and to engage with the HImP in its broadest sense. There are five key areas involved in developing the HImP (Arora et al 1999):

- Health needs assessment
- Resource mapping
- Identification of priorities for action
- Strategies for change
- Service and financial framework for the NHS.

At first glance, some of these areas may seem beyond the normal remit of nursing, but assessing need, interagency planning and health promotion are everyday aspects of nursing practice. Nurses also need to keep abreast of the National Service Frameworks and guidance issued by the National Institute for Clinical Excellence (NICE), as these will have a key role in influencing local strategy. NICE is a special health authority established as part of the modernisation programme, to collate evidence and review research about best practice, as a resource and guide for those planning services.

Chapter 6 sets out ways of profiling health needs in a local area. Most community practitioners already know what the major health needs are in their area, even if they may not articulate it in the same language as a HImP document. What is important is that they have a voice and a means of conveying their knowledge. There are some key issues that are likely to occur in many areas, and which could be incorporated into a local strategy for health improvement if the need exists. Some local information could usefully be sought about:

- Child poverty
- Parenting skills
- Teenage pregnancy
- Inequalities and social exclusion
- Emotional well-being
- Offending behaviour
- Prevention – early intervention
- Child protection
- Inclusive education
- Poor-quality housing
- Homelessness
- Children looked after by the local authority
- Substance misuse
- Mental health.

All of these are relevant to the development of a local health plan, and are well within the knowledge base and experience of most local community practitioners. Steel (1999) and Collinson (2000) argue that nurses bring a personal dimension and a human touch to their work, which may not be apparent in other areas such as medicine. This could be debated, but as nurses we must not forget that this factor allows us a rare insight into the lived experience of local people. This could be a major contribution; but the skill lies in being able to transfer that personal knowledge into a sound, evidence-based plan of action.

Interestingly, a recent study of Health Improvement Programmes found that very few of them highlighted the needs of children or broad issues such as housing, but concentrated on accidents and coronary heart disease. These are all laudable and excellent initiatives, but may suggest that the health needs assessment undertaken has not included the wider views of community nurses or other agencies in their data collection. An emphasis on prevention, early intervention and full participation of the local community and sectors other than the health service is often lacking. It seems there is still some way to go to achieve the paradigm shift required to move away from the selective, medically-oriented approach explained in the first half of this chapter, towards the fully comprehensive and integrated approach to primary health care envisaged in the 'New NHS' white paper (Department of Health 1997).

NURSING KNOWLEDGE AND POWER

The new-agenda public health emphasis on addressing health and social inequalities through a holistic approach gives increased legitimacy and recognition to nurses and health visitors working in the primary care sector. However, these emerging developments require nurses to exercise greater accountability and to be more proactive (Lomax & Wright 1997). The shift in thinking, within policy at least, from the domination of a medical public health model to recognition of the need for a community development, bottom-up approach, should allow health visitors and nurses with public health skills to find their true position of influence.

Knowledge of policy and an ability to synthesise information about health needs, the views of the local community and the way that services can help to address those needs are all crucial attributes if nurses are to contribute effectively at a strategic level. Similarly, it is important to be able to use research in a way that will influence policy. Local research can be influential and needs to be more focused on what the clients need rather than be service-led. Nurses may feel they have no contribution, perhaps even being unaware of major policy changes or of the connections between policies, which could have a direct impact on both their position and the people they work with. However, when staff are informed and involved the information they hold can be harnessed and used effectively.

One important spin-off of the shift to PCGs has been the establishment of local community nursing groups, variously known as 'nursing networks' or 'nursing forums' through which nurses, midwives and health visitors working across a local area meet with board nurses, usually monthly, for mutual support, information-giving and planning purposes. These were set up to ensure the wider community of nurses could contribute, with local communication groups below board level being recognised as crucial. This would give the board nurse more power and influence, and there will be a sense of ownership from within the primary care field. However, nursing forums are not easy to facilitate and have sometimes been viewed as a threat to other PCG members. It is worth noting that GPs are both well-represented and organised by local medical committees (LMCs) (Singer 1998). Given the significance of nursing in terms of workforce numbers and planning, it is important for their forum to be regarded in a similar light to that of the LMC, and for sufficient time to be made available for nurses to attend meetings and support the board nurses in rising to the challenge of providing relevant information to the PCG.

Billingham (1998) suggests that, 'nurses involved in health needs assessment, multiagency planning, community development, research and evaluation should be well placed to meet the challenge'. However, it is not that simple; nurses and health visitors still find it difficult to have their voices heard and feel that they have an influence. Suggestions that this is the 'fault' of the nurse or health visitor are unhelpful and may undermine the confidence of individuals still further. Argyris (1985) argues that individuals resort to a number of defensive routines, particularly in situations where staff feel undervalued and disempowered in organisations, and discouraged from taking risks. One response to this is a constant drive to seek autonomy and to be recognised. Unchallenged, defensive routines can lead to a less reflective and innovative practitioner, who becomes frustrated and demotivated, unwilling to contribute to local objectives.

This leads to the conclusion that possessing the right balance of practice skills and public health knowledge means that nurses can now take up the challenges. There are constraints for practitioners within primary care, which are not always recognised by those in non-clinical positions, and which require new models of leadership to challenge them. The constraints are not insurmountable but are more connected to the culture of organisations. They may also be a manifestation of the difficulties experienced by organisations as they attempt to move from one agenda to another.

Organisational culture and priorities are also significant in ensuring the sustainability of public health approaches (Community Practitioners and Health Visitors' Association 1999). It has argued that organisations must adopt a public health ethos, that is a bottom-up approach to change allowing the cultivation of appropriate skills, and that nurses must capitalise on the effects of policy changes. It is certainly the case that the policy framework can be used to take forward a number of initiatives that had not been acknowledged as a priority before (Walters 1999).

LEADERSHIP

Leadership and leadership development are seen as crucial in enabling nurses to contribute in the present rapidly changing health care system. It is not enough to have excellent grass roots knowledge and to be at the sharp end of practice. There is a need for the development of leadership skills at a grass roots level and a structure within organisations which allows leaders to emerge. Collinson (2000) has recently articulated the need for nurses to develop entrepreneurial skills and this emerges in other literature.

If practitioners are to grasp the opportunities, they need a capacity for leadership that differs from the skills needed to operate in traditional organisation and management structures. Indeed, people who have difficulty working within traditional hierarchical systems are often the very practitioners who are most comfortable operating on the 'margins' of the organisation and possibly working with the most marginalised groups. In turn, they may have a great deal to contribute to local policy, being practitioners who operate at the interface of policy and yet have remained within the clinical arena, committed to the practice of community nursing or health visiting.

The concept of leadership is closely related to the transformational skills of inspiring and motivating others (Young & Antrobus 1998). The RCN had already stated this in a series of lectures (Andrews-Evans 1997). Kanter (1979) and Rafferty (1993) argue that there are two types of leaders; the visible and those who are less visible. The less-visible leaders are excellent facilitators and effective as leaders because they enable others, delegate and are not afraid to put 'subordinates' in powerful positions. This is the bottom-up approach to leadership, the 'hidden' leaders (Rafferty 1993) who are often seen as provocative and difficult within organisations, but whose risk-taking challenges and innovative initiatives are so badly needed now.

The leadership model advocated perhaps covertly within the 'New NHS' (Department of Health 1997) seems to suggest a move to this bottom-up approach, with its emphasis on partnership, collaboration and multidisciplinary working. However, the structure of the PCG board, with its built-in medical majority and veto over election of the chair, does not support this notion. Even so, board nurses can still exercise great influence.

Rafferty (1993) refers to hidden leaders whose role is to inspire and facilitate, but who have no formal leadership position. These are often seen as 'nonconformist' and even deviant (Rafferty 1993) as they challenge the status quo of the organisation. The present policy agenda provides an ideal framework for this bottom-up transformational style of leadership, but there is a tension between the culture of existing NHS structures that are still based on a hierarchical, perhaps paternalistic, model.

The new agenda is an attempt to empower both the users of the services and workers within them to influence and drive the need for change. However, the empowerment model is the antithesis of the paternalistic model that has dominated statutory services. The former top-down approach of needs assessment and intervention has not improved the conditions of those experiencing the most disadvantages in our communities. Empowerment, which is discussed at some length in Chapter 8, becomes the key to overcoming cultural barriers resistant to preventive approaches. Empowerment within and for nursing holds the key to unlock the potential for nurses to influence local initiatives. This is linked to the need for both leaders and leadership skills.

Executive skills

The key question is: what do nurses need to function effectively at board level themselves, and to enable other nurses to contribute effectively? This question, about the skills needed by PCG nurses, is similar to those being asked in the early 1990s, when NHS trusts were being established with a requirement for all trust boards to have a nursing member. The circle may seem complete when the PCGs have all been transformed into PCT's with a major difference being the flattening of the hierarchies and opportunity for nurses to contribute strategically while maintaining a base in practice. 'Success' will be reflected (or not) in the individual nurse's ability to transfer his or her clinical knowledge base to the strategic planning table. Only then can real improvements in the population's health be envisaged and the contribution of nurses far exceed existing boundaries.

Nursing representation takes on a different meaning in this context when it is seen as being concerned with the health of the whole population. It is this ability to translate individual needs into a collective population view, which is vitally important. The nurse is required to move up and down the ladder from strategic to operational levels. It is clear that combining a caseload with strategic work is a major challenge, not least because of the personal cost involved, because the 2 days per month allocated are not adequate to cover the PCG workload (Sackman 1999).

Despite the frustrations, and in some cases limited support, nurses are contributing enormously to the planning and delivery of HImPs and clinical governance, often taking the lead within PCGs in these issues. Clearly, more work needs to be done in this area, particularly with the transition to PCTs. There is also the ever-present danger that, as nurses develop and move from 'novice to expert' (Benner 1984), they will lose sight of the reason for their representation, which is to contribute a grass roots perspective and be an advocate for the community. The development of shared governance will hopefully play a major part in producing nurse leaders who can step beyond what has been called the 'doctor–nurse game'.

LEARNING ORGANISATIONS

Moving again into the arena of leadership stresses the need for learning organisations (Senge 1990). Within a learning organisation people are encouraged to challenge the status quo, take risks and learn from their mistakes. We need to nurture these people and the appropriate skills of 'entrepreneurial competence' (Collinson 2000) if we are to fulfil the challenges in 'Making a Difference' (Department of Health 1999b). Collinson identifies six key areas for nurses to consider:

- Networking
- Marketing
- Influencing
- Negotiating
- Business planning
- Self-managed development.

Steel (1999) has also described the need for political awareness as a prerequisite for influencing and negotiating, as well as having media training. It may also be necessary to consider new educational programs for nurses to meet the twenty-first century challenges of nursing. In all of this development of new skills, we must not forget who we are and remain focused on the needs of clients; the diversity encompassed by community nursing is a strength that helps our contribution to planning local policies. There is a danger that we could lose the public health focus of looking at local health needs as we, as nurses, begin to move into areas traditionally dominated by managers.

OVERCOMING THE BARRIERS

Boards were expected to settle quickly and begin contributing to Health Improvement Programmes, selecting local targets, and selecting representatives for clinical governance and commissioning. The pace of change was very rapid, which may have contributed to the impression in many areas that this was a medically-led decision-making process, with little challenge from the members who were just finding their feet in a new, difficult role. In some areas there was the issue of appropriate nursing representation, with GPs protesting that 'their' practice nurse was not represented. Thus, it is apparent that nurses on boards had a whole range of both hidden and explicit agendas to deal with, as well as trying to represent both their colleagues and users of the services.

Singer (1998) argues that the change called for enlightened GPs who understood the views and roles of nurses more clearly. However, there may be some underlying difficulties in the relationship between GP and board nurse which can affect the board dynamics and function. It may be necessary for some GPs to develop better committee skills in order to move more appropriately into the shared governance procedures that will assume greater significance as PCGs assume trust status. As it was, the period of change and settling-in led to many GPs feeling threatened and demanding more control from the government (Beecham 1998, Shapiro 1998). The government response, which ensured an inequitable balance of power within the PGC boards, inevitably had a knock-on effect on the remaining board members. Increasingly, board nurses referred to themselves being a token presence (Shapiro 1998, Sackman 1999), feeling that their influence was not as great as they had expected.

Steel (1999), in her critique of the white paper from a US perspective, argues that far from marginalising nursing there is a potential for a new relationship between doctors and nursing. Nevertheless, collaboration implies partnership and experiences to date suggest that the relationship is not on an even keel. Steel (1999) argues for a higher level training course to prepare nurses to stand on an equal footing with doctors. This may appear logical, but may in fact reinforce the subservience of nurses, while we surely should be celebrating our diversity.

Clarke (Santry & Clarke 1999) described what happened to PCG board nurses in one English region, outlining the selection process at length and concluding that there was little literature to inform the process. It became clear that medical issues and interpersonal relationships were not the sole problem responsible for all difficulties. Among the numerous other issues to be considered, three are of great significance:

- Different definitions of public health, from within and external to nursing
- Differences and diversity within nursing, midwifery and health visiting
- Time.

The different definitions and meanings attached to 'public health' are discussed at length in this book, with Chapters 1–3 focusing especially on the meaning for nurses and health visitors and in relation to health promotion. Those chapters point to the debate that has been unfolding over the last 10 years or so in these fields. However, the debate about what public health means in relation to primary health care, and indeed the different meanings attached to that term (outlined at the start of the chapter) add to the confusion.

The second point, differences across the nursing fields, came more sharply into focus after the government conceded that GPs were to maintain a majority voice on PCG boards. When first floated, the idea was that a board comprised of primary care workers, with added lay and social services representation, would be best placed to know the needs of local population, and how best to serve those needs. The board members were never, therefore, intended to serve a professional representative function in the way that happens in, say, trade union negotiations. Their collective role was always to represent the population's needs, bringing a practice knowledge and perspective to planning and developing the most appropriate services to meet those needs.

However, once one occupational group gained a position of power, it became almost almost inevitable that the remaining community groups would want to be represented. Many hospital staff and therapy professions too, felt diminished and threatened by what seemed to be a privileged position offered to community nurses. In most instances, this initial wrangling has been settled as the various committees and forums provide opportunities for all nursing voices to be heard, and the original purpose of the boards is reasserted. Indeed, in some cases, the amount of time taken to contribute to the committees and nursing forums that feed into the PCG/PCT board seems so prohibitive that committee positions are no longer greeted with much envy.

Lack of time is the third key issue; it is one of the major obstacles for nurses in contributing effectively to the public health agenda in primary care. The role of board nurses is demanding and time-consuming. It is, of course, highly exciting; if not frustrating at times. But here lies a further tension. The practitioner working within a caseload is required to attend board meetings, sub-groups, nurse forums, to read papers and to become an overnight transformational leader! Some enlightened areas have enabled this process by providing cover for nurses, but this is by no means a consistent model (Sackman 1999).

The job description of board nurses is fascinating, and one wonders how anyone could meet such challenging criteria and not already function as an executive nurse. In many ways, it removes the grass roots appeal of the practitioner and moves away from the white papers' emphasis on the contribution of practitioners 'working together in new PCGs to shape services ...' (Department of Health 1997). However, many policy makers sitting on HImPs and other such strategic planning initiatives are not practice-based and welcome the broad knowledge offered by the nursing contribution. In the author's experience, and in discussion with other board nurses, it takes a while to feel able to contribute and to be comfortable in a new culture. However, it is also apparent that nurses should not be expected to totally conform to a different culture, but should be encouraged to be themselves; after all, it is the nursing knowledge and skill that is valued.

CONCLUSION

There are a number of challenges facing nurses in primary care at this time. The key challenge is the identification and development of nurse leaders who will influence and manage the change process needed in the transition to primary care trusts. The creative leaders in nursing, midwifery, and health visiting are already there: the risk-takers who have a clear long-term vision. They have the ability to bridge gaps between organisations and to realise a vision for nursing, as well as the communities they work with. A further and essential challenge for these nurses is to ensure that all nurses in their locality are both informed and engaged. Only then will local experiences and real health needs information be used to inform local planning and strategy. Then, at last, we can truly say that we have contributed in some part to improving the health of the local community: providing a public health voice within primary care.

DISCUSSION QUESTIONS

- How far have the new structures gone toward developing a truly comprehensive version of primary health care in your own area?
- Find out how each of the following groups can contribute to the health plan in your local area: community nurses, hospital-based nurses, midwives, voluntary organisations, housing officials. Who is your own immediate contact person?
- What is meant by 'leadership' in relation to serving on a PCG board, nursing forum or committee that contributes to the Health Improvement Programme?

FURTHER READING

Blanchard K & Johnson S 1996 The One Minute Manager. Harper Collins Business, London

Blanchard K, Oncken W, Burrows H 1994 The One Minute Manager meets the Monkey. Harper Collins Business, London.

Blanchard K, Zigarmi P, and Zigarmi O 1994 Leadership and the One Minute Manager. Harper Collins Business, London

Blanchard K, Carlos J, Randolph A 1998 Empowerment Takes More than a Minute. Berett-Koehler Publishers, San Francisco
'One minute' series, renowned for accessible and easy reading style. Full of useful tips for coping with the everyday demands placed on managers and leaders.

Dixon M & Sweeney K (eds) 2001 A Practical Guide to Primary Care Groups and Trusts. Radcliffe Medical Press, Oxford
A collection of bite-sized chunks of personal wisdom gained in the first year of operating primary care groups in England. Covers a wide range of practical 'implementation' issues, giving tips, checklists and resources.

Macdonald J 1992 Primary Health Care: Medicine in its Place. Earthscan Publications Ltd, London
Strong, but positive, critique that challenges the idea that medical practice should lead in primary health care.

Peckham S, Taylor P & Turton P 1998 Public Health Model of Primary Care: from concept to reality. Public Health Alliance, Birmingham

Largely completed before the recent policy changes, but full of useful explanations and practically-based ideas about incorporating a public health perspective into primary health care.

Senge P 1990 The Fifth Discipline: the art and practice of learning organisations. Doubleday, New York
Explains and unravels the issues involved in systems change.

REFERENCES

Andrews-Evans M 1997 The leadership challenge in nursing. Nursing Management 4(5):8–11

Argyris C 1985 Behaviour in organisations. In: Pugh D S (ed) 1990 Organisational Theory, 3rd edn. Penguin, London

Arora S, Davies A, Thompson S 1999 Developing Health Improvement Programmes – Lessons from the first year. King's Fund, London

Beecham L 1998 GPs have continuing concern over primary care groups. British Medical Journal 316:1481

Benner P 1984 From Novice to Expert. Addison-Wesley, Berkeley, California

Billingham K 1998 Getting in on the Act. Nursing Times 94(10):24

Collinson G 2000 Encouraging the growth of the nurse entrepreneur. Professional Nurse 15(6):365–367

Community Practitioners' and Health Visitors' Association and Office for Public Management 1999 Leading and Future. Published and edited by T G Scott, London

Department of Health 1997 The New NHS: Modern, dependable (Cmnd 3809). The Stationery Office, London

Department of Health 1999a Saving Lives: Our Healthier Nation (Cmnd 4386). The Stationery Office, London

Department of Health 1999b Making a Difference: a strategy for nursing, midwifery and health visiting. Department of Health, London

Department of Health 2000 The NHS Plan: a plan for investment; a plan for reform (Cmnd 4818). The Stationery Office, London

Kanter R M 1979 Power Failure in Management Circuits. In: Pugh D 1990 Organisational Theory, 3rd edn. Penguin, London

Lomax H & Wright J 1997 Community Health Practitioners: Their Public Health Role. Public Health Resources Unit, Oxford

Macdonald J 1992 Primary Health Care: Medicine in its place. Earthscan Publications Ltd, London

National Health Service Executive (NHSE) 1994 Developing NHS purchasing and GP fundholding: towards a primary care led NHS. EL (94)92. NHS Executive, London

Rafferty A M 1993 Leading Questions: A Discussion Paper on Nursing Leadership. King's Fund Centre, London

Sackman T 1999 Personal communication: Conversations at a Community Practitioners and Health Visitors' Association Training Day

Santry H & Clark J 1999 Primary Care Groups: Nurses on Board. Nursing Standard 14(5):34–39

Senge P 1990 The Fifth Discipline. Doubleday, New York

Shapiro J 1998 Fighting for a seat at the table. Health Service Journal 108(5623):20–21

Singer R 1998 Opportunity knocks. Community Practitioner 71(4):130

Steel J 1999 Primary care for the 21st century. Journal of Nursing Management 7:67–69

Walters S E 1999 Keep your eyes on the prize. Nursing Times 95(50):60–61

World Health Organization 1978 Primary Health Care: Report of the International Conference on Primary Health Care, Alma-Ata, USSR. WHO, Geneva

World Health Organization 1999 Health 21: Health for all in the 21st century. European Health for All series No. 6. WHO, Copenhagen

Young L & Antrobus S 1998 Strategic skills in primary care. Primary Health Care 8(5):6–8

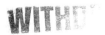

6 Profiling health needs

Jennifer Billings

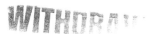

KEY ISSUES

- Profiling assists with the identification and prioritisation of health needs through the collection and comparison of health data within caseloads and communities. This helps practitioners to take part in decision-making processes about service provision, by enabling them to articulate public health priorities for proactive health promotion activity that can address inequalities in health.
- There is no standard health profiling procedure due to the variation in health data availability. It is recommended that a wide range of health data is aggregated, to counter the geographical and chronological anomalies that exist within different service and public sources. Seen as a complex, analytical process, profiling is best conducted within a multidisciplinary team or supported as a seconded project.
- Incorporating the consumer perspective is important, to counter the largely normatively defined, illness-focused statistical data. Care must be taken to avoid 'tokenism' and to ensure that views are representative of the wider community.
- Five stages to the profiling process are put forward:
  1. clarifying the purpose of profiling
  2. defining the boundaries
  3. getting support
  4. identifying, collecting and analysing the data
  5. developing and implementing strategies to meet need.
- Information technology is playing an increasing role in health needs profiling. A large range of information in now collected in acute, primary and commissioning settings, although coordination and retrieval of this data for profiling purposes is still problematic. Geographical software that permits the mapping of data is also becoming more accessible.

INTRODUCTION

In recent years community nurses have witnessed many changes to their working practices and organisational structures as a result of the implementation of successive government policies (Department of Health 1990, 1992, 1997, 1999). More recently, the representation of nurses on primary care groups and trusts has provided the opportunity for them to take part in the decision-making processes concerned with the identification of appropriate local services and Health Improvement Programmes (Department of Health 1997). For others, responding to these changes through new ways of working has provided opportunities for community nurses to expand and develop their roles.

This chapter seeks simply to assert the fundamental value of needs assessment, and to assist community nurses in redefining their position within public health care delivery. By providing a comprehensive review of approaches to needs assessment and profiling, it intends to equip community nurses with working models that may help them to provide the evidence needed to re-evaluate their work and prioritise their service.

There is considerable variation in approaches to assessing needs, depending on the professional, client and organisational requirements. Accordingly, there can be no universal prescription for health profiling, as methods must reflect the individual aims and function of the process. There have been several published accounts of profiling from a variety of community nursing and team perspectives, which have led to new strategies and/or innovative services. This chapter will therefore include examples of approaches to needs assessment used in the field from reported or published accounts. These examples will highlight methods of data collection, analysis, resulting service changes or strategies, and any strengths or weaknesses of the approaches. The purpose of this is to provide a variety of working models for use in practice.

There are certainly things to be learned from the practical application of profiling. Importantly, the overriding message appears to be that, to be successful, needs assessment and profiling requires commitment and support throughout the organisation. It is no longer viewed primarily as a task allocated to individual community nurses, but as a team activity, ideally undertaken in liaison with commissioners and purchasers. Increasingly, specialist roles are recruited for the purpose of facilitating and developing needs-assessment proforma, in recognition of its complexity. But this ideal is not attainable for many practitioners, so the examples offered here may provide a means to initiate discussion with colleagues, managers and others involved in health care provision.

The chapter begins by explaining the main terms involved, before reviewing the relevance of profiling to current community nursing practice, and evaluating its use above other forms of needs assessment. The consumer perspective is also examined and described. This is followed by a more detailed explanation of profiling, including a summary of its main strengths and weaknesses, and by an account of the process of profiling. This incorporates data-source identification, the teamwork approach, and a review of previous research on the subject. Examples of profiling in practice will include community, general practice and caseload profiles, as well as uni-professional and team approaches.

CLARIFICATION OF THE TERMS

Need

Need is a complex and contentious term to define, and open to differing interpretation. Within the context of needs assessment, the focus is generally thought to be the client, but in reality there are often political, professional and lay conflicts between the needs of various people involved. For example, profiling exercises often reveal resource deficits and training needs, which must be

BOX 6.1   *Definitions of 'need' (Bradshaw 1972)*

- Normative needs are those defined by professionals or experts according to their own standards.
- Felt needs are those perceived by an individual or a community.
- Expressed needs are felt needs that have progressed to a demand.
- Comparative needs are identified when a community sees that it lacks services/resources which another area has.

addressed before the health needs of the population can be tackled. As it is not within the remit of this chapter to provide a comprehensive discussion of the issues, readers are referred to texts published elsewhere (see Appleton & Cowley 2000). For the purposes of clarification, Bradshaw's (1972) interpretation of need will be used (Box 6.1). His taxonomy of normative, felt, expressed and comparative need remain relevant to those delivering and receiving health care.

Health needs assessment

This is a broad term concerned with a description of those factors which must be addressed in order to improve the health of the population. This definition allows for the delineation of the range of factors which make up the concept of need.

Health profiling

The health profile is a method by which needs are assessed. It has been identified in its widest sense as:

'The systematic collection of data to identify the health needs of a defined population, and the analysis of that data to assess and prioritise strategies in health promotion.' (Twinn et al 1990 p 2)

Health profiles use mainly quantitative health data, such as statistical information, but qualitative health data, such as individual assessments and client perceptions, can also be incorporated to form a more holistic picture. They are snapshots of the health of a given population at any one time, and should be updated annually to monitor health trends. Increasingly, profiling is seen as an interprofessional or multiagency venture, capitalising on existing skills, resources and information.

Three levels of profiling will be described: community, practice and caseload profiling. Some debate has taken place over the terms 'community' and 'caseload', and this has impeded agreement over meaningful definitions. However, the aim here is to provide basic clarification only, and to give further illustrations of these profiling approaches through the examples provided throughout the text.

- Community profiles refer to the assessment of need within a neighbourhood, district or town.
- Practice profiles refer to the collection of health data and assessment of need within the general practice population: that is, those clients who are registered with a practice.
- Caseload profiles refer to the assessment of need within the community nurse's caseload: in this instance, those clients and/or families for whom the community nurse has a designated responsibility.

These levels of profiling are not separate from each other. Community profiles, for example, may include general practice and caseload information. Practice profiles will need some community-wide information for comparison purposes. Compiling a profile should be seen as an important first step towards developing a programme of health care based on the needs of the population. It has the potential to provide the information to assist interagency collaboration and community participation.

THE RELEVANCE OF NEEDS ASSESSMENT AND PROFILING

Needs assessment has always been relevant to community nurses, for whom an assessment of individual, family and community is fundamental to ensuring that the health needs of the most vulnerable sections of society are met, and matched to the appropriate services (Cowley & Appleton 2000). The Council for the Education and Training of Health Visitors (1977) has specified that the search for health needs and a stimulation of their awareness were to be principle objectives within health visiting practice. Considering the challenges faced by today's practitioners, including social deprivation and poverty, inequalities in health and the growing morbidity from heart disease and AIDS; these principles are as relevant today as they were for community nurses in the 1970s (Acheson 1998).

From a broader, more pro-active perspective, profiling in health visiting can be viewed not only as the mechanism to assist with prioritising work with clients, but also as the means for all community nurses to influence local policy and policy-makers, and private sector and independent organisations (Carey 1999). Building alliances with people who are in a position to tackle environmental, social and economic factors may have an impact on local people's health and well-being.

Needs assessment is clearly recognised as important within government health policy, and policies stress that all decisions about health care should be based on an assessment of needs. Without doubt, the contract culture between purchasers and providers engendered by the 1990 NHS and Community Care Act provided further impetus for community nurses to look more closely at how they can articulate the value of their work. In the current climate, this momentum continues with the recognition of the part community nurses can play, in working through primary care groups to determine service requirement, to address public health concerns such as inequalities in health (Lock 1999). Hence, needs assessment and profiling continue to be a vital tools for providing the evidence upon which to plan public health practice.

APPROACHES TO NEEDS ASSESSMENT

Epidemiological perspective

The epidemiological perspective is the approach most used in public health departments. This defines need in terms of lives lost, morbidity, and loss of social functioning. So, for example, collection of data primarily concerned with birth, morbidity and mortality rates is required to assess the fertility of a population and the level of ill-health present. By providing standardised measures such as average birth and death rates and standard mortality, incidence of death and disease can be compared across the country. However, Chase and Davies (1991) observe that such statistics lose their impact in assessing a population's health when used in isolation. They state that this is particularly so when the death rates are low, as by implication the majority of the population remain alive in various states of health. Epidemiological information from public health can provide a comprehensive picture of health need for some populations, but is unable to provide information about the stresses of everyday life which may lead to illness. This 'normative', professionally-defined information is therefore restrictive to nurses in the community who deal with less morbid clientele, or people who may become ill in the future. In addition, health need from an epidemiological perspective is constructed within a medical model, with the focus being on disease. Lightfoot (1995) raises questions about the definition of health within this context, which appears to contradict the increasing importance attached to primary health care at both national and international policy levels (World Health Organization 1985, Department of Health 1997).

Indicators of deprivation are also used, based on census data. Variables such as numbers of single parents, ethnicity and elderly people living alone are measured, combining social and material deprivation into a composite score. This provides a valuable means of ranking geographical areas, such as electoral wards, according to their disadvantage or affluence. Jarman's (1984) score to determine underprivilege is the system most widely used to compare areas. However, there are some problems in validating deprivation measures. For example, Jarman's underprivilege score has been criticised for its bias towards elderly people. Other authors have pointed out that the scores may hide deprivation within electoral wards. For example, a small disadvantaged council estate within a larger affluent area would not be detected by the Jarman score (Chase & Davies 1991). There are also contradictions between different deprivation scores. Jarman, for example, asserted that the most deprived local authorities were in London, with none in the north, while Townsend and his colleagues suggest the opposite (Townsend et al 1985). These problems may be overcome by choosing only indicators of material deprivation such as the proportion of households with no car, or unemployment rates, and by incorporating other methods such as 'grass root' surveys and practitioner caseload information to check statistical results (Hawtin et al 1994).

A further major problem with the epidemiological perspective is the potential of this approach to stereotype groups of people as 'in need' when this may not necessarily be the case (Stalker 1993). This point is of particular importance to community nurses; for example there is much evidence in the academic literature testifying to the hardship endured by low-income groups, especially lone parents (Billings 2000). However, as indicated by Cowley and Billings' (1997) health needs research, what may be perceived to be a challenging environment by professionals may not be viewed as such in the context of the lived experience of the client. This highlights the relevance of client-centred approaches to needs assessment and practice intervention. Despite this caution, while restricted in their ability to assess need in isolation, epidemiological data are an important ingredient in any profile.

Health economist perspective

The health economist perspective defines need in the context of effectiveness, supply and demand. The main thrust of this approach is that areas of need are relative and, in the context of limited resources, can be 'traded off' against each other (Donaldson & Mooney 1991). The health of the community can be defined in terms of quality adjusted life years (QALYs); authors argue that more resources should be allocated to treatments with marginal cost per QALY, and fewer resources to more expensive treatment. An example would be to expand a chiropody service and reduce dialysis, as more QALYs could be produced with less expenditure (Bryan et al 1991). In a study of school-leavers with significant educational needs, Thomson and Ward (1994) evaluated QALYs as a useful method of considering value-added benefit in provision to people with disabilities. Although this viewpoint may rationalise service provision, and is popular within political circles, it has been strongly criticised for its unethical stance in relation to the quality of life in illness (Smith 1995), and runs counter to the philosophy of a consumer-oriented service.

Rapid appraisal

The aim of this approach to needs assessment is to gain some insight into a community's own perspective of its main needs, in order to translate these findings into action. Furthermore, one purpose is to set up a continuing relationship between those commissioning services, professionals delivering the service and local communities (Murray et al 1994). The framework is based on the World Health Organization's 'Health For All' philosophy, with the focus on deprived areas. Need is defined within the context of inequalities of health: those living in relatively disadvantaged areas having greater need. The approach has often been referred to as 'participatory' appraisal, as its central source is the community itself. 'Rapid' refers to its ability to be conducted in two weeks, but only if outside researchers are used.

Information is collected on nine issues, in an 'information pyramid' (Figure 6.1). The bottom layer defines the structure and composition of community, how it is organised, and its capacity to act. The second layer is concerned with the socioeconomic factors which influence health. The next layer looks at the resources in the community, their accessibility and acceptability. The effectiveness of current services can be evaluated to identify what improvements need to be made. The top layer is concerned with national, regional and local health policies. In particular, information is sought as to the commitment of the political leadership to community participation in health. Data are collected on three areas: existing written records about the neighbourhood; interviews with a

| FIGURE 6.1 | *Rapid appraisal information pyramid (Murray et al 1994).* |

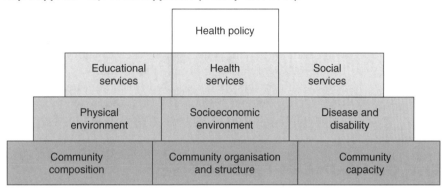

range of informants; and observations made in the neighbourhood or in the homes of interviewees. An example of this approach is provided in the case study below.

CASE STUDY 1

Community health profiling by Murray et al (1994).

Method

The project was carried out in Edinburgh, on a council estate of 670 homes. The team consisted of a GP and health visitor from one general practice, a community educationalist, and two social workers. The study was conducted over three months, with members of the team giving about four hours each week to the project. A part-time secretary was also recruited. A semi-structured interview schedule was developed with the assistance of World Health Organization training material. Key informants included people with professional knowledge of the community, community leaders, shopkeepers, voluntary workers, transport officials and youth groups: a total of 24 individuals and four groups of interviewees. In addition, 17 residents were selected. Interviews were conducted by two team members: one interviewing and one taking notes. Data were allotted to the blocks of the planning pyramid, and interview data were separated into ten separate areas and allocated to each file. Census data were also included. Feedback meetings were arranged with the informants to present and validate the findings.

Strengths

This approach helps to identify strength of feeling in the community about key issues; enables GPs to respond to the immediate needs of their clients; offers a practical way of involving local people in making decisions about their health service.

Weaknesses

Involves considerable time and commitment from team members.

How it was used

Examples include re-routing of buses through the estate; new mental health group; information courses for home helps to inform elderly people of local services; provision of toys for the waiting area in the practice; collection facility for repeat prescriptions.

More recently, the rapid participatory appraisal method has been used to assess young people's sexual health needs and was felt to be useful in the identification of achievable health targets in this area of need (Lawlor et al 1999). In general though, difficulties with this approach are centred around identifying clearly what sorts of data to collect within each category, which can be a lengthy procedure. Also, obtaining a sample representative of the population causes problems, as informants are not selected at random. Instead, they are chosen because they are thought to be in the best position to understand the issues in the community. Getting the 'consumer view' is outlined more fully below.

THE CONSUMER PERSPECTIVE

The rapid appraisal method highlights how client views can be incorporated into the needs assessment process. Increasingly, community nurses are becoming involved in this process, or are working with the results of surveys conducted in their areas. However, this process is not straightforward. There are strengths and weaknesses, and it is important to be able to review approaches to these surveys critically, in order to evaluate first their potential contribution to the overall picture of health needs, and secondly the extent to which results can influence strategy. This section of the chapter will provide an overview of this approach and critically review methods to obtaining the consumer perspective as well as combining data into local policy.

Overview

Public consultation to obtain the consumer viewpoint appears to be a feature of needs assessment that is attracting considerable interest, both within the population and among professionals (Lawlor et al 1999). It offers an opportunity for the community to make its needs known and, theoretically, ensure that these needs are adequately addressed within plans. For example, Clark (1997) ensured the views of users and carers living in a rural community were secured and considered in a joint planning exercise. The outcomes of this study revealed the considerable geographical and cultural difficulties in service provision that were heard by health care planners. The community profile has been accused of being limited in its ability to provide a picture of health needs because it is restricted to the collection of existing information from a service point of view (Peckham & Spanton 1994). The current wave of interest in client opinion has not come from a sudden development of socially-conscious managers. Phillips et al (1994) state that the government's policy of controlling public expenditure and encouraging a mixed economy of care has introduced a strong element of enterprise culture into public service organisations. Central policy thus demands greater choice and independence for service users.

Approaches to consultation

Reviewing the various approaches to consultation, Cooper et al (1995) highlight several ways in which this can be achieved: client feedback via forums, public meetings, and consumer representation on user groups. Local interviews, postal or telephone surveys of views and satisfaction surveys have been used also (Roberts & Magowan 1994). The use of focus groups has also been put forward as a valuable method of exploring perceptions of need, and has proved enlightening when used in this context (Cowley et al 1996). Consultation is not without its difficulties, however. Focus groups, for example, are generally characterised by small numbers, which raises questions about the reliability of the results. To overcome this problem, some studies have used a combination of techniques to obtain an improved picture; Munday's (1996) research, which describes a peer research approach to needs assessment among young people, is a case in point.

Satisfaction surveys are a common method of obtaining consumer views. As with all questionnaires, they are able to target a wide population and are seen as more cost-effective (Robson 1993). However, the constraints of satisfaction surveys in the health care setting have long been recognised, not only with regard to poor response rates, especially from disadvantaged and disabled people, but in relation to how the questions are designed (Avis 1994). In reviewing the evidence, Avis states that people are notoriously reluctant to criticise their health care, due in part to lack of comparative health care experiences and deference to health care workers. The use of 'global' questions (e.g. 'In general, how do you rate the service?') and leading questions (e.g. 'Are you happy with this service?') urge the consumer to reply positively. This does not assist in service improvement, and allows organisations to presume that all is well (Avis 1994). Using more face-to-face methods may overcome these obstacles.

A weakness common to all approaches to consultation concerns reliability of sample selection. Rodgers (1994) suggests that, where researchers do not strive to gain equity of response, there will be a tendency for the more articulate, less-burdened consumer's voice to be heard loudest. Consultation, therefore, has the potential to reinforce inequalities in service provision, rather than address them. This was also found by Clark's (1997) research with rural communities, where geographical barriers further confounded access to user involvement.

Combining the data

Once data from the consumer have been compiled by a chosen method, consideration must be given to their synthesis, with broader health information, into local policy. In an analysis of community plans, Richards (1991) noted that, while most of them emphasised the importance of aggregation of data, few practical proposals for achieving it were made. This becomes increasingly significant when considering the depth of information obtained by community nurses through individual needs assessment. Incorporating such information into meaningful policy statements can be onerous. For example, unless the total population within an area can be targeted, bias may be an inevitable consequence and 'felt' need never fully identified (Lightfoot 1995). However, focusing on small groups within a locality, such as carers or families of physically challenged children, may converge areas of need in a more meaningful way (Richards 1991). The section on 'analysing data' gives further ideas about how such information can be aggregated.

Wistow et al (1992) suggest that public consultation may be nothing more than 'tokenism' in some areas. In their analysis of 22 English community care plans they discovered that, where consultation had been employed, methods differed considerably across regions. The extent to which the results of the exercises had influenced the completed strategy documents was far from clear. Respondents in a study reported by Cowley et al (1996) were not convinced that their views were respected, both at an individual level and as part of a service-planning exercise.

The role of the community nurse as advocate in this context is clear. By influencing or taking part in the development of satisfaction surveys, or ensuring representative participation in consultation procedures in their trusts, community nurses can do much to enable the views of their clients to be represented as fully as possible. An example of obtaining the consumer perspective in practice is given below.

CASE STUDY 2

Community health profiling reported by Craig (1996).

The Kendoon community health profile was carried out in Drumchapel, Glasgow and used a community development process to increase residents' participation in community health activities, and gather local perceptions of health. It was initiated by fieldworkers in response to the need for a more community-led agenda in the area.

Method

A profile group was formed consisting of seven local residents, seven workers from Glasgow Healthy City Project, and representatives from health promotion, health visiting, the local volunteer centre, community work, housing and an addictions project. This group was responsible for planning and executing the process. The residents included representatives from tenants, groups, active community members and volunteers. Data from residents of Kendoon were gathered by structured interviews, using a questionnaire developed by the profile team. Most interviews were carried out by the community members of the groups, and a response-rate of 97% was achieved. In the analysis, the epidemiological and demographic profiles of Drumchapel were noted, but the health profile focused on the real-life experiences of health and illness of around 100 residents and their families.

Strengths

Involvement and participation by the community; used a range of expertise; identified real health concerns in the local population.

Weaknesses

Found to be lengthy and time-consuming, requiring considerable commitment; difficulties persuading the relevant organisations to respond to the recommendations; difficulties in accessing funds; community health needs not seen as a priority for health and social services funding; methods criticised for not being sufficiently representative of the population.

How the profile was used

Production of a video to highlight issues in Drumchapel to local residents and policy makers, and for training purposes; a community health library; research and campaigning on children's play areas and street safety; a women's health network; counselling and complementary therapies; a range of self-help and support groups; initiation of a project (now called 'Drumming Up Health') which included the secondment of a health promotion officer and a health visitor. Recommendations used for health promotion activities and to increase access and responsiveness of local health services.

PROFILING HEALTH NEEDS

Although the methods of needs assessment mentioned above help us to identify and interpret some areas of health need, it is the profiling approach that allows their collective value to become evident. The framework offered by the profile with its multiple data sources allows a comprehensive picture of health needs to emerge. Although a consumer perspective cannot always be obtained by community nurses, the profile has the ability to emphasise the unique contribution practitioners can make to this knowledge. This is by the accumulation of 'soft' data relating to families, so adding to and enhancing statistical information (Cowley & Appleton 2000). 'Soft' data are also useful to identify the range of need within the context of Bradshaw's (1972) taxonomy.

The strengths and weaknesses of the profile

In some areas, needs assessment and profiling have become an integrated part of the community nursing service as the Case Studies indicate. Boxes 6.2 and 6.3 summarise the main strengths and weaknesses of profiling.

BOX 6.2	*Strengths of profiling*

- Identifies and prioritises community, practice, group, family and individual need
- Identifies population, group and individual characteristics and trends
- Identifies areas for research and development, and staff training
- Identifies and corrects gaps between needs and service delivery
- Sets targets for health promotion and illness prevention
- Provides evidence with which to justify additional resources such as health promotion programmes
- Provides a method by which the public can become involved in decisions about healthcare. Provides information for primary care groups/trusts, NHS trusts, workers and users of the services, to assist in making informed choices about health
- Provides information with which to determine the direction of community nursing services and the setting of aims and objectives
- Provides a method of improving partnerships within and between disciplines/teams, agencies and clients
- Annual compilation and measurement helps to assess and evaluate health interventions for health and health promotion activity

BOX 6.3	*Weaknesses of profiling*

- Data collection and analysis for profiling is time-consuming, and requires commitment and skill
- Data sources are sometimes difficult to locate, and information may not be reliable
- Profiling may be competing with other types of data-gathering procedures within trusts, and its value may be lost
- Social needs may be revealed that cannot be fully acted on or resolved easily (such as poverty and housing problems)
- Strategies resulting from the profile may not be compatible with trust strategies, primary care group or health authority requirements
- Lack of managerial or commissioning support may prevent professionals from changing practice in response to profile results
- There are ethical problems associated with the gathering of personal data from people who may not benefit from new services
- Loss of confidentiality for clients is a risk if data are collated in a format that can be traced back through, for example, individual computer identification numbers or post-code data
- Profilers are often unable to include the consumer perspective, which is a challenging task
- As profiling methods vary across the country, cross-comparison of need in a meaningful way is often not possible

Despite the many advantages of profiling, the weaknesses inject a note of realism to the process. The difficulties of matching need with resources have long been recognised. Goodwin (1995) has noted the potential for the profile to cause frustrations and disillusionment for both provider and recipient, raising concerns about professional accountability where needs cannot be met. Cernik and Wearne (1992) suggest that, unless all primary health care workers are prepared to change their attitudes to working practices, the profiling exercise will have been a waste of time. As shown in Box 6.3, consideration of the ethical issues involved in obtaining information about a community from both statutory and informal sources appears to be largely absent from the literature (Cowley & Billings 1997). This 'invasion of privacy' increases in significance if a large percentage of the population from which data is being obtained will not benefit from any service provision. Coupled with this, the often-perceived unequal relationship between professionals and those receiving care may mean that clients are placed in compromising situations when revealing personal details for the purposes of a profile. A balance must be achieved between a desire to locate and provide for unexpressed needs and the right of citizens to maintain their privacy.

As Box 6.2 demonstrates, however, the profile has potential marketing value by revealing working patterns, effectiveness and outcomes, at a time when clinical effectiveness is high on the NHS agenda. Information from profiles allows practitioners to reflect on practice and to be pro-active in making improvements (Billings 1996). Further, use of profiles to justify action accords with the quest for evidence-based practice. In addition, Carey (1999) stresses that profiles provide a positive opportunity for community nurses to influence decision-making at the primary care group level. It is important to acknowledge the shortcomings of this approach, but the range of examples in this document demonstrates that profiling can be helpful in many cases.

CASE STUDY

Community heath profiling researched by Donnolley and Shepherd (1996).

The Bristol Community Health Profiling Project was launched in 1993, as a joint health authority, FHSA and trust initiative. It involved the identification, collection, collation and reporting of health-related information from the area served by the United Bristol Healthcare Trust.

Method

Quantitative information about the demographics and epidemiology of the area was supplied by the health and local authorities. Qualitative information about resources and deficits came from the health professionals working in the communities. Health visitors were chosen to coordinate the process, as it was felt that they provided their own valuable perspective on local needs. The whole project was collated into a standard format by a health visitor seconded to the public health department. The 1991 census data were processed using general practice lists as the basic unit. The core area served by each practice was identified, and the practices were merged into neighbourhoods. Census data were broken down into districts, and census profiles of the neighbourhoods were built-up. This was supplemented by further information from health visitors about the health needs of the community, service deficiencies, and constraints on service delivery, using caseload information and knowledge of the area.

Strengths

This study recognised the restrictive nature of epidemiological information when used in isolation. By collecting qualitative information from those people who work most closely with service users, such as GPs and community nurses, it was possible to get a more complete picture of local health needs. It was also successful in combining the skills of healthcare workers on both sides of the commissioning and providing interface, and demonstrated the importance of cooperation in needs assessment.

Weaknesses

There were considerable overlaps between neighbourhoods and difficulties in matching the data. Presence of branch surgeries tended to distort the core area served, as did single-handed practices (which tended to serve large areas), and a village situated some distance from its service base.

How it was used

Publication of the full profiles was achieved about two and a half years after the beginning of the project. The profiles have been used as a resource for health service commissioning and provision of services.

THE PROCESS OF PROFILING

As previously indicated, evidence from published and reported sources shows that there is variation in how, where and why profiles are compiled and what data are used. This will depend on many factors such as who is doing the profiling, what data is easily available, and how the process is funded, and these factors may influence its perspective. For this reason there cannot be a prescriptive model for the process of profiling. The intention here is to provide an overview and examples of what happens in practice. For those community nurses unfamiliar with profiling, the following outline of the main stages may help. Many of the points are illustrated in the examples provided.

Stage one: clarifying the purpose

Embarking on a profile requires commitment and enthusiasm. It is essential to have clear aims and a sense of direction before starting, so that energy is not wasted. Questions need to be asked about why the profile is being undertaken, and how the results will be used.

Stage two: defining the boundaries

It is important to be clear about the area being profiled (e.g. town, electoral ward, practice or caseload), as this will help to focus the data-collection process and keep it relevant. With caseload or practice populations which are widely spread, it may be helpful to plot random samples of clients on maps to identify 'clusters' in each electoral ward. This will be useful when using ward-based information such as census data. Such information will be more applicable to the client population when numbers are high.

Stage three: getting support

From a nursing perspective, whether profiling in isolation or with a team, it is vital to get support and agreement from nurse managers, primary care groups and health authorities. This may include negotiating allocated time and resources such as information technology and local expertise. Getting support will also help with accessing data and avoiding duplication and may facilitate implementation of the resulting strategies.

Stage four: identifying, collecting and analysing data

These issues are further elaborated later, but it is important to collect data that are relatively easy to access and relevant to the aims and objectives of the profile, in order to avoid wasting time and becoming frustrated. Fruin (1978) suggests that data should be collectable, correct, complete, comparable and concise. It is also helpful to note where and from whom the data were obtained;

this will help with the annual up-dating of profiles. Identifying computer expertise in stage three will also be useful for analysing data.

Stage five: developing and implementing strategies to meet need

Having analysed the data, a range of health needs that are amenable to health promotion work will become evident. These may range from the development of a new service, such as community development work, to increasing the scope of an existing service, such as a clinic, or simply justifying the maintenance of an existing service, such as an opportunity play group for children whose parents do not speak English as a first language. Prioritising potential projects will depend on many factors. There will be competition between politically-set health targets, client/professional preferences, organisational requirements and, most critically, available resources. There is no easy solution, but gaining support prior to profiling and making effective use of the evidence collected through profiling will act as powerful levers. The following points may help the profiler win recognition for their work:

- Projects should be outlined in a written report stating aims and objectives, duration of project, and how it will be evaluated. The profile data should be used to justify your proposals.
- Projects also need to be costed, including staff time, resources such as photocopying and video, hiring a room, drinks/food and so forth. Help may be forthcoming from your NHS trust to cover the expenses.
- Find out what other local statutory, voluntary and community organisations are doing in health promotion. You may be able to link with existing projects and share the costs and resources.
- Take your ideas to the public and colleagues, to trust managers and other services providers (social services, for example) to find out their priorities. Public consultation could take the form of displays at clinics or surgeries, press coverage in local papers, or meetings with local community groups. Presenting ideas to colleagues at staff meetings will provide useful feedback. More formal presentations to primary care groups should also be considered.

IDENTIFYING DATA SOURCES

Identifying information that will help community nurses to profile their areas or caseloads is described within the literature. Most authors appear to agree that the data required will depend on the particular focus of the profiler and the special features of the locality. For example, a poverty profile as outlined by Blackburn (1992) may be appropriate for practitioners working in deprived areas. Also, as data collection progresses areas of relevance warranting more detailed attention may emerge. Guidance also varies on the kinds of information which should be collected. Hawtin et al (1994), for example, describe an extensive collection of data relating to housing, environment, health and resources, including a survey of the community. They suggest that this information be obtained from published sources such as census material, interviews and questionnaires in the community, 'streetwork', or casual observation, thereby combining quantitative with qualitative approaches. Their guidance about the practical application and measurement of these components is equally extensive, but may be more useful for practitioners without full caseload responsibilities.

Equally comprehensive suggestions for the content of a community health profile appear to be offered by Luker and Orr (1992). These are given from a health visiting perspective, but are pertinent to all community nurses. Twelve topics are selected, ranging from organisations and power and leadership information to health status of the community and health action potential. The authors say they have drawn on knowledge from sociology, psychology, epidemiology and social policy for this selection. They also suggest a range of local informal and formal sources of data (housing, social service and voluntary departments), and official sources such as census data. Despite this extensive range of components, specific guidance on how to actually interpret the criteria is limited, making evident the skill involved in completing a profile.

The practitioner choosing this approach should be selective, and not over-ambitious. Other measures such as the health profile (Twinn et al 1990), a school health profile (Health Visitors' Association 1991) and the GP practice profile (Royal College of Nursing 1993), are abridged versions of the above, but with different perspectives. Care must be taken, however, when collecting data, as the profiler can become overwhelmed with them. Maintaining a focus upon distinct aims and objectives for the project may help. Conversely, data may be difficult to obtain, due to difficulties with accessing key individuals in organisations for example. Godden and Pollock (1997) also state that the increase in private health care provision means that there is a loss of data on the population and this must be acknowledged.

Regarding the caseload profile, the components suggested by health visitors in Cowley and Billings (1997, 1999) action research project included information about the size of the household, number of children, single parents, families with disabled persons, and types of social support. In addition, the numbers of families assessed as having multi-focal problems and children at risk were also documented. This project formed part of a larger study concerned with family health needs assessment. The work undertaken with health visitors is elaborated upon in the following case study.

CASE STUDY 3   This was part of a larger project concerned with family health needs assessment conducted between 1994 and 1996 in Hastings and St Leonards (Cowley & Billings 1997).

Method

A group of health visitors was formed to work with the project researchers. Work began by brainstorming ideas. The challenge was to identify data relevant to community nurses, purchasers and commissioners, to provide a picture of health visiting work, and information with which to prioritise work. Development took place over six months within an action research cycle of planning, testing, evaluating/reflecting and planning, and a schedule was agreed. It was clear that the schedule had developed in a way that allowed it to replace existing birth books. This had the added bonus of reducing the amount of paperwork. The schedule was widely circulated for comment, and some modifications made. Headings included personal details (name, address, age of mother, other siblings); status (married/employed), housing; other local classifications concerning vulnerable families, feeding details (including weaning), accident rates, date and outcome of assessments, and an immunisation record. There were two further sections to collect coded data about a range of child and family-health issues, and to record basic outcomes. An analysis sheet to count and record yearly numbers was also constructed. Training sessions are now under way. A health visitor in each locality from the initial group is available if individual implementation problems arise. Information presentations to purchasers and commissioners have also taken place. The tool and guidelines will be re-evaluated after one year of use.

Strengths

This method has allowed the development of a professionally owned measure that has wide-ranging, detailed, continuing relevance for those involved with needs assessment. Such a method will also allow cross-case comparison.

Weaknesses: Time commitments were often problematic. Developing guidelines with shared meanings was difficult, and reflected the subjective nature of health visiting. This requires further evaluation.

Further developments: This process has been completed with other groups of community nurses: namely, practice nurses, community midwives, community psychiatric nurses, district nurses and school nurses.

Drennan (1990) suggests components for analysing district nursing caseloads which are described in the following case study.

CASE STUDY 4

This project was initiated in Islington health authority to investigate the information needs of managers and practitioners (Drennan 1990). It was prompted by the decentralisation of community nursing services in the area, and the need to make decisions about staff resource allocation. The purpose of the project was to look at information needed to examine district nursing workloads, to determine a method of comparing them, and to establish a system which could readily be used by practitioners.

Method

A working group of managers and practitioners was set up, supported by a professional development officer. Brainstorming sessions were held alongside literature searches, which culminated in the drafting of detailed forms for the collection of data. Information included the total number of patients; characteristics of clients (e.g. age, gender, ethnicity, housing, financial difficulties); relationship to nursing services (e.g. dependency level on nurses and carers, frequency of contact, type of nursing activity, length of time on books); discharges and admissions over a three-month period; reductions in nursing care over the previous three months; staff in the nursing team; clinics; other work roles; geographical aspects of areas that cause stress; neighbourhood areas covered; any other factors that added to the workload. The profile was completed for every district nurse team seven months after the initial sessions, each profile taking about half a day to complete. The profiles have provided information about the demography of the area, nursing practice, access to and use of the service and concerns of practitioners.

Strengths

The data have produced tangible evidence to support the perceptions of field staff and managers, and have provided a means to raise questions about service provision, nursing practice, relationships with other agencies and future developments.

Weaknesses

Not all teams were able to complete their profiles promptly, due to unfamiliarity of the exercise, time commitments and constant interruptions.

How the profiles were used

The information prompted further investigation and research concerning leg-ulcer treatment and help with hygiene, and practice policy has been developed as a result. Information from caseloads is given to new staff. The profiles were used to develop a weighting system. They also acted as a catalyst for a range of work undertaken in the community unit.

It must be stated that the amount and quality of the data that can be obtained from caseload notes will vary between practitioners. Also, with some areas currently adopting client-held or parent-held health records, retrospective analysis of data may be made difficult by limited access to information.

RESEARCHING THE PROCESS OF PROFILING

The process of profiling has itself been a subject of investigation, particularly with respect to data collection for community profiles in the context of the NHS reforms. The next case study describes such an investigation, looking at sources of data and issues relating to the accessibility of the data and its usefulness to community nursing (Billings 1996). This study also highlights the overwhelming and contradictory tendency for 'health' data to be focused on disease, with positive indicators of health, other than screening uptake, less easy to identify at community level.

CASE STUDY 5

Method

A community and GP practice profile were compiled to identify family health needs for service development. This project provided the opportunity to isolate local and national data sources, and to examine data in relation to access, relevance to health needs identification, and reliability and validity (Billings 1996). Luker and Orr's (1992) framework provided initial guidance to data collection, and local data were obtained through networking with a range of statutory and voluntary agencies. Data that were difficult to access, irrelevant or invalid/unreliable were not incorporated into the profile.

Findings

The local health authority information unit, family health services authority (pre-merger) and public health department proved to be useful and easily accessible sources of epidemiological data, including Jarman scores (although not available in post-coded areas) and service use. Several health surveys and service reviews were also available. Local authority departments also provided a wealth of local information on census data, accident figures, and housing. Information was less forthcoming from hospital trusts, more difficult to access, potentially costly and largely invalid. GP practice information was problematic to access because of the recent installation of new computer software. Differences in coding of health information between practice staff led to concerns about the validity of the data, but practitioner caseloads held a rich source of concurrent health and social data about the practice population. Information which could not be obtained despite attempts included DSS benefits uptake, population-wide morbidity, and voluntary sector data; the latter due to lack of databases. There were also difficulties obtaining data relating to positive health from a community perspective, although this was more evident in health visiting caseloads (e.g. social support). Other findings that rendered identification of GP practice health needs difficult included: large geographical differences between data (e.g. census data is available per electoral ward, mortality data per health authority, practice population per town); significant chronological differences between data (e.g. census 1991, mortality 1992, practitioner caseload 1994); lack of comparative data between GP practice and health authority (e.g. no mortality statistics available at the practice).

ANALYSING THE DATA

If the profile is to have any influence on professional practice, the multiple sources of data require careful interpretation. There is very little clear guidance in the literature to undertake this analysis, and this would appear to be the weak spot of profiling. The task is made more difficult by the issues raised by Billings (1996) concerning the geographical and chronological differences between health data. Thomas (1997) states that, when carrying out data analysis and interpreting findings, it is important to consider possible sources of bias, and undue prominence should not be given to problems which confirm beliefs and values. She also emphasises the importance of gathering a wide range of data to assist in recognising different perspectives and agendas. The analysis of data will be facilitated by developing caseload profiling measures such as those previously described. A simple number-crunching process will enable some comparative description of trends in caseloads to be seen.

Billings (1995) has investigated ways of analysing a range of profile data and has developed a method from Yin's (1994) case-study design. The general strategy was to develop a case description through matching themes identified within each piece of data, and building patterns. For example, a columned schedule was drawn up and, taking each data source in turn, the predominant themes were entered in the columns. This process enabled sources to be cross-referenced for similarities or patterns and trends, which allowed the data to explain the health situation in the community, and its impact upon individual families. The data were also mapped, which facilitated visual pattern-matching.

This method has been useful in making sense of multiple data sources and in the identification of broad indicators of need. However, the process was complex and time-consuming and conducted largely without the assistance of computer software. Geographical mapping programmes are now available in some areas (health authorities and universities), which could prove useful in the analytical process. There a general need for further research in this area to generate a more manageable data-analysis processes for practitioner use.

TEAMWORK AND PROFILING

The important relationship between teamwork and profiling is increasingly acknowledged (Billingham 1995, Lock 1999). Profiling can be conducted in teams for the mutual sharing of data collection and analysis, in recognition of the time and commitment difficulties facing practitioners who profile in isolation. This can also demonstrate a more rational use of community nursing time, which is important when identifying and prioritising strategies for service delivery.

Profiling can also be used as a central feature of developing primary health care teams (Cook 1996). The aims here are to gain an appreciation of the different roles of team members and to build a coordinated, flexible and more efficient service, based on identified health needs.

The need to develop methods of practice profiling has been conclusively argued by Billingham (1995), in response to the growing responsibilities and involvement in needs assessment of all members of the primary health care team. This method recognises the importance of devising a tailor-made tool through a team approach, using local sources of data. Through facilitation via the Premier Health NHS Trust primary care development unit (PCDU) and the former Family Health Services Authority (FHSA), the process started with a multidisciplinary group of GPs, health visitors, managers, district nurses and practice nurses. A tool was developed for the entire team which fitted with existing information systems, such as health promotion banding and child health, while being relatively simple and not too time-consuming. It drew together information that would inform the team of the health status of the practice population, uptake of preventive services, and factors influencing population health. The process was designed to ensure maximum ownership and commitment by all the project members.

All the practices introducing the method had workshops organised for them by the PCDU. Flexibility was important, however, as teams had variable experience with and knowledge of profiling. Thus, support programmes were designed to suit the needs of each primary health care team. The PCDU also provided public health information, research reviews, and advice to individuals and teams.

This method has shown itself to be a useful method for practice profiling, with strengths including devising a public health perspective in primary care, a focusing on the needs of the practice population, and enhanced communication between team members. However, drawbacks include the difficulties of developing a pro-active view of health when reactive practice can become the norm; the inability to obtain the consumer perspective; the flexibility of profiling tools making comparisons difficult, and the variability of information systems that are not always suited to needs assessment.

The team approach to profiling has also been undertaken by nursing staff in Runcorn. Gardner (1996) concurs that at present the procedure is viewed as more important than the product with respect to mutual learning and team-building. Differences between social and biomedical needs identified within the practice have meant that GPs have difficulties being as fully motivated and participative as the other team members, however willing they are. Gardner also notes that the skills of the facilitator are paramount in the profiling process, in order to motivate and enthuse team members. It is seen as inappropriate to identify one individual as solely responsible for the profile, as this seems to give other members tacit approval to abdicate from the process. Gardner stresses that, unless all team members share responsibility for profiling, a sense of collective ownership will not be achieved, which may cause conflict when prioritising and implementing strategies.

An additional system of primary care team health needs assessment has been developed by Hooper and Longworth (1998). It purports to take teams through a systematic decision-making pathway seen as action-focused. The authors state that this decision-making can be passed to the primary care group and then on to the health authority for the development of the health improvement programme for future years. Other team approaches to profiling are illustrated in the following two examples.

CASE STUDY 6

This was an 18-month pilot project designed to equip ten general practices in the Leeds health authority area with the necessary tools and skills to undertake a health needs assessment of their practice population. The results were intended to identify changes needed in service provision and purchasing decisions, and to inform local policy-making (Watson 1996).

Method

The project consisted of a project manager, a steering group (three directors from public health, primary care medicine and contracting/planning, and the project manager), and a project implementation team (project manager and a range of other health authority personnel recruited for specific skills). The project manager offered support to the project practices in the development of needs-assessment approaches. Various programmes were designed and developed, including formal and informal workshops based on the King's Fund community-oriented primary care framework (Gillam et al 1994), and the rapid participatory appraisal technique (Murray et al 1994). All programmes were tailor-made to suit individual practice teams' needs by a consultation process between the project manager and practice team members.

Strengths

The practice-led nature of the project meant that the practice team determined its priorities within a local/national framework; the involvement of all primary healthcare team members increased commitment and understanding of respective roles.

Weaknesses

Practice time was at a premium so funding was obtained for three practices to allow protected time to undertake the practice-based health needs assessment programme.

Outcome

Information for the initial community health profile was geographically organised by enumeration district, and has allowed the teams to identify local needs, disease-group needs, and age-group or general health needs (e.g. mental health). This helped to inform local strategy and purchasing requirements to meet the health needs of the population.

CASE STUDY 7

A system of practice profiling was initiated in Milton Keynes by two working parties of health visitors and district nurses (Hugman & McCready 1993). This was facilitated and coordinated by two clinical practice development nurses (CPDNs) with backgrounds in each of the disciplines, employed specifically for this project.

Method

The CPDNs provided workpacks on profiling. Profiling began with health visitors and district nurses collecting practice population age and sex data, geographical information, amenities available, epidemiology, demography, mortality and morbidity about each patch, and waiting-list information. Details of their caseloads were also collected. The CPDNs were on hand for guidance and to encourage involvement of all practice staff including GPs. The district-nurse data included dependency levels of each patient, calculated using an activities of daily living score (e.g. incidence of incontinence, leg ulcers, chronic disability/disease). The health visiting data included numbers of single mothers under 18, homeless families, mothers breastfeeding from birth, at six weeks and six months, families transferring into the area, and numbers of mothers seen in the antenatal period.

Strengths

The completed practice profiles enabled community nurses and managers to take a snapshot view of their localities, with details of target areas for health promotion and services.

How it was used

No-smoking initiatives; pressure-sore prevalence study and the development of a prevention policy with the acute unit; breastfeeding initiatives; development of school nursing standards; peer-group review of professional standards; profiles used to establish clinical audit by determining levels of performance throughout the practice, and to evaluate caseloads.

PROFILING AND INFORMATION TECHNOLOGY

Information technology has rapidly expanded in the field of health care in recent years. The advent of GP fundholding was partly responsible for the prolifer-ation of computers in practices, to gather health information and generate patient databases. The use of information technology in profiling is being realised in some areas. Studies are emerging that are developing methods to enable more accurate analysis and synthesis of multiple sources of data to identify needs and prioritise services. In addition, some areas are using geographical information systems which allow demographic data to be reproduced in a visual form in a locality (Young & Haynes 1993). These systems do require considerable financial investment.

However, for many community nurses, access to terminals at their workplace is still problematic. Coupled with this, the rapid computer growth in GP practices has occurred unchecked, in the absence of a coordinated strategy in most cases. This has meant that most individual systems cannot be used for inter-agency communication of health data, which has been a singularly lost opportunity. Casey (1996) adds from a trust perspective that much of the early impetus to develop information systems for the community came from a management need to measure community nursing activity. These systems cannot now be adapted for use in profiling. She states that one of the main barriers to development has been the difficulty faced by suppliers in identifying the information technology requirements of community nurses. Without this understanding, information technology developers cannot build systems to support practice, and do not provide direct benefits to clients and practitioners. Current government initiatives are, however, targeted at addressing these problems and rectifying the IT interface problems that have developed (Department of Health 2000).

Organisations such as the national Nursing Professions Information Group (NPIG) are concerned with monitoring and developing better communication and information systems for nurses. Community nurses are adapting current software programs at practice level to input and extract health-related data for needs-assessment purposes, but as yet there are no systems in existence specifically for profiling.

CASE STUDY 8

Health visiting activity and caseload analysis using programmes of care and information technology (Hurley 1996). Funded by the Welsh Office, Focusing Community Services aimed to introduce methods of managing information that would improve the efficiency and effectiveness of health visiting services. Objectives included the development of descriptions of activity and outcomes, and a means of collecting information that supported the health visitors' work.

Method

A project team was formed (senior nurse, health visiting, clinical nurse specialists, liaison and generic health visitors). Five programmes of care were drafted and circulated to all health visitors and other professionals involved. The project health visitor then visited groups to discuss the work, after which redrafting took place. The eventual programmes comprised:

- Routine child and family health – antenatal review, five periodic pre-school assessments, transfer into area, well baby clinic
- Supplementary child health – behaviour problems, care of next infant, child protection, children with special needs, feeding/eating problems, non-attenders, post-accident contact, sick child, speech and hearing problems
- Supplementary family health – bereavement visit, breastfeeding, crisis visit, housing problems, relationship difficulties, maternal stress, postnatal depression, parental anxiety, teenage parents, vulnerable families
- Adult health – screening, monitoring accident rates, coronary follow-up, group work
- School health – entry health assessment, health education, immunisation, counselling.

Hand-held computers for data collection were purchased and linked to larger computers in five clinics, from which inputted data could be taken by health visitors. Codes used for data collection related specifically to the programmes of care. One central computer was set up to transfer information between sites using a modem.

Strengths

The involvement of all health visitors enabled smooth uptake; health visitors are now able to provide managers and purchasers with caseload information for activity planning and costing.

Weaknesses

Time required to implement software systems; difficulties developing watertight coding specifications; need for greater hands-on technical expertise; information about health visiting activity restricted by the IT system, so significant compromise necessary.

CONCLUSION

This chapter has attempted to provide community nurses with a range of profiling models to help them undertake an assessment of need in their area. To acknowledge the very different communities with which community nurses work, many of the examples have concentrated on the process of profiling. But it is important to remember that profiling is not solely concerned with the collection and interpretation of health-related information. It is about translating identified needs into service provision. With profiling, community nurses have the tools, the information, and the evidence to influence decisions about local health services.

DISCUSSION QUESTIONS

- Practitioners have an important part to play in the identification of 'soft' health needs data within families. How could these be more formally identified for measurement in your caseload?
- What health information is readily available for practitioners to help with profiling? How could practitioners influence the dissemination of health data for practice?
- How could practitioners in your area influence service planning using evidence-based strategies developed from the profile? Investigate the organisational routes you would need to take.

FURTHER READING

Needs

Appleton J & Cowley S (eds) 2000 The Search for Health Needs: research for health visiting practice. Macmillan, Basingstoke
A collection of research illustrating some of the complex skills used and variable interpretations of the term 'health needs'.

Robinson J & Elkan R 1996 Health Needs Assessment: theory and practice. Churchill Livingstone, Edinburgh

Detailed explanations of the different types and levels of needs assessment, with accompanying practical details and applications drawn from nursing and health care.

Epidemiology

Ashton J (ed) 1994 The Epidemiological Imagination: A Reader. Open University Press, Buckingham
Leading epidemiologists were asked to contribute a paper of work they had been involved in themselves and one classic paper that seemed to them to convey the potential and excitement of the epidemiological approach. The resulting collection provides a selection from the masters and the classics.

Mulhall A 1996 Epidemiology, Nursing and Healthcare: A new perspective. Macmillan, Basingstoke
Demonstrates how 'epidemiological thinking' is relevant across nursing in acute and community setting.

Profiling Process

Billings J 1996 Profiling for health: the process and practice. Health Visitors' Association, London
A booklet that covers much of the information in this chapter, but includes a larger range of practical, worked through examples.

Guidelines for developing a general practice profile are available in 'worksheet format' from http:www.nottingham.ac.uk/chdgp/guidelin.htm

Use of profiles: caseload weighting

Horrocks S, Pollock J, Harvey I, Emond A & Shepherd M 1998 Health visitor understanding and rating of 28 health and social factors used as part of a health visitor caseload weighting system. Health and Social Care in the Community 6(5):343–352

Shephard M 1992 Comparing need with resource allocation. Health Visitor 65(9):303–306

Shephard M 1996 Poverty, health and health visitors. Health Visitor 69(4):141–143
Three papers that illustrate how the researchers are working towards the use of caseload weighting based on profiles of health need.

APPENDIX 6.1 FURTHER EXAMPLES

CASE STUDY This model for the development of a primary care nursing team was devised in North Staffordshire Health, in the recognition that effective teamworking does not automatically follow the creation of primary health care teams (Cook 1996). An important facet of this model was the need for team-building through health needs profiling and service planning. The goal of the programme was to provide a coordinated nursing service through a practice-based nursing team, to meet the needs of the practice population. Other aims included encouraging the mutual understanding of the roles, function, skills and experience of each person in the team.

Method

A pilot project involving three nursing teams was set up as a joint venture by the FHSA and the Combined Healthcare NHS Trust. A nursing team development model was devised by primary care facilitators and a training and development officer. This model placed practice population profiling as the first step to identify needs, review nursing skills and needs, implement action, and adapt roles accordingly. The model was put into action over two separate sessions. The nursing teams met away from the practice and addressed methods of profiling and the use of professional profiles to identify skills and interests. Before the next session, team members assembled a range of health and social data about caseloads, practice demography, morbidity and mortality, and information about screening and immunisation programmes. This information was used in the subsequent session to identify nursing needs and to formulate an action plan. Each team's practice profile was written up by the facilitators, including a list of identified needs and plans.

Strengths

Involvement of the entire nursing team; effectiveness of the model; FHSA and trust collaboration; managerial support (cover for absent staff was supplied); low-cost process (trust facilities used); has generated interest; model can be adapted for use by other practices and teams.

Weakness

Insufficient preparatory information available; team development aims not always understood by practices.

How the action plans were used

Implementation of action plans is under way, and includes the production of a database of information on pain control in palliative care in order to share expertise with the whole team, and the development of health promotion packs about accident prevention for vulnerable groups. Evaluation of the model has taken place and weaknesses have been addressed.

CASE STUDY   This community profile of an area was compiled as part of a two-year public health nurse project based in a general practice in Castlefields (Wearne 1992).

Method

The principles of rapid appraisal were adopted, namely, identifying and collecting relevant information, and involving the community in devising strategies to meet identified health needs. The primary health care team at the surgery was also closely involved. Three processes were undertaken:

1. Getting to know the area. This involved learning about the history, culture and practices of local people by networking and listening to their concerns and those of other agency workers.
2. Identifying information sources. Data sources included small area database (based on the census and available from the health authority); general practitioner data (annual practice report, practice protocols, medical service data available from the health authority); cancer register (available at electoral ward level); community trust services (operational data, access to child health

computers); previous studies and annual reports (including an external report on local consumer views). The information was collected on word processing and graphic software packages.

3. Identifying other health profiles via a literature search. These sources were less productive than directly contacting the researchers or nurses involved. When analysing the data, accuracy, relevance, importance and usefulness were considered.

Findings were discussed with other members of the primary healthcare team, agency workers, councillors and local people. Priority areas to target were chosen on the grounds of shared concern and available resources.

Strengths

The process produced closer collaboration with other agencies, which resulted in joint funding of initiatives; involvement of the community in defining need resulted in more appropriate initiatives and consequent use of local community volunteers; team profiling was a learning experience, and helped to establish good communication, shared goals and joint working strategies.

Weaknesses

The incompleteness of information, the lack of suitable comparisons, and lack of availability of some data proved to be problematic.

How it was used

Appointment of a nurse practitioner; 'Look after your heart' community projects; Castlefields Health Forum and volunteers in general practice initiative; highlighted the need for training in data management, public health epidemiology.

CASE STUDY

In October 1991, a working party of five school nurses launched a pilot study to develop a profiling format to enable school nurses to build a health profile of each school in the district (Neylon 1995). The intention was to computerise the information to render it more detailed and more accessible to other health agencies. Funding for the project was obtained from the trust.

Method

Assistance was sought from the literature and through a journal advertisement. Liaising with a quality assurance facilitator and an IT expert, a draft was printed, circulated widely and adjusted. The format consisted of data on schools (nurse working hours, numbers of pupils and significant members such as special needs and health promotion people); detailed information about special needs children (on the child protection register, statemented, needing extra help); children with identified health problems (social, physical, behavioural, emotional); details about accidents; availability of public transport (obtained by a one-day snapshot view); access to community and health care facilities; school nursing health education activity; annual requirements. A software programme was selected and monitored by the research expert. Seven infant schools were selected for the pilot study. Data were recorded manually on the printed sheets using guidelines. Information was entered into the computer database and individual reports were issued. Profiles were implemented across the district in 1992 following training. Caseloads were weighted according to numbers of problems.

Strengths

Improved distribution of resources; computer use enabled easier handling and analysis of data, as well as achieving greater accuracy of recording; training needs have been identified.

Weaknesses

The validity of the profile depended on the accuracy of data recording at the schools, which was found to be suspect for both accidents and asthma.

How the profiles were used

Training programmes have been set up for school nurses to improve the reporting of asthma incidence; meetings with education authority about the recording of accidents resulted in a review policy; school nurse caseloads have been redefined; education programme have been set up to identify needs of the nurses.

CASE STUDY

For the past three years, health visitors at Guild Community Healthcare Trust have been profiling their caseloads (Sissons 1996). Profiling was initiated to demonstrate health visiting effectiveness by identifying good practice, to target resources more precisely, and to contribute towards the evaluation of specific initiatives.

Method

The initiative was started and organised by working health visitors, and took a bottom-up approach. Categories to measure and client groups to be targeted were agreed by all health visitors, including care outcomes and social factors. It was decided that every client on the caseload should have an individual form for health visitors to code health information, effectively anonymising it. The forms were developed to be read electronically once completed, thereby rendering the data easy to handle and analyse. Following a preliminary audit, each health visitor received a print-out of caseload information, such as area averages, clinic performances, and outcomes for specific groups such as homeless children. This information was subsequently shared with the borough council, health promotion and public health departments. An annual snapshot of caseloads is compiled each year, and is compared with achievements from the previous year. Profiling in this way is now supported by the trust, with monies allocated for coordination and analysis, although the management of the project is still fully controlled by field workers.

Strength

Good for assisting structured reflection about practice, such as helping health visitors discuss what does and does not work; assists with targeting work and the evaluation of service developments; helps to show the effect on vacant caseloads; makes health visiting work visible and assists with marketing; provides the basis for practical discussions within primary healthcare teams to improve specific areas of practice.

Weaknesses

The process is time-consuming; categories can only be drawn from easily-audited sources, which limits the profile to children and families where professional records are used, and to categories where there is consistent recording.

How the profiles have been used

To plan and target health-visiting work; to contribute towards skill-mix evaluations; to target cross-disciplinary breastfeeding initiatives; to contribute to evaluations of changes in service establishment; to assist with resource allocation in disadvantaged areas; to hold workshops with minority ethnic groups about service provision.

ACKNOWLEDGEMENT

This chapter develops and updates material first used in Billings (1996) (Billings J 1996 Profiling for health: the process and practice. Health Visitors' Association, London) with thanks to the Community Practitioners' and Health Visitors' Association for permission to use this material and reproduce the case study examples from that booklet.

REFERENCES

Acheson D (Chair) 1998 Independent Inquiry into Inequalities in Health. The Stationery Office, London

Appleton J & Cowley S 2000 The Search for Health Needs: Research for Health Visiting Practice. Basingstoke, Macmillan

Avis M 1994 Satisfying solutions: a review of issues in measuring patient satisfaction. Paper presented at the RCN annual research conference, Hull

Billingham K 1995 Progress with Profiling. Premier Health, Burton-on-Trent

Billings J R 1995 Investigating the potential of the profile in needs assessment and contracting. Unpublished MSc thesis. Department of Nursing Studies, King's College, London

Billings J R 1996 Investigating the process of profile compilation. Nursing Times Research 1:270–283

Billings J R 2000 Lay perspectives on health needs. In: The Search for Health Needs: Research for Health Visiting Practice. Macmillan, Basingstoke pp 102–131

Blackburn C 1992 Improving health and welfare work with families in poverty. Open University Press, Milton Keynes

Bradshaw J 1972 The concept of social need. New Society 30:640–643

Bryan S, Parkin D & Donaldson C 1991 Chiropody and the QALY: a case study in assigning categories of disability and stress to patients. Health Policy 18:169–185

Carey L 1999 Using health profiling as a tool for needs assessment. Supplement: Learning Curve. Nursing Times 95(5):S6–S7

Casey A 1996 Nursing terms and the need for community systems. The British Journal of Healthcare Computing and Information Management 13(3):19–21

Cernik K & Wearne M 1992 Using community health profiles to improve service provision. Health Visitor 65:343–345

Chase H D & Davies P R T 1991 Calculation of the underprivileged area score for a practice in inner London. British Journal of General Practice 41:63–66

Clark A 1997 Community participation in determining the needs of users and carers of rural community care services. Health Bulletin 55(5):305–308

Cook R 1996 Paths to effective teamwork in primary care settings. Nursing Times 92(14): 44–45

Cooper L, Coote A, Davies A & Jackson C 1995 Voices Off. Tackling the Democratic Deficit in Health. Institute for Public Policy Research, London

Council for the Education and Training of Health Visitors 1977 An investigation into the principles of health visiting. Council for the Education and Training of Health Visitors, London

Cowley S & Appleton J V 2000 The search for health needs. In: The Search for Health Needs: Research for Health Visiting Practice. Macmillan, Basingstoke pp 1–24

Cowley S & Billings J R 1997 Family health needs project: final report. Department of Nursing Studies, King's College, London

Cowley S & Billings J 1999 Implementing new health visiting services through action research: an analysis of process. Journal of Advanced Nursing 30:965–974

Cowley S, Bergen A, Young K & Kavanagh A 1996 Establishing a framework for research: the example of needs assessment. Journal of Clinical Nursing 5:53–61

Craig P 1996 The Kendoon community health profile. University of Glasgow, Glasgow

Department of Health 1990 Working for Patients (Cmnd 555). HMSO, London

Department of Health 1992 The health of the nation (Cmnd 1986). HMSO, London

Department of Health 1997 The New NHS: Modern, Dependable (Cmnd 3809). The Stationery Office, London

Department of Health 1999 Saving Lives: Our Healthier Nation (Cmnd 4386). The Stationery Office, London

Department of Health 2000 The NHS Plan: a plan for investment, a plan for reform (Cmnd 4818). The Stationery Office, London

Donaldson C & Mooney G 1991 Needs assessment, priority setting and contracts for health care: economic view. British Medical Journal 303:1529–1530

Donnolley J & Shepherd M 1996 Using profiles in dialogue with purchasers. United Bristol Health Care Trust/Avon Health Authority, Bristol

Drennan V 1990 Gathering information from the field. Nursing Times 86(39):46–48

Fruin D J 1978 Analysis of need. In: Brown M J (ed) Social issues and social sciences. Charles Knight, London

Gardner L 1996 Notes on practice profiling by nursing staff at Castlefields Health Centre, Runcorn. Premier Healthcare, Burton-on-Trent

Gillam S, Plamping D, McClenahan J & Harries J 1994 Community-oriented primary care. King's Fund, London

Godden S & Pollock A 1997 Everybody counts. Health Service Journal: 30–31

Goodwin S 1995 Commissioning for health. Health Visitor 68:16–18

Hawtin M, Hughes G & Percy-Smith J 1994 Community profiling: auditing social needs. Open University Press, Buckingham

Health Visitors' Association 1991 Profiling school health. Health Visitors' Association, London

Hooper J & Longworth P 1998 Health needs assessment in primary health care teams. Calderdale and Kirklees Health Authority, Huddersfield

Hugman J & McCready S 1993 Profiles make perfect practice. Nursing Times 89(27):46–49

Hurley A 1996 Focusing community services. Welsh Office, Cardiff

Jarman B 1984 Underprivileged areas: validation and distribution of scores. British Medical Journal 289:1587–1592

Lawlor D, Marsden C & Sanderson J 1999 Rapid participatory appraisal of young people's sexual health needs. Health Education Journal 58(3):228–238

Lightfoot J 1995 Identifying needs and setting priorities: issues of theory, policy and practice. Health and Social Care in the Community 3:105–114

Lock K 1999 Meeting the need. Community Practitioner 72(6):157–158

Luker K & Orr J 1992 (eds) Health visiting: towards community health nursing. Blackwell Scientific Publications, Oxford

Munday C 1996 Voices: A peer research approach to needs assessment. Young People Now 88:28–29

Murray S A, Tapson L, Turnbull J, McCallum J & Little A 1994 Listening to local voices: adapting rapid appraisal to assess health and social needs in general practice. British Medical Journal 308:698–700

Neylon J 1995 Computerised school health profiles: implementing a new system. Nursing Standard 9(25):35–38

Peckham S & Spanton J 1994 Community development approaches to health needs assessment. Health Visitor 67(4):124–125

Phillips C, Palfrey C & Thomas P 1994 Evaluating health and social care. Macmillan, Basingstoke

Richards J 1991 Consumer-oriented planning. In: Community care plans – the first steps. Department of Health, London

Roberts H & Magowan R 1994 Local sensitivities. Health Service Journal 104(5393):30–31

Robson C 1993 Real world research. A resource for social scientists and practitioner-researchers. Blackwell, Oxford

Rodgers J 1994 Power to the people. Health Service Journal 104(5395):28–29

Royal College of Nursing 1993 The GP practice population profile. Royal College of Nursing, London

Sissons C 1996 Profiling health visiting caseloads. Guild Community Healthcare Trust, Preston

Smith K 1995 Quality adjusted life years in the NHS – health care for all? Care of the Critically Ill 11(2):82–85

Stalker K 1993 The best laid plans ... gang aft agley? Assessing population needs in Scotland. Health and Social Care in the Community 2:1–9

Thomas E 1997 Community nursing profiles: their role in needs assessment. Nursing Standard 11(37):39–42

Thomson G & Ward K 1994 Cost effectiveness and provision for special educational needs. Mental Handicap Research 7(1):78–95

Townsend P, Simpson D & Tibbs N 1985 Inequalities in health in the city of Bristol: a preliminary view of statistical evidence. International Journal of Health Service 15:637–663

Twinn S, Dauncey J & Carnell J 1990 The process of health profiling. Health Visitors' Association, London

Watson Y 1996 Practice-based health needs assessment project. Report brief. Leeds Health Authority, Leeds

Wearne M 1992 A report on a two year pilot project to explore the role of a public health nurse in a general practice. Mersey Regional Health Authority, Liverpool

Wistow G, Leedham I & Hardy B 1992 A preliminary analysis of a sample of community care plans. Department of Health, London

World Health Organization 1985 Targets for health for all. WHO Regional Office for Europe, Copenhagen

Yin K 1994 Case study research: design and methods, 2nd edn. Sage Publications, California

Young K & Haynes R 1993 Assessing population needs in primary health care: the problem of GP attachment. Journal of Interprofessional Care 7:15–27

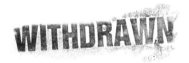

7 Understanding effectiveness for service planning

Peter Griffiths

KEY ISSUES

- Direct evidence of effectiveness for public health interventions is often lacking, and decisions must often be made on the basis of a range of available evidence.
- Evidence that is available is often ignored.
- The effectiveness of a service is its ability to achieve desired outcomes.
- Evidence for effectiveness should not be confused with efficacy: the impact of an intervention in ideal circumstances, as opposed to in everyday practice.
- The evidence-based healthcare paradigm identifies the randomised controlled trial (RCT) as the strongest form of evidence for service effectiveness.
- The reality of complex healthcare interventions means that RCTs may only provide evidence of *efficacy* in all but the simplest cases.
- RCTs may sometimes be impossible for public health interventions.
- The decision about the ideal type of evidence for many public health interventions is more complicated than it is for simple drug treatments.
- The idea of a clear hierarchy of evidence must be disputed.
- *No* form of evidence (qualitative or quantitative) can be rejected out of hand when determining the effectiveness of public health interventions.
- *Any* form of evidence must be critically appraised rather than taken at face value.

INTRODUCTION

Surely effective public health care is good health care? It does what is intended to do, which is to restore or promote health or to prevent illness. The difficulty arrives when it comes to deciding the appropriate outcomes, the appropriate ways of defining them and the appropriate way of determining whether the desired outcome has been achieved. This is the problem of determining effectiveness. It is often at its most problematic when dealing with complex, multi-faceted interventions, which have multiple outcomes and operate through complex mechanisms. Many public health interventions, especially those undertaken by public health nurses, are of this type. Nurses and health visitors are increasingly expected to contribute to service planning too, perhaps as the board nurse on a primary care group, or in a working group for one or more aspects of a local Health Improvement Programme (HImP). How can they choose which services will best meet the health needs? Those seeking evidence to use in planning public health services need to consider the type of evidence needed and the value of that evidence very carefully, prior to putting any intervention into effect.

Much of the debate about effectiveness is fuelled by competing approaches to scientific enquiry and arguments about the nature of human knowledge and experience. Those who are tempted to paddle in these turbulent philosophical waters are advised to bear in mind that at the heart of the effectiveness debate lies a simple endeavour. To put it most plainly, we wish to determine whether our actions had an effect and whether that effect was that which we intended. For public health interventions the desired effect is 'health' construed in its broadest sense to encompass a range of human experiences from the relief of physical illness through to positive aspects of well-being in individuals or groups.

We begin with a definition of effectiveness drawn from the emerging discipline of evidence-based health care, going on to examine this paradigm and the approaches to determining effectiveness. The chapter then moves on to an examination of approaches to evaluation, beginning with a consideration of the role of experimental/quasi-experimental approaches. After examining the limitations of the experimental approach, alternative and complementary approaches to evaluation will be examined, which in turn emphasise the need to consider the full complexity of public health interventions when seeking evidence for effectiveness. Finally, we will consider the role of guidelines in the delivery of effective public health.

DEFINING EFFECTIVENESS

Muir Gray (1997) offers a simple definition of effectiveness. The effectiveness of a health care service or professional is the extent to which desired outcomes are achieved by it. Effectiveness is distinguished from quality, which is seen as the adherence to (best) standards of care delivery. Although we would generally expect that standards of care be set in order to deliver the most effective care possible, this is frequently not the case. One reason for this is that the effectiveness of many health care interventions is simply not known. In many cases (perhaps all) the goal is not the most effective care possible for a specific problem, but that which yields the best effect within parameters which are dictated by financial resources and decisions about allocating resources across a range of interventions for a variety of problems. Effectiveness must also be distinguished from efficacy, the impact of an intervention in ideal circumstances, as opposed to everyday practice.

Should the distinction between quality and effectiveness seem unconvincing, it may help to consider an alternative framework for defining quality in health care. According to Donabedian, a health outcome is, '... the effect of care on the health and welfare of individuals or populations' (Donabedian 1988 p 177). Donabedian's work distinguishes outcome from process ('... care itself') and structure ('... the characteristics of the settings in which care is delivered') (1988 p 177). Although the validity of any quality indicator is predicated upon a relationship between that indicator and some dimension of patient health or well-being, it is frequently the case that this relationship is hypothetical (Donabedian

1966). Quality in the structures and processes of care is not necessarily based on a proven link to outcomes, i.e. effectiveness.

A hypothetical example might illustrate these differences. Suppose that we designed a fall-prevention programme for elderly people. We choose to implement it through individualised visits to people identified as at-risk by a specially trained health visitor. The programme consisted of an assessment of risk in the home, advice on exercise and feedback to the GP about any risks to the individual from their medication regime and the need for any further medical assessment.

A research programme demonstrates that the programme dramatically reduces the number of falls experienced by the target group when compared to an appropriate group, and it is deemed a success. Such a research programme would almost certainly have at its core a randomised controlled trial in which clients are randomly allocated to receive the fall-prevention programme or a control intervention which would probably be simply GP follow-up. At this point the programme has been identified as having efficacy since it has worked, albeit in these special circumstances. A range of such studies have in fact been done, which provide some evidence for a focused assessment in preventing falls (Gillespie et al 1999) although research has not generally examined the specific contribution of public health nurses.

The health authority therefore identifies this service as representing quality care for at-risk elderly people. The quality of a health visiting service for elderly people might now be judged in part by whether practitioners offered this programme.

Unsurprisingly, when the intervention is implemented in everyday practice its effectiveness is not nearly so dramatic as identified in the original research. The intervention is but one of many activities undertaken by health visitors. Often district nurses undertake it, as relatively few health visitors specialise in elderly people. None of those involved has had specific training and the clients they see are not so carefully assessed prior to referral as were those in the pilot site. We will return to these distinctions between aspects of quality later, but for the moment the important points are that neither quality services nor evidence of efficacy necessarily guarantee effectiveness.

EVIDENCE-BASED HEALTH CARE

Evidence-based medicine has been defined as '... the conscientious, explicit and judicious use of current best evidence in making decisions about the care of individual patients' (Sackett et al 1997 p 2). The approach is not, however restricted to decisions about medical care nor to the care of individual patients. Evidence-based health care (EBH) is more broadly defined in terms of decision-making about the health care of individual patients, groups of patients and populations (Muir Gray 1997) and it is this broader term which is used here. Although the particular set of practices and principles which represent the current evidence-based health care movement emerged into the mainstream of practice only during the mid 1990s, its advocates claim illustrious ancestors.

Origins in public health practice

The link between public health practice and evidence-based health care is firmly established. Authors in the area often seek to establish its lineage by tracing its roots to the pioneering epidemiological work of Semmelweiss and Oliver Wendel Holmes, both of whom identified the role of health care practitioners in causing puerperal fever through lack of basic hygiene (Rangachari 1997). Systematic observation allowed Holmes to discern that incidence of puerperal fever seemed to be in clusters associated with particular physicians. Semmelweiss' comparison of infection rates in women cared for by doctors (who did not wash their hands when attending to women after post-mortem examinations) and midwives (who were not contaminated in this way) is held up as an early prototype for today's randomised controlled trials (RCTs).

If Holmes and Semmelweiss are claimed as its grandfathers, Archie Cochrane, an epidemiologist who worked on the earliest RCTs conducted by the Medical Research Council in the UK, could be said to be the father of today's evidence-based health care movement. After a lifetime spent working on studies of effectiveness he complained, 'It is surely a great criticism of our profession that we have not organised a critical summary, by speciality or subspecialty, adapted periodically, of all relevant randomised controlled trials' (Chalmers 1997). For Cochrane, an unbiased synthesis of evidence from good-quality studies is the true endpoint of health research. He campaigned for effective health care to be free in the National Health Service (NHS), but equally argued that interventions with no evidence of effectiveness should not be offered outside of well-designed research programs.

USE OF EVIDENCE

At the heart of the evidence-based health care movement lie two simple premises. Many interventions lack evidence of effectiveness and much existing evidence of effectiveness is not put into practice. For practitioners and policy makers alike, the most significant aspect of this problem will be the identification and utilisation of existing evidence, since action can rarely be delayed until new research is commissioned to answer a question. Even where the main action is to undertake or commission research or implement pilot projects to be evaluated, it is to be hoped that such action would be based on an appraisal of the existing evidence-base (or lack thereof).

Muir Gray (1997) reduces the problem of identification and utilisation of evidence of effectiveness to a simple algebraic formulation (which I suspect he would not wish us to take too literally). In his formulation the decision-maker's performance as an 'evidence-based decision-maker' is proportional to motivation (to utilise evidence) and competence (in identifying, appraising and interpreting evidence). It is inversely related to barriers which, in Muir Gray's account, are lack of resources for accessing evidence (Box 7.1).

BOX 7.1	*Algebraic account of research utilisation* (after Muir Gray, 1997)

$$\text{Performance} \; = \; \frac{\text{Motivation} \times \text{Competence}}{\text{Barriers}}$$

Muir Gray's term 'motivation' covers a complex set of cognitive processes which are often touched on in studies of research utilisation. In the extreme case it has been frequently argued that practitioners will simply disbelieve or disregard evidence if it does not accord with pre-existing beliefs (Hunt 1996, Jones 1997, Rodgers 1994). Within the paradigm of evidence-based health care these complex factors are essentially irrational, in that they will tend to lead the individual toward making an incorrect decision (or to be sufficiently unmotivated as to make no decision at all).

The experiences of the early pioneers Semmelweiss and Wendel Holmes illustrate that the power of rational argument alone is not enough to ensure that evidence is implemented. Semmelweiss was eventually dismissed from his job and returned to his native Hungary, after failing to find further work in Vienna. Wendel Homes was the subject of considerable scorn from eminent practitioners for many years, before his findings were finally accepted. One detects a whiff of anti-semitism in the treatment of Semelweiss and it is clear that the perceptions of the messenger have considerable impact upon people's willingness to listen to the message. This is a complex topic, and one which is well outside the remit of this chapter.

There is, however, one issue of substantive import which must be addressed prior to moving on. I would not wish to ally myself to an extreme relativist position on knowledge. Absolute relativism has little place in a practice discipline where all parties must accept (if only on pragmatic grounds) that individuals do not completely construct their own realities. Events such as survival and death are of universal significance and subject to external verification. However, this does not necessarily mean that the evidence available for rational scrutiny is not subject to interpretation. What one party may perceive as useful evidence may not necessarily be seen as such by another.

Much of the research on research utilisation implies that disbelieving the evidence of research is always an essentially irrational phenomenon. Certainly, experience suggests that a blanket refusal to believe research evidence based on a sophisticated rational appraisal of its limited utility is rare. However, the distinction between effectiveness and efficacy identified earlier should serve as a warning that the implications of a particular piece of evidence for practice in a particular setting are often far from clear. Thus, lack of motivation might in part be a product of the lack of utility practitioners find in evidence offered to them for making decisions about effectiveness. We will return to this later when considering the formulation of evaluations.

For now we will consider the model decision-maker who is motivated to find evidence for effectiveness and is willing (at least in principle) to implement it. What follows is based squarely within the evidence-based health care paradigm. The reasons for this are two-fold.

First, the literature on evidence-based practice clearly describes the basis on which many health care policy and practice decisions can be, and are, made.

| BOX 7.2 | *The UK's NHS strategy for identifying effective intervention* |

In the UK, a number of initiatives were developed to provide evidence for practice and health care management. Key to these initiatives was making information readily available to 'consumers' of research. The worldwide web (WWW) has been used as a mechanism for disseminating information on effectiveness and the initiatives themselves. The WWW addresses for four of the key initiatives are:

- Centre for Reviews and Dissemination – http://www.york.ac.uk/inst/crd/
- National Electronic Library for Health – http://www.nelh.nhs.uk/
- National Institute for Clinical Excellence – http://www.nice.org.uk/
- Health Technology Assessment programme – http://www.hta.nhsweb.nhs.uk/

Indeed, although by no means ubiquitous (see Sheldon et al 1996), the evidence-based health care model is probably the dominant one in current health services research and policy. Certainly, the majority of initiatives which have resulted from the UK's NHS research and development and information strategies (e.g. the Centre for Reviews and Dissemination, the National Institute for Clinical Excellence, the Health Technology Assessment programme and the National Electronic Library for Health – Box 7.2) seem to adhere broadly to the tenets of the model. The second reason is that the model's critique of many aspects of current (evidenceless) practice is compelling, as are some of the solutions offered. The following sections will describe the nature of the evidence which the evidence-based decision-maker is urged to use in order to ensure patients and clients receive the most effective health care.

HIERARCHY OF EVIDENCE

Imagine we wish to implement a programme to control head-lice in children. In the first instance the question appears to be a simple one. What is the most effective treatment of head-lice? Clearly, in order to determine the relative merits of any one treatment we would wish to compare it with the alternatives (including non-pharmacological approaches). The treatment that led to the highest number of children being free of head-lice would be the most effective. So a carefully controlled comparison is what we require.

In evidence-based practice the ideal single study design for answering this form of question is the (well-conducted) randomised controlled trial (RCT). There is a clear and explicit hierarchy of evidence. There is some discussion of the relative merits at the lower end of the hierarchy but for a single study there is no serious debate as to the superiority of the RCT.

A physicist is able to create a vacuum in order to control extraneous factors, such as air resistance, to determine whether the acceleration of a pebble subjected to gravity is the same as that of a feather (it is!); no such parallel vacuum exists in health care interventions. Since in health care we cannot remove extraneous variables (differences in the characteristics of people), the RCT allows variation arising from these factors to be dealt with by distributing the groups of people who will receive the interventions to be compared randomly to different treatment groups. The probability of any differences between groups prior to the intervention is precisely modelled by probability theory, as are individual variations in response to treatments. Statistical-significance testing allows chance variation to be quantified and discounted (certainly over repeated replications).

The problem of using non-random groups to compare the effectiveness of interventions is clear when considering a hypothetical comparison of two head-lice treatments. Imagine treatment X is the most expensive pediculocide on the market. If we simply compared those children whose parent bought and used treatment X with those who received the extremely cheap treatment Y it is difficult to determine what caused any observed differences in louse infestation. Treatment X may appear more effective because it is more diligently applied by parents who have invested heavily in treatments. Treatment Y might appear more effective because it tended to be bought by parents who thought they ought to treat 'just in case' but had in fact seen no lice. The permutations are endless but just about any pattern of outcomes could be accounted for by explanations other than differential effectiveness in treatments.

Only when treatment X is compared to treatment Y in a well-conducted RCT can differences between the two groups be confidently attributed to the treatment itself. In the paradigm of evidence-based health care the ideal form of research evidence for answering a question such as this is thus the RCT. This, then, is the type of evidence which decision-makers should seek in order to answer their effectiveness questions.

However, evidence from RCTs is not always available. In some cases randomisation to groups may be practically or technically impossible. In these cases, other comparative designs such as cohort studies (where outcomes of comparable groups with and without exposure to the intervention are compared), case control studies (where known cases, e.g. those exposed to an intervention or experience, are compared to matched controls) or 'n of 1' trials in which an individual (or group) is exposed to one or more interventions intermittently, may be considered. Our natural experiment on head-lice treatment would constitute a (rather poor) cohort study. Studies of disease causation must generally be cohort studies, since randomisation to the causal agents of disease is frequently impossible and almost never ethical. The individual case report, or series of case reports, where the effectiveness of the intervention is illustrated by a change in status before and after exposure to an intervention or agent, with no comparison whatsoever, is seen as evidence which is so weak as to be negligible.

Many public health interventions are delivered at a level of service organisation where randomisation of individuals to receive 'treatments' would not be possible. For example, if one wished to investigate the impact of aspects of a recent reorganisation of a health service on the health of the public within the catchment area of newly-formed primary care group (PCG), randomisation of individuals would be impossible. If the policy change had been introduced gradually, it might have been possible to compare cohorts of people in PCG pilot sites with appropriate cohorts of people whose GPs were fund holders in similar localities, for example. An 'ideal' design here would probably be one in which the unit of randomisation was the locality grouping and effectiveness was measured in terms of population outcomes rather than at the individual level. However, like the PCGs, widespread policy initiatives are often implemented without piloting. In such cases, it may be that the only available comparison is with a historical cohort prior to the implementation of change.

In cases where non-randomised studies are conducted, a judgement on the quality of the evidence produced is generally made upon the extent to which the study has managed to control bias. A study on the effectiveness of PCGs might attempt to adjust (in statistical terms, 'control') for differences in the age and socioeconomic status of individuals in the lists of practices involved in the study.

Complex techniques of design and analysis are deployed to improve the validity of results from such non-randomised (quasi-) experiments (Cook & Campbell 1979). All are essentially designed to control for the effect of extraneous causes which might lead to differences between groups, and thus to increase the confidence with which cause can be attributed to the intervention under investigation. In essence, the endeavour is to make the quasi-experiment as much like the RCT as possible. Thus, alternative study designs represent no shift in the paradigm. Rather they represent best fixes for technical problems that mitigate against the use of an RCT.

Nonetheless, two of the leading authors in the field offer the following observations:

> 'With the data usually available for such studies, there is simply no logical or statistical procedure that can be counted on to make proper allowances for uncontrolled pre-existing differences between groups.'
> (Lord 1967 p 305 cited in Cook & Campbell 1979)

In other words, nothing really beats a good RCT, a point emphasised by Muir Gray (1997):

> 'The main abuse of a cohort study is to assess the effectiveness of a particular intervention when a more appropriate method would be an RCT.' (p 92).

Yet, as we have seen, in some cases the *only* available design to measure effectiveness is in fact a quasi-experiment. The criticism of the quasi-experiment and associated analysis techniques is offered here largely to establish their inherent imperfection and associated uncertainty. Unlike the true RCT such uncertainty cannot be precisely quantified and thus the influence of other factors cannot be discounted simply by replication, and reduction of the probability of 'random' error accounting for the findings.

CRITICAL APPRAISAL

The first step in seeking evidence of effectiveness is thus to seek reports of appropriate primary research (or ideally systematic reviews of all such research – see below). In general this will be from a randomised controlled trial (Dickersin et al 1995) or, for complex interventions such as many public health initiatives, a cohort study or occasionally a case-control study.

Clearly, having identified studies that can provide answers to questions of effectiveness, it is important to assess the validity of the studies themselves. Not all RCTs are properly conducted and reported. Most texts on evidence-based practice provide critical appraisal guidelines for varying types of study designs.

Those given by Greenhalgh (1997) and Muir Gray (1997) are both typical and usable, with details of how they should be applied. Box 7.3 gives an outline of key points to be considered.

BOX 7.3   *Critical appraisal for studies of effectiveness*

Appropriateness of design

In identifying evidence for effectiveness, the first stage is to determine whether or not a particular study design is appropriate to answer a question about effectiveness. Clearly there must be some form of comparison.

In general, the study design should be the strongest possible. Cohort studies are viewed as weaker evidence than RCTs and case-control studies as weaker still. Although we question the absoluteness of this hierarchy later in this chapter it is still important to consider. If the design is not appropriate there is no point in reading the study.

The paper should then be scrutinised to identify the description of the intervention under study and what it is to be compared with. Adequate description is essential in order to determine if the evidence is useful.

Finally it is crucial to identify the actual outcomes studied and how they were measured. If a paper claims an intervention is 'effective', it is important that it is clear that a reader knows precisely *what* it is effective for.

Applicability

A study report should be scrutinised in order to identify the particular population studied. An intervention which was tested on one group or in one setting may not work in another. Evidence that cervical screening programmes are effective in university students says little directly about the effectiveness of a similar programme in a council estate. It is also important to consider the 'control' condition to which an intervention is compared. Crudely, an intervention which improves health, compared to no services at all, cannot be assumed to be effective compared to some other services.

Bias

In appraising any comparative design it is vital to establish that comparison groups were similar in every way but their exposure to the treatment. In an RCT this is achieved through properly concealed randomisation, complete follow-up and analysis of outcomes on the basis of the groups to which people were randomised to (irrespective of treatment received) – so-called intention to treat analysis. In non-randomised studies possible bias must be discussed and the authors must demonstrate that groups did not differ in terms of all important prognostic factors.

Outcomes assessment

Outcomes should ideally be assessed by someone with no knowledge of the intervention received by an individual or group (although this is not always possible). For retrospective studies, there are additional problems associated with identification of both the outcome and the exposure or otherwise to the intervention. In these cases it is vital that both outcome and intervention are assessed using a standardised approach which uses clearly-defined criteria.

ACCUMULATION OF EVIDENCE INCREASING PRECISION

At the pinnacle of the hierarchy of evidence is the systematic review, which should represent an unbiased synthesis of all the (valid) evidence available for the effectiveness of an intervention. In a classic paper Antman and colleagues (1992) criticised the traditional 'review' article for providing biased accounts which fail to properly represent the current state of evidence. Thus, the emphasis of the evidence-based health care movement on the use of systematic reviews might at first seem perplexing.

The word 'systematic' is key. The systematic review should contain an explicit statement of its objectives and methods. This should include the techniques used for searching the literature and identifying all relevant studies, the criteria for selecting studies for the review, a description of how the criteria were applied and an explicit method for synthesising the findings of the studies. The systematic review is conducted with the rigour expected of primary research and the validity of a review is judged by similar criteria (Mulrow 1995).

The logic of the systematic review is to eliminate the effect of 'random' variation between different settings and participants, in order to determine a precise, numerical, estimate of 'true' effect. However, while the RCT allows precise quantification of uncertainty, the lack of control over extraneous variables intrinsic in other study designs means that quantitative estimates of effect from systematic reviews of other types of study implies a rather spurious confidence in the success of statistical control. Nonetheless, the systematic search and appraisal of all relevant research studies, which is at the heart of the systematic review, clearly represents a major advance from selective reviews, which can present a significantly misleading picture of the weight of evidence in a particular area (Mulrow 1995).

STUDIES OF EFFICACY VS EFFECTIVENESS

The emphasis of the evidence-based practice approach to determining effectiveness is on determining that observed differences between groups are caused by the intervention rather than by chance. This is an important component of any answer regarding a question of effectiveness. Indeed, it may ultimately be the most important answer. However, confidence in the answer comes at a price, which may considerably reduce its utility. A quick review of our hypothetical RCT for head-lice treatments can illustrate one way in which such utility is limited. Even in the case of such a simple question, which can be reduced to one of treatment effect, it is far easier to answer the question of 'efficacy' than truly answer the question of 'effectiveness'.

In an experimental study, the factors that lead people to participate in the study may make them more or less likely to utilise the treatment in a particular way. In the earlier example of an RCT of head-lice treatments I hypothesised that the expensive treatment might induce a particular diligence among parents using it. The circumstances of an RCT may often mean that the application of an intervention is in many ways atypical. The factors which determine the success (or lack of it) of the interventions may be masked by the very act of experimental control, which deals with 'extraneous' factors by attempting to balance the probabilities of them occurring in each group to be compared. Even where such balance is successfully achieved there is no guarantee that the extraneous factors do not interact differently with different treatments to produce different effects.

In an RCT application, regimes will be strictly standardised to ensure proper control and a fair comparison. But our expensive treatment X may have a less noxious odour than treatment Y. Under the controlled conditions of the study this may have little effect, as people adhere to the application-regime specified, but may well lead to ineffective use of Y in other circumstances. Thus, application of Y will be improved by inclusion in an RCT while the use of X would be much the same in or out of it. The very fact that efficacy and effectiveness are not the same thing should point to a need for a wider consideration of the mechanisms through which interventions operate.

The evidence-based health care paradigm is thus subject to a bias wherein questions of effectiveness are in fact often answered by information about efficacy. Quasi-experiments may in fact be more suited to addressing real-life situations through use of pre-existing groups and patterns of behaviour or intervention, but are associated with an unquantifiable imprecision and susceptibility to bias. There seems to be an inevitable conflict between the internal validity associated with an RCT and the high external validity but lower internal validity of the quasi-experiment.

A well-designed study can strive to minimise bias and grapple squarely with the question of effectiveness. However, it is unlikely that RCTs (or quasi-experiments) alone can fully answer these questions even in the simplest medical treatments. Most public health interventions are not at all like simple medical treatments. Evidence about efficacy should only be accepted in the absence of direct evidence of effectiveness. In some cases, this may mean accepting weaker evidence of effectiveness over and above more robust evidence of efficacy.

We will now move on to consider the determination of effectiveness from the perspective of a body of applied research that examines programmes in action – evaluation. Evaluation as a discipline holds a promise to both broaden our focus on outcomes, as we attempt to assess the value of those outcomes, and to directly address effectiveness, since evaluation research is generally associated with programmes of care targeted at individuals or populations, rather than the efficacy of specific treatments.

EVALUATION AND PUBLIC HEALTH INTERVENTIONS

Øvretveit (1998) outlines four different evaluation perspectives. The experimental perspective focuses on establishing cause – effect relationships and predictable patterns of outcome. Its model research design is the RCT although, as we have seen above, alternative quasi-experimental approaches exist, wherein pre-existing groups are used for comparison and to determine the effect of the intervention.

The economic perspective focuses on the use of resources. Although Øvretveit differentiates between the experimental and economic perspectives, in reality the essential difference between the two lies in the chosen outcome

BOX 7.4	*Types of economic evaluation*

- Cost minimisation – the cost of two interventions is compared to see which is cheaper

- Cost effectiveness – a cost is put upon improvements in an outcome associated with the intervention for example cost per life saved for a cancer-screening, programme

- Cost-utility – the outcome is given a value, so rather than simply measuring lives saved a measure of quality of life is introduced and costs are set against a measure such as a 'quality adjusted life year' or 'health day equivalent'

- Cost-benefit – a monetary value is attached to both the intervention (cost) and the outcome (benefit). Since both benefits and costs are measured in the same terms, it is theoretically easy to see if the benefit is greater than the cost. The reality of putting a monetary value on (for example) a year of life is somewhat more complex

measures. Evaluations range from simple costing exercises and cost-minimisation (where the cost of two interventions is compared to see which is cheaper) through to more complex approaches aimed at combining costs and some measure of effectiveness (Box 7.4).

Øvretveit's (1998) remaining evaluation perspectives are the 'developmental' and the 'managerial'. The developmental perspective sees the purpose of evaluation as guiding change and developing or improving the interventions that are the subject of evaluation. The role of the evaluator is as much to feed back information to guide the development of the intervention process, as it is to accumulate generalisable evidence. The managerial perspective focuses on the implementation of policies and processes defined by those with a supervisory or regulatory function.

These distinctions are, in my opinion, somewhat arbitrary. However, they do serve to introduce the idea that there may not be one single answer to the question of effectiveness. Rather it may depend on precisely what question is being asked, which may in turn depend upon who is asking it. Øvretveit also identifies a range of possible 'stakeholders' such as patients (or recipients of interventions), practitioners, managers, politicians and health researchers.

The priority, indeed value, ascribed to a given outcome (effect) may differ according to the position of a given stakeholder and thus the views of the effectiveness of a programme may differ. It is in the nature of public health interventions that there are a potentially large number of stakeholders including (but not limited to) all those mentioned above. A naive 'scientific' approach does not at first seem compatible with accommodating these perspectives. Science seeks truth, not opinion; facts, not values. A sweeping critique of experimental perspectives made by Guba and Lincoln (1989) not only reiterates the limitations in determining effectiveness outlined above, but adds an inability to accommodate multiple perspectives to the charge.

Guba and Lincoln (1989) reject experimental evaluation as a tool for exploring the perspectives and values of stakeholders. They argue for the need to accommodate qualitative, descriptive and interpretative methods to answer such questions. Clearly there is considerably more to evaluation than the s determination of an 'effect'. The context of any action in the social world (including public health interventions) is usually a complex one and the effect of the intervention will be valued differently by different parties. More significantly, interventions themselves will be mediated by individual values and perceptions, as well as the social (and economic) context the individual finds themself in.

For example, campaigns aimed at promoting breastfeeding which are based solely on the beneficial effects for the baby may be successful in some contexts but fail in others, due to a failure to address the competing motivations which lead some women to choose not to breastfeed and others to give up in the face of adversity. The results of the experimental evaluation of head-lice treatments described might be very different if conducted in an area which introduced a campaign to involve the whole community in 'bug-busting' techniques (Fee et al 2000), which involve encouraging everyone to routinely wet-comb their children's hair at each wash to reduce the spread of infection. Even if all parents were not persuaded to change their children's hair-washing routine for the duration of the study, it would be extremely difficult to unravel whether the changes in infestation rates were simply due to application of one treatment or another, or were dependent on reduced exposure to head-lice because of changes in prevalence in the surrounding area.

However, this critique does not in itself negate the value of experimental approaches in determining differences between groups in terms of achieving (particular) goals when subject to different interventions. Qualitative research approaches can ask participants direct questions concerning effectiveness, but if the aim is to determine the effectiveness of one intervention relative to another, any evidence obtained this way must be weak in terms of our certainty that any differences in effect are indeed caused by the intervention.

Nonetheless, Guba and Lincoln's critique raises a vital counterpoint to the experimental approach. Questions of effectiveness are essentially questions of how to achieve change. A broader range of approaches are needed in order to explore the context and mechanisms which lead people to make particular decisions or choose particular behaviours in the face of public health interventions. There is an apparent contradiction here. Approaches to evaluation that can shed light on *how* something works appear to be weak in determining *whether* something works. However, determining effectiveness using the experimental perspective will generate little knowledge of the mechanism through which change occurred (or why it failed to).

A resolution to this apparent contradiction is proposed by the advocates of 'realistic evaluation' (Pawson & Tilley 1997). Essentially, they argue that a range of research techniques are valid and necessary in order to evaluate fully the context, mechanism and outcome of social interventions. Although their work is primarily based upon research in the area of penal reform, the arguments can easily be transferred to a public health context. An ideal realistic evaluation would explore all aspects of context, mechanism and outcome. It is necessary to understand how programs affect people ('mechanisms') and under what circumstances ('context'), in order to fully understand how to achieve a particular effect ('outcome'). This daunting endeavour may perhaps be moderated by an analysis of what is already known in relation to each of the three components, in order to determine the priorities for any given evaluation. Where little is known about effectiveness (outcome) however, it is difficult to avoid the need for some kind of comparative (quasi-experimental or experimental) study. Nonetheless, lack of knowledge about outcomes does not remove the need to evaluate other aspects of a programme. In some cases the priority may reasonably be on examining mechanisms (or to return to Donabedian's framework, process) because the link between process and outcome is well-established.

The true value of a realistic evaluation is in allowing an accumulation of knowledge on effectiveness that has sufficient context and mechanism information to allow the selection of appropriate interventions for particular circumstances. Where generalisation is not a prime concern, outcome information may be all that is required and the experimental approach alone may be appropriate. However, given the limitations associated with experiments and quasi-experiments identified earlier, it becomes harder to promote these as the sole means for assessing effectiveness in the absence of detail on the setting in which the study is carried out.

However, more fundamental limitations can arise from taking a purely experimental perspective. Of even more concern to the limits of knowledge generated from RCTs is the danger of limiting interventions to those which can only be evaluated by this 'gold standard' measure of effectiveness. In order to develop an RCT the outcomes of interest must be measurable. The measurable effect of the intervention must occur over a time-scale within which it is realistic to run an experiment. Finally, it must be possible to deliver the intervention to individuals or discrete clusters of individuals so that randomisation to comparison groups can be achieved. While this may be technically possible for any intervention which is targeted at individuals, it is simply not achievable in the case of many public health interventions where the programme may be diffuse (such as an advertising campaign) or be anticipated to have effects over a long period which may not be discernible at an early stage (for example Sure Start – see Box 7.5). While it may seem farcical to neglect potentially beneficial interventions simply because they cannot be evaluated by an RCT, this phenomenon has been observed in a number of settings, for example AIDS education programmes in Australia (Kippax & Van De Ven 1998).

In seeking to accumulate evidence for effectiveness, it is important to start from the interventions which are to be tested rather than shaping interventions to research designs. The nature of the intervention and existing knowledge about it should define the information which is most important to determine in evaluations, and the range of possible methods to be deployed in gaining it.

THE ROLE OF GUIDELINES

Guidelines, or rather (clinical) practice guidelines, are defined as systematically developed statements to assist in making decisions about appropriate health care for specific circumstances or problems (Field & Lohr 1992, Sackett et al 1997). Sackett goes further in his definition by insisting that a guideline should bring together the best external evidence to guide decisions (Sackett et al 1997). Since we would not wish to advocate anything less than the best evidence, clearly Sackett's definition should be taken. However, the evidence which is to be admitted into clinical guidelines by the adherents of evidence-based practice

BOX 7.5	*Sure Start*

In the UK in the late 1990s the government launched the 'Sure Start Programme', which aimed to support families with young children and reduce social exclusion. The key to the programme was to provide early interventions aimed at preventing later difficulties and thus to provide the children with a 'sure start'. Rather than identifying a single intervention or set of interventions the programme invited 'trailblazers' to develop packages and approaches to care which adhered to a number of key principles. These included delivery of a service which involved all families within a locality, provision of long-term support (rather than 'one off' interventions), parental involvement, coordination and streamlining of services and improved access to services (Department of Education and Employment 1999).

Some of the research on which the programme was based has been the source of considerable controversy within the world of education. In the USA a number of 'Headstart' programmes were set up, to prepare children for school through various activities such as pre-school groups, sometimes combined with family support through home-visiting and other activities (Cowley 1999). Early studies using rudimentary quasi-experimental designs led to ambiguous results, which could be analysed in a number of ways to show either a positive effect, a negative effect or no effect (Cook & Campbell 1979). Later RCTs seemed to show a positive early effect on school performance which then tailed off over time (Barnes McGuire et al 1997). Thus the programme was scaled back, as long-term benefits were not demonstrated. However, later reassessments showed that by the time the children came to leave school it appeared that fewer of those who had received the Headstart package had dropped out or were identified as 'delinquent' and more went into jobs (Lazar & Darlington 1982). The programme may have had the ultimately intended effect; but the presumption that this could be measured by sustained performance in school tests was erroneous.

This of course presents a significant problem for evaluating 'Sure Start' since it may be that the benefits are not easily measured in the short term. Furthermore, the insistence on universal involvement in a defined area rules out randomisation of individuals, while the absence of a prescribed single intervention makes randomisation of 'clusters' impossible since a particular programme will exist in only one site. The variation in programmes over localities provides ample opportunity to explore 'context-mechanism-outcome' configurations as advocated by Pawson and Tilley but necessitates the acceptance that ultimately the evidence on outcome cannot be as strong as would be provided by an RCT. Of course, the alternative would be no evidence on outcome, since such a programme ultimately cannot be evaluated by an RCT.

is of course limited to that which is recognised as valid by that paradigm. Sackett is perhaps rightly sceptical of guidelines that are based simply upon expert opinion, insisting instead that they be developed and reported with the same rigour that is demanded of systematic reviews.

The previous discussion in this chapter suggests that the nature of the evidence that should be admitted into guidelines for public health may differ markedly from that which might be regarded as legitimate for medical-treatment guidelines. Where there is good evidence from randomised controlled trials or quasi-experiments then these should form the core of any guideline. However, the utility of any such evidence for public health interventions can only be assured if it is 'be accompanied by information of the context and associated mechanisms.

Public health interventions are generally multifaceted and complex. It will rarely be possible to prescribe the precise way an intervention should be delivered to ensure success, and thus it is important to include information from a range of research perspectives in a guideline, in order to guide practitioners and policy-makers to the nuances and detail which may be vital in ensuring success, or which may suggest that one strategy rather than another would be most appropriate in their particular circumstances.

Guidelines may represent the best available accumulation of evidence of effectiveness, but a lack of evidence on mechanism and context may limit their utility in determining the best approach in a particular situation. Thus, although systematic reviews of effectiveness and synthesis of evidence into single estimates of effect may seem appealing, it is also vital to explore the reasons for and nature of variation across studies, in order to understand the necessary conditions of success. Such evidence must come from a range of appropriate research designs.

If such contextual information seems to be a nicety which in truth could be dispensed with, consider the following example drawn from the history of public health. In 1854 there was a major outbreak of cholera in London that was centred on an area close to Covent Garden. The area was supplied with water by means of a pump at Broad Street. Suspecting this to be the source of the infection, a local doctor, John Snow, removed the handle from the pump and miraculously ended the outbreak. If we disregard for a moment everything learned since 1854 about the mechanism of transmission of cholera, consider the evidence for control of cholera which John Snow's act provided. To end an outbreak of cholera, one must remove the handle from a water pump.

This evidence (not provided from an RCT) was quite compelling. Although there have been few outbreaks of cholera in London in recent years, I would speculate that this strategy would no longer work and so John Snow's remarkable achievement is confined to history. However let us add the context: the pump was people's prime water supply. A mechanism: cholera is transmitted by water. More context: nearby water sources were not infected. While neither the mechanism nor the context are in themselves evidence for effectiveness, it is this information *and only this* which allows John Snow's evidence of effectiveness to have a broader utility. The context and mechanism information tells us precisely the circumstances where exactly the same intervention would still work (where water is supplied from a contaminated pump but nearby sources are clean). Perhaps even more importantly, it gives us a very good idea of how one might go about planning effective interventions in quite different contexts. We should not assume their effectiveness (human capacity for ingenious self-harm being what it is) but we may be confident in using the knowledge to guide us.

Perhaps there is a danger in utilising such an extreme example. However, I believe it is not absurd, in particular since the contexts and mechanisms for social change are, if anything, even more changeable and context-bound than Victorian water supply. With a continuing improvement in the overall health of the population and the increasing implication of complex social structures (as opposed to simple material deprivation) in determining relative health disadvantage, it is likely that public health interventions will resemble Sure Start more often than John Snow's elegant solution to the cholera epidemic.

A short note on the philosophy of science

For the 'positivist', true scientific knowledge enables the scientist to exercise precise control over future events by the knowledge of predictive laws. These laws:

> '…enable one to know what will happen under specified conditions, so that what is wanted may be brought on … by making sure the necessary circumstances do come about.' (Pratt 1978 p 76)

Such theories are evaluated not by their ability to describe a reality, but merely by the accuracy of their predictions. It is important to note that it is the accuracy of the predictions, not the assumptions, which lead to scientific credibility under this model (Pratt 1978), since the key to positivist science is control, prediction and manipulation.

Precise prediction and control leading to universal 'laws' are increasingly seen as redundant by many social scientists (Gergen 1982). Since public health services (and researchers) are unlikely to achieve such precise control over antecedent variables to allow the consummate control implied by positivism to come about, it may be time to abandon the pure endeavour of positive science in this arena too. Even in the case of such concrete and controllable interventions as removing handles from water pumps, the nature of the intervention is changed as the world changes around it. In this regard it is worth remembering that all health services are essentially transient historical constructs.

However, this is no reason to abandon the attempt to differentiate chance associations from real ones and hence the rejection of the RCT specifically, and empirical research generally, in no way follows from this shift. Following Gergen's proposals for social science, research should serve to point out influences on behaviour, expose assumptions which have not proved useful and enlighten us as to possibilities and probabilities. Much of the evidence for effectiveness in public health practice will be in this form, rather than universal scientific laws. Experimental and quasi-experimental studies are still crucial. However, with this changed perspective they provide but one part of the necessary evidence, not all of it.

CONCLUSION

The effectiveness of a service is its ability to achieve desired outcomes. Evidence for quality of a service does not necessarily establish that it is effective unless there is an established link between a particular care process and a particular outcome. This is frequently not the case. Evidence for effectiveness should also be distinguished from efficacy: the impact of an intervention in ideal circumstances as opposed to everyday practice. This distinction is particularly relevant to many public health interventions which are complex and multifaceted.

The evidence-based health care movement has developed in response to an increasing recognition that many health care interventions lack evidence for their effectiveness, and that many decisions about health care are made without recourse to evidence, even when it is available. A clear hierarchy of evidence suggests that the best evidence for effectiveness stems from a randomised controlled trial. However, many public health interventions are not readily subjected to an RCT and so other types of research evidence must be sought. In this chapter we also suggested that in fact the RCT may be better suited to providing evidence for *efficacy* rather than *effectiveness*. Decisions about the ideal type of evidence for many public health interventions is more complicated than it is for simple drug treatments. Evidence for the relative effect of one intervention compared to another will come from a suitable comparative design, but the ideal design will be different for different types of intervention. In some cases the superior external validity of a non-randomised study may give it precedence over a randomised study. In other cases randomised studies may be impossible. In all cases the research must be critically appraised rather than simply taken at face value.

In order to be truly useful in making decisions for public health interventions, any evidence for effectiveness will need to be accompanied by descriptions of the context and mechanisms which are thought to be relevant to the programme's success (or lack of it). It is only with this information that informed decisions about generalisation of evidence can be made in a complex and changing social world. Thus, while comparative empirical research must form a crucial part of the evidence for effectiveness, it is but a part of the necessary evidence. We would ultimately question the idea of a rigid hierarchy of evidence. However, the evidence-based health care paradigm does provide much useful guidance for those seeking to determine what services are effective. Perhaps most importantly it urges us to do so!

DISCUSSION QUESTIONS

- Are health policies made on the basis of evidence? Discuss with reference to a recent policy development that affects your area of practice.
- How could evidence for the effectiveness of a universal health visiting service be obtained?
- Can evidence of effectiveness be obtained without a comparison group?

FURTHER READING

Elkan R, Kendrick D, Hewitt M, Robinson J, Tolley K, Blair M, Dewey M, Williams D & Brummell K 2000 The effectiveness of domiciliary health visiting: a systematic review of international studies and a selective review of the British literature. Health Technology Assessment 4(13):1–339
A systematic review of evidence for health visiting that illustrates the merits of using diverse sources of evidence while maintaining the rigour of a systematic review. The report discusses the difficulties of generalising evidence across widely differing health care settings. This is interesting and important reading,

both as a direct source of evidence and as an example of how to bring together evidence for complex interventions.

Gomm R & Davies C (eds) 2000 Using Evidence in Health and Social Care. Sage, London
A good general introduction to the use of evidence in practice and for planning services. The text deals with a wider range of issues than most introductory texts. Its focus on health and social care makes it more relevant to public health practitioners than many evidence-based medicine texts.

Greenhalgh T 1997 How to read a paper. The basics of evidence based medicine. BMJ Publishing Group, London
An extremely readable, user-friendly guide to finding, appraising and using evidence. This book covers all the basic issues of evidence-based health care in a practical manner.

Pawson R & Tilley N 1997 Realistic Evaluation. Sage, London
A review of the history of evaluation research and a description of a new approach, 'realistic evaluation', which offers a solution to the problems of accumulating evidence for complex interventions. The critique of previous approaches is scathing and irreverent and the case for realistic evaluation perhaps overstated. However, anyone wishing to aquaint themselves with the state of the art in service evaluation should start (and perhaps finish) with Pawson and Tilley.

REFERENCES

Antman E M, Lau J, Kupelnick B, Mosteller F & Chalmers T C 1992 A comparison of results of meta-analyses of randomized control trials and recommendations of clinical experts. Treatments for myocardial infarction. Journal of the American Medical Association 268(2):240–248

Barnes McGuire J, Stein A & Rosenberg W 1997 Evidence based medicine and child mental health services. A broad approach to evaluation is needed. Children and Society 11(2):89–96

Chalmers I 1997 Assembling comparison groups to assess the effects of health care. Journal of the Royal Society of Medicine 90:379–386

Cook D C & Campbell D T 1979 Quasi-experimentation: Design and analysis issues for field settings. Houghton Mifflin Co, Boston

Cowley S 1999 Early Interventions: evidence for implementing Sure Start. Community Practitioner 72(6):162–165

Department of Education and Employment 1999 Sure Start: making a difference for children and families. Department of Education and Employment Publications, Sudbury

Dickersin K, Scherer R & Lefebvre C 1995 Identifying relevant studies for systematic reviews. In: Chalmers I & Altman D (eds) Systematic Reviews. BMJ Publishing Group, London

Donabedian A 1966 Evaluating the quality of medical care. Millbank Memorial Fund Quarterly: Health and Society 44(2):166–203

Donabedian A 1988 Quality assessment and assurance: unity of purpose, diversity of means. Inquiry 25:173–192

Fee J, Briault V & Long J 2000 A community approach to reducing head lice infection. Community Practitioner 73(2):477–480

Field M & Lohr K 1992 Guidelines for clinical practice: from development to use. National Academy Press, Washington DC

Gergen J K 1982 Towards Transformation in Social Knowledge. Springer Verlag, New York

Gillespie L, Gillespie W, Cumming R, Lamb S & Rowe B 1999 Interventions for preventing falls in the elderly (Cochrane Review). The Cochrane Library, Issue 1. Update Software, Oxford

Greenhalgh T 1997 How to read a paper. The basics of evidence based medicine. BMJ Publishing Group, London

Guba E & Lincoln Y 1989 Fourth Generation Evaluation. Sage, Newbury Park

Hunt J M 1996 Barriers to research utilization. Journal of Advanced Nursing 23(3):423–425

Jones J E 1997 Research-based or idiosyncratic practice in the management of leg ulcers in the community. Journal of Wound Care 6(9):447–450

Kippax S & Van De Ven P 1998 An epidemic of orthodoxy? Design and methodology in the evaluation of the effectiveness of HIV health promotion. Critical Public Health 8(4):371–386

Lazar I & Darlington R 1982 Lasting effects of early education: a report from the consortium of for longtitudinal studies. Monographs of the Society for Research in Child Development 47:2–3, serial number 195

Lord F 1967 A paradox in the interpretation of group comparisons. Psychological Bulletin 68:304–305

Muir Gray J 1997 Evidence Based Healthcare: how to make health policy and management decisions. Churchill Livingstone, London

Mulrow C 1995 Rationale for systematic reviews. In: Chalmers I & Altman D (eds) Systematic Reviews. BMJ Publishing Group, London

Øvretveit J 1998 Evaluating Health Interventions. Open University Press, Milton Keynes

Pawson R & Tilley N 1997 Realistic Evaluation. Sage, London

Pratt V 1978 Philosophy of Social Science. Methuen, London

Rangachari P 1997 Evidence-based medicine: old French wine with a new Canadian label? Journal of the Royal Society of Medicine 90:280–281

Rodgers S 1994 An exploratory study of research utilization by nurses in general medical and surgical wards. Journal of Advanced Nursing 20:904–911

Sackett D, Richardson W, Rosenberg W & Haynes R 1997 Evidence Based Medicine: How to practice and teach EBM. Churchill Livingstone, New York

Sheldon T A, Raffle A & Watt I 1996 Department of Health shoots itself in the hip. Why the report of the Advisory Group on Osteoporosis undermines evidence based purchasing. British Medical Journal 312(7026):296–297

8 Effectiveness and community empowerment

Anne Graney

KEY ISSUES

- Major philosophical shifts in health are occurring globally. They are pushing health practitioners to refocus their efforts more towards the environmental and economic influences on health, and the use of community-empowering approaches to tackle the resulting inequalities in health.
- Community empowerment and social capacity-building theories offer practitioners useful frameworks to assist in exploring and evaluating the effectiveness of their public health practice.
- Community practitioners must carefully consider their philosophical approaches to practice, so that they can predict outcomes and choose appropriate research methods to measure achievements.
- A wide range of methodological approaches to evaluation are available; each will measure success in different ways, use different tools and contribute different data to the evidence bases.
- Evaluation of community-empowering approaches to practice is often very difficult and the methods used are often considered unacceptable as they do not produce hard data.

INTRODUCTION

Public health decisions need to take into account whether planned strategies and treatments can reasonably be expected to do what they set out to do. Evidence of efficacy and clinical effectiveness are very important in informing such decisions. The methods used to determine clinical effectiveness are mainly designed to evaluate technologies or treatments used for single individuals with a particular condition or illness. These methods have origins which are based upon positivistic scientific theories and philosophy, where facts and values are separated, and where knowledge regarding effectiveness is based upon observations of effects, as in the randomised controlled trial (RCT). However, these methods are considered less suitable for evaluating complex community-based initiatives and the kind of 'empowerment practice' aimed at by grass roots public health practitioners. This was acknowledged by the government when it announced the establishment of the Health Development Agency (HDA) (Department of Health 1999) from April 2000. Among its duties, this organisation is to maintain an up-to-date map of the evidence base for public health and health improvement, and strengthen the evidence base in areas where action programmes are required to improve health and tackle inequality. Despite this acknowledgement at government level, there remains limited awareness and a lack of acceptance of the different philosophical positions and theoretical frameworks that can be used for evaluating effectiveness in public health practice.

The post-positivist schools of thoughts suggest there are many approaches to acquiring knowledge. Their philosophical position is that knowledge is tentative, it may change, for example, with time or because of cultural and social determinants. This evidence is based upon consensus rather than actual observations of cause and effect. A whole range of approaches can be used to determine effectiveness and build up an evidence base. It depends upon the philosophical position and the associated theoretical framework chosen as to what exactly is going to be measured and by whom. Feminist theory, interpretivism, structuration theory, critical theory and paradigmatic theory, although separate, are overlapping (post-positivist) theories, each giving an opportunity to create unique and important knowledge which can be used to build an evidence base for any public health intervention.

This chapter aims to explore some of the reasons why the traditional (positivist) methods, discussed in Chapter 6 and most often used for measuring effectiveness, may be unsuitable for community-based public health work. Examples of such approaches to public health work will illustrate how different philosophies of health affect measurement procedures, how work with communities requires a range of methods of evaluation, and how a practice focus based upon empowerment philosophies and theories can be appraised through a range of suitable methods.

PHILOSOPHICAL CLARITY IN RELATION TO OUTCOMES IN PUBLIC HEALTH NURSING

Much of the 'effectiveness debate' is linked to changing world health philosophies. Such philosophies are changing beliefs in what constitutes effective public health or community practice, and how we determine evidence and outcomes. The political context in which practitioners find themselves is also paving the way for great changes at the start of a new century. The new emphasis in public health practice incorporates empowering approaches which address inequalities in health and take targeted community or population perspectives, as in community development. This reflects a movement away from concentrating only upon the medical and the individualistic approaches which have been traditional in Western societies during most of the twentieth century. The nature of evidence and effectiveness in this chapter is thus largely based upon community empowerment models and theories, their associated outcomes, and the tools practitioners may use to evaluate such approaches in their practice.

Initial consideration must be given to public health effectiveness in terms of gaining philosophical and conceptual clarity. This is the essence of successful evaluation, it is an essential and yet often neglected starting-point in the evaluative process. The dominating concept of public health in western society reveals changes over the course of the last century, with different eras being identified, for example, the sanitary era at the turn of the century has very different concepts of public health than those which we discuss today. Effectiveness, as such, is also a dynamic concept, encapsulated within our own cultural, political, historical and health-belief systems.

FIGURE 8.1   *Approaches to health (Seedhouse 1986).*

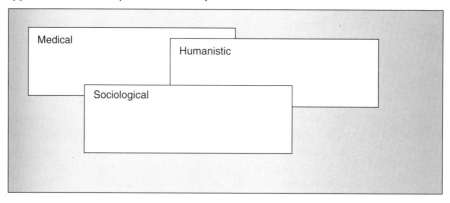

Just as our concept of what constitutes public health changes, so does the way in which we evaluate it. The great philosophical shifts in world health-beliefs are resulting in changing values and new emphasis being placed upon the varying concepts of health and disease. The three main philosophical approaches used today to define western health are medical, sociological and humanistic; they all overlap and inter-link as shown in Figure 8.1.

These approaches are not seen as alternatives to each other, rather a mixture of philosophies are recommended (Seedhouse 1986). However, until quite recently, it was a commonly-held view that all health improvements were made as the result of a medical approach (Ashton & Seymour 1988). The blanket use of the medical model has been widely criticised in recent years, as it does not always take account of the difficult circumstances in which many disadvantaged people live (Ryan 1976); these limit life choices, adversely affect their health and ultimately contribute to health inequalities.

CHANGING PHILOSOPHIES IN PUBLIC HEALTH

The new shift is towards the use of sociological and humanistic approaches to improving health. The World Health Organization (WHO) has greatly influenced this thinking, changing global philosophies to focus on health, not just disease, thus reducing health inequalities through economic, political and social changes. Benefits of advances in medical care are well recognised (WHO 1999), but the new philosophy incorporates a population or community development approach, with empowerment as its goal, and identifies primary health care as its cornerstone (WHO 1978, 1981, 1985, 1986a, 1986b).

The Healthy Cities movement (WHO 1987, 1988), designed to focus upon the health impact of environments in which people live, is also pushing practitioners to think more collectively and move away from individualism. The challenge is to move towards considering the health of whole communities, towns and cities, and basing public health practice upon sound ecological principles (Ashton 1992). This shift is basically about changing local policies in order to create a health-enhancing environment (Hancock & Duhl 1986). The implementation of new healthy public policy shifts the focus from individualised priorities to collective issues which affect health, such as environment, housing, food, energy, justice and economic development (Evers et al 1990).

New public health philosophy is more concerned with environmental issues, incorporating social, physical and psychological environments, than with therapeutic and personal preventative measures (Ashton & Seymour 1988). It recommends a multisectoral focus, which involves industry and local government agencies, as public health is no longer regarded as belonging solely within the NHS. In this movement, community health initiatives which use community-empowering, bottom-up approaches have been identified as an essential part of developing and shaping health policies. The promotion of public health is becoming more accepted as being necessarily a political process, in that the development of local healthy public policy is regarded as an essential to meeting new public health needs (Draper 1991).

In the UK, the policy context of public health at the turn of the century is mirroring these images. The English public health green paper 'Our Healthier Nation' (Department of Health 1998) went further than any previous government document in identifying environmental and social factors as major concerns to public health. Poverty, employment and social exclusion were all cited as major factors affecting health. This consultation paper was followed in due course by a White Paper with specific targets (Department of Health 1999) and similar public health papers emerged in Scotland, Wales and Northern Ireland (Department of Health and Social Services 1999; Scottish Assembly 1999; Welsh Office 1998). All extended the previous understanding of public health beyond the medical model; treatment of individuals and diseases remains important but is now seen as only one part of a wider field. Health Improvement Programmes (HImPs), health action zones, healthy living centres, healthy schools, workplaces, and neighbourhoods for older people flagged up in the consultation paper in 1998 are becoming a reality. New targets, new groupings and new ways of thinking and working all require new methods for evaluation. Government directives have started to reorientate evaluation to focus more specifically on outcomes and quality, away from previous measures of quantity and frequency (Department of Health 1997, 1998, 1999, 2000).

Most of the measuring in community nursing in the past has focused upon individual practice methods, which has been and still is generally reflected throughout the NHS (Cowley 1994). The individualistic orientation in community nursing has failed to recognise the importance of family, group and community-health approaches, which are essential in the evaluation of new public health practice. Nor has quality ever been satisfactorily measured (Luker 1992). Growing political, economic and professional challenges are being faced by all health practitioners, now that there is a greater need to provide evidence of effectiveness. This must be undertaken with colleagues across agencies, making the business of evaluation more complex. However, despite this multiagency thrust for evaluation, it is still important for practitioners to be able to articulate exactly what their particular contribution to the overall public health jigsaw is going to be, and how they will evaluate their contributions. The outcomes for health achieved using this new type of approach are inevitably very different from those seen with individual and traditional approaches.

BOX 8.1	*New public health developmental outcomes (Evers et al 1999)*

- Developing food cooperatives
- Decreasing lead contamination in a town
- Supporting self-help groups
- Assisting women in employment discrimination

The example drawn in Box 8.1 describes the type of results or developmental outcomes which practitioners can expect to achieve using the new public health philosophies and approaches to practice. They illustrate achievements that are made through an ongoing process and sought through a focus on the community, that will make a difference to people's lives and the choices they are able to make. This is an essential basis for empowerment, of which more later. These shifts in global thinking toward community empowerment and creating healthy public policy present a great challenge for all community health practitioners, in terms of addressing changes in their practice philosophies, work methods, networks with other agencies, and what is to be valued and defined as 'public health gain'.

CLARIFYING PRACTITIONER AND COMMUNITY VALUES AND GOALS

It is increasingly recognised that whichever public health definitions or approaches are chosen and agreed by professionals, it is also essential that the definitions, the values and the goals of the communities being worked with are equally considered. If this process is undertaken, success in public health is much more likely, as it will naturally tailor the public health initiative more sensitively at the local level (Liss 1993). This sensitivity is a skill which many community nurses have, but which needs developing and making explicit. Thus, the understanding of community values and goals will essentially shape the type of practice approach taken and the overall practice framework for every aspect of public health practice. An Australian health team, when using community work methods, found that having an understanding of the social view of health within their team, in common with the community and other agencies they were working with, gave more legitimacy to their community health roles. They became more accountable to their professional colleagues and to the community as a result; they could also plan and monitor more effectively (McWaters et al 1989). This is not always an easy step to take, as shown in the example in Box 8.2, where a number of difficulties in evaluation arose because of continuing changes in the perception and the original purpose of the project.

Thus, to critically examine the effectiveness of public health nursing interventions in terms of meeting the new public health agenda, we must first be clear about our philosophical positions, the range of approaches which are available to be used, and why we have chosen to use those approaches in

BOX 8.2	*Evaluating the effects of a community alcohol action programme in New Zealand (Duignan 1989)*

Difficulties experienced in relation to identifying values and goals:

- Defining the real problem was difficult, as it is was perceived differently and changed with time, e.g. the programme started because of a perceived problem with drink driving, then moved to encompass all alcohol-related problems.

- It was unclear whether the initiative really stemmed from the community and its own priorities.

- The aims were unclear generally.

- Solutions were usually multifactoral, but often only one intervention was chosen as a focus for evaluation.

- The programme had unrealistic expectations, it was over-ambitious and seen as a panacea for all social problems.

- Control of confounding variables in the community was difficult to establish.

particular. Secondly, we must also be clear about their value and acceptability for the communities being worked with. This initial clarification allows practitioners to know what achievements and resulting outcomes they can realistically expect from their chosen practice approaches, and which tools are the most appropriate to measure such outcomes. Before community practitioners even begin to think of public health nursing effectiveness and associated outcome measures, there are three important steps they first need to consider (Figure 8.2)

FIGURE 8.2	*Steps towards defining public health nursing outcome measures.*

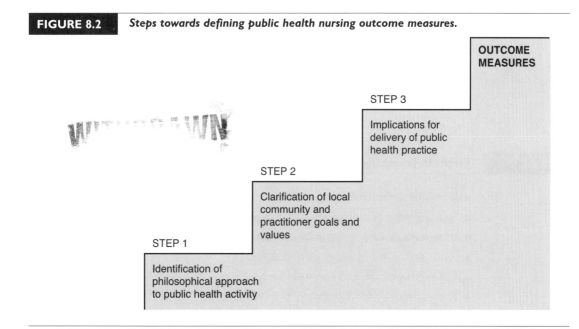

OUTCOME MEASURES

STEP 3
Implications for delivery of public health practice

STEP 2
Clarification of local community and practitioner goals and values

STEP 1
Identification of philosophical approach to public health activity

EMPOWERMENT THEORIES, GOALS AND OUTCOMES

If philosophical clarity is achieved, it is then much easier to predict the type of outcomes expected. Practice approaches and the range of theories supporting those approaches will also become more valid and acceptable to the practitioner, the community, and others associated with the intervention.

Empowerment theories offer a range of frameworks which can be used to help to explore and explain some of the issues surrounding the use of collective approaches to public health nursing and the process of evaluating them. Empowerment is a controversial concept, but it is widely used in the health field today, both in terms of work with individuals and with communities. There is a vast range of literature indicating that increased individual empowerment and the associated high levels of self-esteem are considered absolutely necessary to achieve maximum health gains (Tones & Tilford 1994). More recently, it has been realised that community empowerment is as important in the process of achieving optimum health status as individual empowerment. Most models now recommend that a distinction is made between the individual 'psychological' and the collective 'community' empowerment frameworks, each having different goals for evaluation. The goals and possible endpoints for evaluation using community empowerment frameworks are discussed in more detail using the following models.

In Rissel's (1994) model, the endpoints for the evaluation of community empowerment (which incorporates individual empowerment) are shown in Box 8.3. Although endpoints are identified it is accepted that each is part of an ongoing developmental cyclical process, each component contributing to the overall achievement of health gain.

Freire's (1972) empowerment model is based upon the belief that people are collectively able to problem-solve for themselves and find their own solutions to their concerns. Freire's work is very influential in the health field and often serves as a comprehensive guide to the process of community empowerment and development. The idea is to facilitate the community in moving from just feeling needs to perceiving the actual causes of their needs and then taking action. This is done through critical consciousness-raising and reflection of thought, which leads to empowerment and ultimately action. The action expected to be taken is to change the surrounding structures causing

---

BOX 8.3	*Endpoints for evaluation of community empowerment (From Rissel 1994)*

- Increased personal development
- Establishment of mutual support groups
- Issue-identification and community organisation
- Participation in organisations and advocacy
- Collective political and social action
- The community gaining control over resources

the needs. Each stage in the process is regarded as an outcome. However, the ultimate goal is action to change the structures which affect people's lives and thus their health. Therefore, the possible outcomes using this model would be:

- Establishment of trust and dialogue with the community
- Identification of collective agreement of locally felt needs
- Facilitation of consciousness-raising activity
- Promotion of individual and community empowerment
- Action by the community and professionals to change structures and remove barriers so as to promote health.

Although the stages in Friere's model will appear unfamiliar to some health practitioners, research demonstrates that health visitors using community development approaches to practice are adamant that this process fits perfectly with the principles of health visiting, if applied on a community-level basis, rather than at an individual or family basis. The principles of health visiting were first identified by the Council for the Education and Training of Health Visitors (1977). They are: the search for health needs; the stimulation of an awareness of health needs; the influence on policies affecting health and the facilitation of health-enhancing activities.

Health Visitors continue to use the principles, but apply community empowerment theory to direct their approaches to public health practice, which results in the need to then evaluate practice in different ways (Graney 1996).

As empowerment models have evolved, so has our understanding of the levels of empowerment. Three main levels now being recognised are:

1. The individual level
2. The community level
3. The organisational level.

Each level plays an essential part in the overall process of promoting public health, each having different goals to achieve, with lots of overlapping as well. This is well demonstrated by Israel et al (1994) in their stress model, which has at its centre issues of 'control'. They identify multiple levels of control, for individuals, communities and organisations. This model also incorporates the relationships between environmental factors, powerlessness, social support, and mental and physical health status into the empowerment process. They define empowerment in the following ways:

1. Individual empowerment combines:

- A positive self-image or personal competence
- A sense of control over one's life
- Individual participation and ability to influence decisions within institutions.

2. Community empowerment is:

- Where individuals and local organisations apply their collective efforts and skills to meet respective needs of the community (this is similar to the neighbourhood empowerment definition which uses capacity and equity to achieve the same goals).

3. Organisational empowerment is:

■ The ability of organisations to empower their own members, share power and function democratically, which in turn influences and empowers the larger community.

This model is particularly useful as it suggests that if the organisations surrounding the community, e.g. religious groups, educational establishments or health services such as a primary care trust, do not work internally towards empowerment, then it will be extremely difficult for changes to occur in the surrounding environment, and for the communities and practitioners living or working there to facilitate changes through a community empowerment process.

However, Israel et al (1994) point out that despite the importance of recognising the interlinked nature of the different levels, most empowerment work continues to occur at the individual level at the moment. The extent to which the personal development of individuals within communities becomes a resource, which is then fed back into the development of the wider community, is largely speculative at present (Cowley & Billings 1999). However, belief in this kind of reciprocity and development of mutual community resources like trust and neighbourliness underpin much community development work. Also, there is a growing theoretical and epidemiological literature about the social environment and its impact on health, which suggests that these matters are particularly important in mediating inequalities in health (Marmot & Wilkinson 1999).

Even in the developed world, much ill-health can be attributed to poverty, but this does not account completely for the patterns and inequalities in health. Health inequalities are more marked in societies that show wide variations across a range of social and economic indicators and where, as in the UK, social exclusion of some groups may be quite marked. These observations have led to the idea of 'social capital' being recognised as an important mediator of health in unequal societies.

'SOCIAL CAPITAL' AND ITS ROLE IN COMMUNITY EMPOWERMENT

Putnam (1993) identified 'moral resources' like trust and cooperation across the whole social system and not just in individuals or families, as significant aspects of what he cumulatively described as 'social capital' (Box 8.4). Much of the interest in this concept for community development workers stems from evidence that community participation is one significant route through which social capital is generated (Gillies 1998). Social capital is an emerging concept and, as with 'empowerment', the exact meaning of the term is widely debated. As the debate unfolds, it can help to identify which aspects of social relationships need to be promoted to enhance health and empowerment at different levels of the community (Campbell et al 1999).

Much of the research that shows the link between social capital and health status has been undertaken on large epidemiological datasets (Kawachi et al

1997, Wilkinson 1996). However, the root source of social capital is widely believed to be in local communities and families, which also demonstrates the significance of the concept to individuals. Early childhood experience, for example, is known to influence matters like self-esteem and ability to trust self and others; in turn this is related to ability to both access and offer help when it is needed (Fonagy 1996, Wadsworth 1999). The extent to which a family is able to generate such resources itself varies for many reasons, including the extent of available support in the local community. Box 8.4 shows how understanding of the concept of social capital was developed through a qualitative analysis of information from two community development projects.

The exact mechanism through which resources like social capital and supportive networks exert a protective effect on health (or their absence, a negative effect) remains unclear. However, there is a burgeoning literature and there have been numerous attempts to define and capture aspects of 'social capital' for measurement (e.g. Cooper et al 1998, Kawachi et al 1997) or to link it with community-based initiatives using qualitative or action-research methods (e.g. Campbell et al 1999, Cowley and Billings 1999, East 1998).

BOX 8.4	*Social capital concepts*

Characteristics of social capital (Putnam 1993)

- The existence of community networks
- Civic engagement: i.e. participation in community networks
- Local identity: a sense of solidarity and equality with other community members
- Norms of trust; reciprocal help and support

Local analysis of two projects (Campbell et al 1999)

- Life challenges
- Local identity: sense of 'belongingness'
- Trust
- Reciprocal help and support
- Attitudes to local government
- Formal and informal group memberships
- Subjective perceptions of 'community':
  - — Respect and tolerance
  - — Gossip
  - — Safety from crime
  - — Children's freedom of movement
  - — Neighbourliness
  - — Reciprocal help and support
  - — Local identity
  - — Living and working conditions

BOX 8.5	*Projected outcomes of work with community (Gilbert 1996)*

- Give the community a voice
- Allow participation
- Sustain the health of their own community
- Influence services
- Improve access to services
- For the community to benefit from more appropriate services
- Benefit from improved interface between services
- Use health services more appropriately

This literature is sufficiently extensive and diverse for it to be clear that, whatever the mechanism, the effect of the social environment on health, and especially on health inequalities, is very strong. As a consequence, there is a new political and strategic recognition of the importance of community-based work, and a focus on changing the disempowering impact of socioeconomic disadvantage. In time, it may be possible to use knowledge about how community-based work develops social capital as a collective resource in robust evaluations linked to changes in health status. In the meantime, it seems that communities that are high in social capital are 'empowered communities'. This opens another fruitful direction for evaluation, especially in terms of identifying goals and measuring levels of community networks and social strengths.

Gilbert (1996) uses a positive health (salutogenic) approach in her practice. In working with the community to identify needs, she not only looks at weaknesses of the community, such as high levels of mental health problems, but also identifies strengths, like a purpose-built community centre which could be used to build upon existing social capacity. Once she has built up a 'picture' of the community she is then able to demonstrate the projected outcomes for her practice (Box 8.5).

Many of the outcomes demonstrated in community development work focus on community empowerment and social-capacity building theories. When health visitors use community development methods in their practice they also describe a similar range of these type of outcomes being achieved (Graney 1996). In this case, and in Hunt's (1987) description of the successful outcomes of her community development project, there is great emphasis on developing community resources from within the community itself. The outcomes are summarised in Box 8.6.

The ideas around what may or may not constitute individual and community empowerment outcomes raise many issues about how we are to measure the success and effectiveness of such goals. Although empowerment theories are complex and highly debated, the practice examples in Box 8.6 make goals and associated outcomes for practice with communities and groups quite explicit. Once goals and values are agreed and established with the community, practice can then be shaped and outcome measures determined more appropriately.

| BOX 8.6 | *Developing community resources – a public health outcome* |

Practice outcomes (Graney 1996):

- Facilitation of food cooperatives
- Development of an Asian women's health group
- Participation of local people with health service policy-makers
- Establishment of self-help groups
- Development of safety equipment home-loan schemes with parents
- Enabling parents to change the policies of a local nursery so that it is more inclusive with the community

Practice outcomes (Hunt 1987):

- Setting up of a tranquilliser support group
- Facilitation of an elderly forum
- Development of a fruit and vegetable cooperative
- Setting up of a women's health club
- Setting up of a food and families group
- Facilitation of a 'compulsive eating' group

MEASURING COMMUNITY EMPOWERMENT OUTCOMES

The fundamental purpose of evaluation is to determine the value or worth of an activity. It is also concerned with *effectiveness*, in that it says whether or not the valued goals have been achieved, and with *efficiency*, in that the action taken to achieve that goal will be measured against alternate actions (Tones et al 1990). The measurement of outcomes using collective empowering approaches is rarely mentioned, other than to highlight how complex it is (Evers et al 1990).

One of the main debates is around whether empowerment is itself a process or an outcome. Mostly, it is argued that it is both process and outcome (Friere 1972, Israel et al 1994). Quoting Zimmerman at length, Fetterman (1996 p 4) explains:

> 'A distinction between empowerment processes and outcomes is critical. Empowerment processes are ones in which attempts to gain control, obtain needed resources and critically understand one's social environment, are fundamental. The process is empowering if it helps people to develop skills so they can become independent problem solvers and decision makers ... Empowered outcomes refer to operationalization of empowerment so we can study the consequences of citizen attempts to gain greater control in their community or the effects of interventions designed to empower participants...'

As the work is developmental, the process is as important as the outcome (Smithies & Adams 1993). However, caution is suggested when using the term 'empowerment' due to the possibility of distortion of the concept by different users, measurement ambiguities, and structural barriers which make

TABLE 8.1	Outcomes and goals in empowerment practice (Adapted from Tones and Tilford 1994)	
	Outcomes	**Goals**
	Ultimate Outcomes	■ Empowerment
	■ Difficult to measure	■ Well-being
	■ Unrealistic and idealistic	■ Health
	Intermediate Outcomes	■ Increase in knowledge
	■ Measures a change but only in terms of associated health benefits	■ Change in beliefs
		■ Increase in self esteem
		■ Increase in motivation
	Indirect Outcomes	■ Facilitate increased levels of community participation
	■ Measures an action which is thought to impact on health	■ Provide health information
		■ Develop social support networks

empowerment difficult to attain (Rissel 1994). A further precaution suggested by Tones and Tilford (1994) is that empowerment as an ultimate outcome should not be used at all, as it is unrealistic in terms of achievement and particularly in terms of measurement. Therefore, intermediate or indirect outcomes are used, as shown in Table 8.1. It is then possible to identify goals that can be measured to show progress towards the empowerment outcomes, instead trying to measure 'the thing itself'.

Another difficulty facing practitioners when evaluating community empowerment and developmental approaches is that this type of measuring does not fit comfortably with traditional positivistic scientific paradigms, as you cannot control the extraneous confounding variables which exist in the community. This is supported by Hunt (1987), who states that the outcomes cannot even be very easily anticipated in advance, therefore it is difficult to prove or disprove, or state your precise theory in advance, as in traditional sciences.

Davies & Kelly (1993) suggest that the type of evaluative research which assesses positive health (salutogenic) approaches must move away from the traditional research paradigms if it is to become more effective and relevant. The relativist stance is thus recommended in that there is no one truth about health, but that it is a quality which should be identified and agreed by individuals and groups.

Labonte (1997) states that epidemiologists are often blind to their own assumptions of science and what constitutes knowledge. He recommends the use of the many social science theories which include education, feminist, economic, ecological and social theories, which are equally valuable to understanding and explaining health, and which are often ignored. Labonte recommends that the 'effectiveness debate' should shift from what constitutes science, knowledge and evidence to asking, 'what are our political and social visions for a just and healthy society?' This type of evaluative research thus remains in its infancy, but the future will bring in theories of change and greater public participation will develop, strengthening the work of the movement, and the evidence bases.

Presently, pressure is often placed upon practitioners by managers and commissioners to use methods and tools from traditional sciences, when they are not necessarily appropriate or useful to the community practice approach. Hunt (1987) found that the qualitative nature of participative evaluation is often less acceptable not only to funders, but to the community, local health professionals, researchers and other community workers, with each group placing their own interpretation upon the measure of successful outcomes.

The difficulties identified by Hunt (1987) in her evaluation of a Scottish community development project, included the realisation that some outcomes may be viewed as both positive and negative, depending upon who is judging them. The evaluation of the development of a tranquilliser support group demonstrated the goals to be reducing drug dependency, which was regarded as the expected successful outcome. However, Hunt describes unexpected negative outcomes also; two women realised why they were depressed and therefore left their husbands and children. This may be regarded as a very negative outcome in terms of social capacity building, especially from the children's point of view. Community development outcomes may have associated outcomes which are perhaps less predictable and more individual than community-orientated. The development of the food cooperative highlighted that this was most successful in terms of usage in the first few months of it running. However, in terms of the individual volunteers running the food cooperative, their skill levels and confidence grew much later. Hunt (1987) describes this as the 'freezing of a dynamic process' to look at varying outcomes at key stages in the overall process, which may be quite long-term and unpredictable.

Graney (1996) found the main difficulty that health visitors experienced when demonstrating their community development outcomes was that most managers, commissioners and colleagues were not able to see the value of these types of practice outcomes, and therefore did not accept them as 'real outcomes'. Nor did many managers place emphasis upon evaluation of this nature. Gilchrist (1995) also supports this view and states that because it is difficult to claim tangible and predictable outcomes from networking, which is essential to the community development process, its value is often underestimated by managers and funders. She sees networking as essential in terms of a method which is used to lay foundations for the work, so as to achieve overall aims. She therefore argues that networks should be evaluated against community development processes and specific goals. The results of networking practice, therefore, should be included in any evaluation (Gilchrist 1995).

Smithies and Adams (1993) stipulate that the challenge is for professionals and their managers to become partners in evaluation and not experts. They discuss the unpredictable nature of outcomes using this philosophy, and the way in which interests may well clash between lay and professional people. In an overview of the possible evaluative research approaches that could be used to make assessments of public health needs, the strongest recommendation for success is to have academics, policy-makers, local people and practitioners working together in the research process (Davies & Kelly 1993). Evers et al (1990) believe that multisectoral training, research and measuring of outcomes, together with the involvement of lay people and politicians, is required to implement successful public health policies. Hancock (1993) sees this level of

BOX 8.7	*Difficulties encountered in identifying healthy community indicators in a Canadian city (O'Neill 1986)*

- Multiagency workshops with local people, politicians and health professionals were set up to look at possible indicators. One of the particular problems discussed was the political nature of the process, which was considered a major difficulty in the research, in that local political conflicts and processes operated against the development of the identification and agreement of indicators

- The initiative was regarded as a project and not as mainstream, and therefore not useful in measuring change.

research as also needing to address the power structures in the organisations that maintain the health inequalities.

One urban area in England made an attempt at identifying the health needs of the public by undertaking a city health-profiling exercise (Ashton & Seymour 1988). The health profile was used to make a community diagnosis and establish public health priorities for the city. However, despite all their greatest effors, the twelve health priorities of the Mersey area were still defined mainly as medical targets, very similar to those defined by the Department of Health (1991) in their 'Health of the Nation Targets', for example, reduction in cancers and suicides, prevention of accidents, and family planning. Although this is disappointing, it does demonstrate the difficulty in measuring health needs and outcomes at this level, and the difficulty which exists in pulling away from the medical-orientated and nationally-led agendas. Although the broader social and environmental issues are discussed and acknowledged, it seems they were lost in the process. The Mersey experience suggests that the debate about what constitutes 'public health needs' did not take place in sufficient depth and the approach was led from the top with little effective community participation. O'Neill (1986) also demonstrates the great difficulties experienced in a Canadian public health exercise to identify community health needs (Box 8.7). This example describes the fragility and the roughness of the evaluative research process, as well as the political problems.

Despite the difficulties highlighted, this does not mean that determining outcomes and evaluative strategies should be disregarded. There are now an increasing number of tools that are suitable for use in this kind of evaluation.

TOOLS USED TO MEASURE COMMUNITY EMPOWERMENT AND DEVELOPMENT

A review of the performance of community development projects in the NHS demonstrates that health visitors, community doctors, primary health care teams, mental health workers and other health professionals are using a wide variety of different methods to evaluate their practice (Beattie 1991). Most methods are qualitative, but Beattie found a move toward using pluralistic evaluations, which incorporate both qualitative and quantitative approaches.

Quantitative approaches and their associated tools for measuring are seen as useful, especially as efficiency and cost-effectiveness are being looked at more closely by managers and commissioners.

Beattie (1995), Drennan (1985) and Stewart-Brown and Prothero (1988) all identify the fact that no one evaluative strategy can demonstrate whether a project's goals are being met; they all suggest a combination of methods and tools is best used. Another recommendation is that any evaluation is carried out both internally and externally to give the best guarantee of validity (Beattie 1991, 1995). However, much of the work around reducing health inequalities using community empowering approaches has been marginal and usually not well-evaluated (Department of Health 1995).

Approaches that involve the community are favoured, because the evaluative process itself contributes to development of local organisations and networks (Fetterman 1996).

So what tools can practitioners use that are appropriate to measure such outcomes? Internal evaluation of such approaches to practice requires tools and measures that reflect the underlying philosophy of empowerment; some examples are shown in Box 8.8.

Community health profiling is essential for determining health needs (Stewart-Brown & Prothero 1988) and tracing changes before and after projects. One tool that can be used quickly and easily is rapid appraisal, detailed in Chapter 6 of this text. This approach was used in one locality in Newcastle upon Tyne, where the thrust of the approach was community participation in the identification of locality need (83 000 population) and the involvement of grass roots workers. It involved a researcher interviewing 50 local community groups and the primary care workers in the area. A locality conference was then

---

BOX 8.8   *Tools for evaluating community empowering practice*

- Community health profiling, e.g. through rapid appraisal
- Surveys carried out by members of the community
- In-depth interviewing
- Monitoring, e.g. participation levels
- Case histories and individual testimonies
- Diaries of thoughts and events
- Audio-visual materials and aids, e.g. photographs of public health needs
- Descriptive evaluative frameworks
- Measures of social support and social networks which may include:
  - size of network
  - type of network (formal and informal)
  - geographical dispersion
  - integration into the network (perceived citizen power)
  - composition of network
  - frequency of contact
  - strength of ties

held to feed information to local people, health professionals and managers, and to then enable a process of prioritisation to take place. The three priority areas were defined in terms of groups in need, rather than the traditional classification of disease and death. The groups identified in this evaluative process were young people, unsupported families and those with mental health issues (Freake et al 1997). It is clear from this example that the way in which needs are originally identified and subsequently labelled changes what gets actioned and ultimately what gets measured as success. In this case, it is the successful development of a family support intervention and the establishment of a new service for young people.

Surveys may be carried out by paid members of the community (e.g. Hunt 1987, Stewart-Brown and Prothero 1988). Semi-structured interviews or questionnaires can be used to find out about residents' and workers, ideas or opinions.

In-depth interviews of individuals (Israel et al 1994, Hunt 1987) may be used to determine perceptions about health needs and what should change to address them, or to find out about changes that have been made in the community and how people are affected by them.

Monitoring can be used to determine levels of participation and the impact of a particular public health initiative on participants (Hunt 1987); this is especially suitable for those engaged in small group work activity.

Individual case histories (testimonies) were recorded by Stewart-Brown and Prothero (1988). These can be followed over a period of months/years and are useful in helping to determine levels of empowerment and the benefit to individuals, their families and the broader community.

Diaries can be kept by workers and residents to show their own and the project's activities, levels of networking, contacts and reflections or thoughts (Hunt 1987, Stewart-Brown and Prothero 1988).

Audio-visual materials and aids like photographs, videos and artwork can be used to involve the community in identifying their public health needs, as well as tracing changes as a result of public health work.

Descriptive evaluative frameworks may be used to describe the goals, processes, and outcomes of a particular intervention. McWaters et al (1989), using such a framework, are able to demonstrate clearly the process of making changes with an identified community goal, i.e. the reduction of feelings of isolation. The process of making changes to the public transport system to reduce community isolation is measured descriptively, as is the way in which the community becomes more and more involved. The differing levels of participation and finally the development of new community management structures and transport systems as a successful outcome are all carefully documented over the years.

Social support and the strength of social networks can be mapped across a local area. There is a wide-ranging literature that helps to explain the analytical links between social relationships and health at the level of the individual, interindividual, organisational, community and macrosocial levels. There are many interactions between these different levels, which are of great interest and provide starting points for assessing the nature of civic engagement (Campbell et al 1999).

Bowling (1991) provides a helpful review of a number of quality of life measures, in the form of scales, some of which may prove useful as tools for

BOX 8.9	*Examples of positive health measures (Bowling 1991)*
	■ Ability to cope with stressful situations
	■ Maintaining strong social supports
	■ Integration within a community
	■ High morale and life satisfaction
	■ Psychological well-being
	■ Levels of physical fitness
	■ Social well-being

measuring individual empowerment levels and social capacity (Box 8.9). Quality of life is defined as being about perceptions of well-being, self-worth and personal satisfaction, and is measured using positive health indicators. Often they are used with individuals and small groups. Another useful tool focusing on positive health is Antonovsky's (1993) 'sense of coherence' scale, which comes in two versions, one being longer than the other. It is particularly helpful because it focuses on positive health and personal resources, rather than on illness and problems.

A simple and easy-to-use scale to measure morale and general well-being, uses 'delighted' and 'terrible' faces (Figure 8.3) to measure feelings, both positive and negative. This is particularly useful where people are not confident with their literacy or have little motivation to fill in a questionnaire.

Although multiple methods and qualitative approaches have much to offer in evaluation of complex community initiatives, there is also great value in 'mining' official data, to see if there have been changes in the local area since the project began. Hospital statistics may reveal whether attendance at the accident and emergency department has changed, for example, or if admissions for a particular disease condition have reduced. Standard epidemiological data are usually available from the local public health department; they may reveal changes in mortality or morbidity, like a reduction in low-birthweight babies or infant mortality. Child protection registers may reveal changes in numbers registered or re-registered in a local area. Crime rates in a local area may give some indication of the success of some local neighbourhood initiatives. Changes in employment or numbers of children excluded temporarily or permanently from school may also give some 'hard facts' to support subjective perceptions of changes in the local area.

FIGURE 8.3	*Delighted–terrible faces scale (Andrews & Withey 1976).*

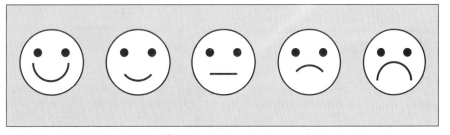

It is important to recognise the sensitive and confidential nature of many of these indicators, that are collated for purposes other than evaluation of community projects. They may be best collected by an external evaluator rather than local residents, who may recognise details of anonymised data because of their own depth of knowledge of the local community. The keepers of confidential records such as child protection registers and school exclusion data will, rightly, need to be assured that care will be taken to respect the anonymous and confidential nature of any information they are prepared to divulge. Caution must also be excercised in that the indicators of success may only partially relate to your project or may not relate to your project or practice at all, they may relate to another variable entirely.

In addition to using these 'ready-made' data, it is also possible to collect a range of research information, using standard methods such as surveys or quasi-experimental procedures to compare effects of activities (Hunt 1987). There are various indices available that can assess levels of empowerment, e.g. levels of control over one's life, or levels of participation within groups, organisations and communities (Israel et al 1994) and levels of self-esteem (Stewart-Brown & Prothero 1988). However, because of the limitations of these survey instruments, it is also recommended that other measures are used in conjunction with them (Israel et al 1994). Self-rating scales are often criticised as being too subjective; a depressed person may be supported, for example, but report feeling unsupported (Procidano and Heller 1983). They are also regarded as subjective and unreliable, in that they depend on individual attitudes and social and cultural factors. Reliability has also been questioned in that indicators for health and well-being are usually based on professional rather than lay concepts (Bowling 1991).

This overview provides only a small selection of the possible approaches which can be used to evaluate collective empowering approaches to public health work. Some of the tools can be used to collate both qualitative and quantitative data. All tools, however, have strengths and weaknesses, which practitioners should bear in mind. Some researchers have found the tools used to measure before and after health status are not ideal, in that they can alienate the community prior to the public health initiative even starting, they are also very open to interpretation (Stewart-Brown & Prothero 1988). However, two of the most important areas to consider in using any measuring scale are:

- Its appropriateness to the community/population you are going to use it with
- The relationship of the scale with other variables which you are not measuring (Hunt et al 1986).

CONCLUSION

In conclusion, there appears to be a general shift in health philosophy throughout the world. A more collective, empowering approach with the greater involvement of people in working towards their own health and health policies appears to be the way forward. It is a radical shift with a greater emphasis being placed upon reducing inequalities in health status. The medical, disease-orientated priorities of the past are giving way to health priorities which are more socially, environmentally and politically orientated. There is a growing body of research evidence suggesting that social and environmental influences are the greatest factors affecting public health today.

The overwhelming evidence suggests that concentrating on medical priorities and individual behavioural changes is not enough to improve health status and reduce inequalities. This shift means that community practitioners will have new opportunities for developing and evaluating collective empowering practice approaches. It also means all practice methods need to be fully evaluated in terms of effectiveness and the changing nature of expected outcomes. This will be no easy task. However, it must be tackled urgently by practitioners, researchers, professional leaders and managers. New tools and a range of methods for evaluating such practice approaches will need to be developed. Public health nurses will need to explore their knowledge and theory bases further than ever before to incorporate the broader social sciences.

The complexity of measuring collaborative (multiagency) 'bottom-up' ways of improving health has not yet been satisfactorily addressed. Research and evaluation needs to change to address the nature of multiagency working and the process of involving local people in this. Goals are different in the new public health movement, addressing the need for structural changes, community empowerment and capacity building, as well as community regeneration and ecological outcomes, which are long-term goals and more unpredictable. Managers, researchers, commissioners and practitioners will need to learn to work in partnership not just with each other, but also with the communities they serve. Equally, health practitioners must examine their methods of practice and find ways to address these philosophical shifts.

The political nature of health and evaluation cannot be ignored. The influencing of policy changes is as essential as any other aspect of health promotion, and appears to be growing in importance. Healthy public policy implementation (locally and nationally) is regarded as essential to the achievement of the environmental, economic and social changes necessary for the achievement of health for all. Public health nursing will need to ensure this is incorporated into practice and its evaluative frameworks. Community participation and empowerment still appears to be very limited in the process of identifying health needs locally and even more limited in the implementation of integrated strategies to address these needs.

With the advent of primary care groups and trusts, (see Chapter 5) local health groups and cooperatives, general practitioners and community nurses now have more responsibility for health promotion and public health needs analysis and policy development. Thus, the acknowledgement and acceptance of new health approaches means that community practitioners must not fear taking on a more political role. Political awareness will be as important as health and ill-health awareness. The challenge is to create a more politically aware and pro-active public health practitioner, who can demonstrate effectiveness through public health improvements, which includes influencing healthy policy making. However, much hinges on the national priority given to health and prevention, not just ill-health. This is not to say that practitioners should stop asking the important questions:

- What steps can I take to influence local health-enhancing policies?
- How will I measure public health processes more clearly?
- How will I involve the community?
- How will I work more collaboratively with other agencies in the community?

There isn't a simple set of philosophies or practice work methods to use in order to meet the public health agenda, nor is there a simple set of tools to use to measure public health changes, but hopefully some of the frameworks and tools discussed here may trigger enthusiasm in evaluating practice methods, where community development is the approach being used. The debate around the value of using traditional research approaches to evaluate collective empowering approaches in practice will continue. The standardisation of variables in the community setting appears impossible, and yet without the use of quantitative tools and frameworks it seems that practitioners evaluations will be doomed to failure in the eyes of some stakeholders. For most practitioners an eclectic approach (a mixture of methods and tools) will need to be used, thus incorporating both qualitative and quantitative research methodologies.

The diversity within nursing practice needs to be valued, recognised and further strengthened in terms of meeting public health needs through community and targeted population approaches in the new century. However, to be successful there needs to be more public health nursing research, and the development and experimentation of new collective empowering practice methods, and tools to measure these approaches.

Understanding research methods is not enough in itself, political and professional agendas must be used to ensure the findings are relevant and valued. Now, more than ever before, the public health and political agenda fits with community health nursing philosophies, it is possible therefore to incorporate the social and environmental determinants of health into measures of health status and outcomes. It is now time to fully recognise the social and political nature of public health nursing, and to find new ways to evaluate and determine the effectiveness of new approaches to public health nursing practice.

DISCUSSION QUESTIONS

- What are the key components of new public health philosophy and how will they shape public health nursing practice and evaluation of its effectiveness in the future?

- How does the shift in public health philosophy effect what is regarded as evidence?

- If public health nursing is to meet the new challenges of influencing local healthy public policies, by working with communities in an empowering way, how will practice be measured at the national and local levels?

FURTHER READING

Connell J P, Kubisch A C, Schorr L B & Weiss C H (eds) 1995 New approaches to evaluating community initiatives: concepts, methods and contexts. Aspen Institute, Washington DC
This collection of papers sets out a theory-driven approach to evaluation, focusing especially on the idea of theories of change. This approach has been popularised in the UK because it is being used by Ken Judge and his team in their current national evaluation of Health Action Zones.

Fetterman D, Kaftarian S & Wandersman A (eds) 1996 Empowerment evaluation: knowledge and tools for self-assessment and accountability. Sage Publications, Thousand Oaks, California
Promotes the ideal that evaluation can be used as a means of enhancing empowerment in individuals and communities.

Guba E & Lincoln Y 1989 Fourth generation evaluation. Sage Publications, Newbury Park, California
Sets out the philosophical case against positivist approaches to evaluation and offers an alternative constructivist method.

Pawson R & Tilley N 1997 Realistic evaluation. Sage Publications, London
Another example of theory-driven evaluation designed for use in complex community initiatives. Written in a humorous and readable style. The authors debunk deep philosophical approaches and propose their own down-to-earth and 'realistic' approach to evaluation.

Shaw I 1999 Qualitative evaluation. Sage Publications, London
Introductory textbook that explains the background debates and gives details about the leading names in qualitative evaluation methods.

Surestart Unit 1999 A guide to evidence based practice, 2nd edn. Department for Education and Employment, London
Collected examples of community-based projects offering approaches to use and ways of evaluating them. Booklet free from DfEE Publications, PO Box 5050, Sherwood Park, Annesley, Nottingham NG15 0DJ.

REFERENCES

Andrews F M & Withey S B 1976 Social Indicators of Well Being: American perceptions of life quality. Plenum Press, New York

Antonovsky A 1993 The structure and properties of the sense of coherence scale. Social Science and Medicine 36(6):725–733

Ashton J (ed) 1992 Healthy Cities. Open University Press, Milton Keynes

Ashton J & Seymour H 1988 The New Public Health. Open University Press, Milton Keynes

Beattie A 1991 Success and Failure in Community Development Initiatives in National Health Service Settings: Eight Case Studies. Open University Press, Milton Keynes

Beattie A 1995 Evaluation in community development for health: an opportunity for dialogue. Health Education Journal 54:465–472

Bowling A 1991 Measuring Health: A Review of Quality of life Measurement Scales. Open University Press, Milton Keynes

Campbell C, Wood R & Kelly M 1999 Social Capital and Health. Health Education Authority, London

Cooper H, Arber S, Fee L & Ginn J 1998 The influence of social support and social capital on health: a review and analysis of British data. Health Education Authority, London

Council for the Education and Training of Health Visitors 1977 An Investigation into the Principles of Health Visiting. Council for the Education and Training of Health Visitors, London

Cowley S 1994 Counting practice: the impact of information systems on community nursing. Journal of Nursing Management 1:273–278

Cowley S & Billings J 1999 Resources revisited: salutogenesis from a lay perspective. Journal of Advanced Nursing 29:994–1004

Davies J K & Kelly M P (eds) 1993 Healthy Cities, Research and Practice. Routledge, London

Department of Health 1991 The Health of the Nation. A Consultative Document for Health in England. HMSO, London

Department of Health 1995 The Health of the Nation. Variations in Health. What can the Department of Health and the National Health Service Do? HMSO, London

Department of Health 1997 The New NHS: Modern, Dependable. The Stationery Office, London

Department of Health 1998 Our Healthier Nation: A Contract for Health (Cmnd 3852). The Stationery Office, London

Department of Health 1999 Saving Lives: Our Healthier Nation (Cmnd 4386). HMSO, London

Department of Health and Social Services 1999 Fit for the Future: A New Approach. Department of Health and Social Services, Belfast

Department of Health 2000 The NHS Plan: A Plan for Investment, A Plan for Reform (Cmnd 4818). The Stationery Office, London

Department of Health and Social Services 1997 Well into 2000 … A positive agenda for health and wellbeing. Department of Health and Social Security, Belfast

Draper P (ed) 1991 Health through Public Policy. The Greening of Public Health. Green Print, London

Drennan V 1985 Working in a Different Way. Community Work Methods and Health Visiting. A Research Project Examining Community Nursing Services. Paddington and North Kensington Health Authority, London

Duignan P C 1989 Evaluating community development programs for health promotion problems illustrated by a New Zealand example. Community Health Studies 13(1):74–81

East L 1998 The quality of social relationships as a public health issue: exploring the relationship between health and community in a disadvantaged neighbourhood. Health and Social Care in the Community 6:149–220

Evers A, Farrant W & Trojan A (eds) 1990 Healthy Public Policy at the Local Level. European Centre for Social Welfare Policy and Research, Westview

Fetterman D 1996 Empowerment evaluation: an introduction to theory and practice. In: Fetterman D, Kaftarian S & Wandersman A (eds) Empowerment Evaluation: Knowledge and Tools for Self-assessment and Accountability. Sage Publications, California, pp 3–48

Freake D, Crowley P, Steiner M & Drinkwater C 1997 Local heroes. Health Service Journal: 107(5561):28–29

Freire P 1972 Pedagogy of the Oppressed. Penguin Books, Harmondsworth

Fonagy P 1996 Patterns of attachment, interpersonal relationships and health. In: Blane D, Brunner E & Wilkinson R (eds) Health and Social Organization. Routledge, London pp 125–151

Gilbert A 1996 A public health nursing post: the tools for getting started. Nursing Times 92(16):32–35

Gilchrist A 1995 Community Development and Networking. Community Development Foundation Publications, Sheffield

Gillies P 1998 Effectiveness of alliances and partnerships for health promotion. Health Promotion International 13:99–120

Graney A 1996 Community Development: A Health Visiting Perspective. Unpublished research, University of Northumbria at Newcastle

Hancock T 1993 The healthy city from concept to application. In: Davies J K & Kelly M P (eds) Healthy Cities, Research and Practice. Routledge, London

Hancock T & Duhl L 1986 Healthy Cities: Promoting Health in the Urban Context. FADL, Copenhagen

Hunt S M 1987 Evaluating a community development project. British Journal of Social Work 17:661–667

Hunt S M, McEwan J & McKenna S P 1986 Measuring Health Status. Croom Helm, London

Israel B A, Checkoway B, Schulz A & Zimmerman M 1994 Health education and community empowerment: conceptualizing and measuring perceptions of individual, organizational and community control. Health Education Quarterly 21 (2):149–170

Kawachi I, Kennedy B, Lochner K & Prothrow-Stith D 1997 Social capital, income inequality and mortality. American Journal of Public Health 87(9):1491–1498

Labonte R 1997 The population health/health promotion debate in Canada: the politics of explanation, economics and action. Critical Public Health 7(1&2):7–24

Liss P E 1993 Health Care Need, Meaning and Measurement. Avebury, Aldershot

Luker K 1992 Evaluating practice. In: Luker K & Orr J (eds) Health Visiting, Towards Community Health Nursing. Blackwell Scientific Publications, Oxford

Marmot M & Wilkinson R (eds) 1999 The Social Determinants of Health. Oxford University Press, Oxford

McWaters N, Hurwood C & Morton D 1989 Step by step on a piece of string: an illustration of community work as a social health strategy. Community Health Studies 13(1):23–33

O'Neill M 1986 Building bridges between knowledge and action. The Canadian process of healthy community indicators. In: Davies J K & Kelly M P (eds) Healthy Cities Research and Practice. Routledge, London

Procidano M E & Heller K 1983 Measures of percieved social support from friends and from family: three validation studies. American Journal of Community Psychology 11:1–24

Putnam R 1993 Making Democracy Work: civic traditions in modern Italy. Princeton University Press, Princeton, New Jersey

Rissel C 1994 Empowerment: the Holy Grail of health promotion. Health Promotion International 9(1):39–47

Ryan W 1976 Blaming the Victim. Vintage Press, New York

Scottish Assembly 1999 Towards a Healthier Scotland. The Stationery Office, Edinburgh

Seedhouse D 1986 Health: The Foundations for Achievement. John Wiley and Sons, Chichester

Smithies J & Adams L 1993 In: Davies J K & Kelly M P (eds) Healthy Cities, Research and Practice. Routledge, London

Stewart-Brown L & Prothero L 1988 Evaluation in community development. Health Education Journal 47(4):156–161

Tones K & Tilford S 1994 Health Education: Effectiveness, Efficiency and Equity, 2nd edn. Chapman & Hall, London

Tones K, Tilford S & Robinson Y 1990 Health Education: Effectiveness and Efficiency. Chapman & Hall, London

Wadsworth M 1999 Early life. In: Marmot M & Wilkinson R (eds) The Social Determinants of Health. Oxford University Press, Oxford pp 44–63

Welsh Office 1998 Better Health Better Wales. Welsh Office, Cardiff

Wilkinson R 1996 Unhealthy Societies: The Afflictions of Inequality. Routledge, London

World Health Organization 1978 The Alma-Ata Declaration. World Health Organization Chronicle 32:28–29

World Health Organization 1981 Global Strategy for Health for All by the Year 2000. World Health Organization, Geneva

World Health Organization 1985 Health Promotion. A Discussion Document on the Concept and Principles. World Health Organization, Copenhagen

World Health Organization 1986a Targets for Health for All. World Health Organization, Copenhagen

World Health Organization 1986b Ottawa Charter for Health Promotion. World Health Organization, Copenhagen

World Health Organization 1987 The Healthy Cities Project. A Proposed Framework for City Reports. Discussion Paper for the World Health Organization Healthy Cities Symposium. World Health Organization, Copenhagen

World Health Organization 1988 Ecological Models for Healthy Cities Planning. World Health Organization, Copenhagen

World Health Organization 1999 Health 21: Health for all in the 21st century. European Health for All series No. 6. World Health Organization, Copenhagen

3 RESEARCH AND POLICY FOR PUBLIC HEALTH PRACTICE

INTRODUCTION TO SECTION 3

Sarah Cowley

Identifying chapter topics for this section was, perhaps, the most difficult of all because of the breadth of public health work carried out by the various grass roots practitioners. It would have been easy to identify fifteen or even twenty worthy topics for inclusion. Indeed, a health visiting/school nursing development project led from the Department of Health in England has identified funding for around 28 short-term (three-year) leadership posts to operate between 1999 and 2002, with a similar number of initiative projects being set up. A staff support network and database linked to the NHS Learning Network and the Our Healthier Nation Website is being coordinated by the Centre for Innovation in Primary Care in Sheffield, to develop a network for innovation in Health Visiting and School Nursing. Many innovation projects are moving closer to the service development and commissioning remit once carried out by public departments in health authorities, and now being shifted into primary care. Others have identified particular vulnerable groups, such as asylum seekers, the homeless population or looked-after children as a key focus, developing specialist skills in a clearly defined area of need.

Public health attention is always directed at health issues that affect the whole of society, singling out individuals for attention not just because their particular needs affect them personally, but because of the effect on the wider population.

Traditionally, this was the basis for contact tracing and infectious disease control, a pursuit that remains significant in these days of HIV, AIDS, variant CJD and a rise again in tuberculosis infections. Vulnerable groups have also been traditionally singled out for attention by public health; the targeting of 'at risk' groups is, again, not solely because their needs matter as individuals. Of course, individual needs do matter; and public health is concerned with the compassionate relief of suffering, just as any other part of the health service is. It is simply that the reason a service exists or is targeted in a particular way lies in the overall health of the population, whether that is defined in local terms (e.g. caselist or neighbourhood) or nationally. An increasing challenge through the twentieth century, however, as increasingly effective treatments for health problems became available, was to maintain a focus on prevention and on health rather than disease.

This remains the key difficulty in health visiting and for community nurses wishing to focus on public health as we enter the new century. Among the many contenders to be the 'biggest health problem' facing the health of the UK at this time, those difficulties that stem from inequalities in health are perhaps the most far reaching. Because the effect of these social and economic health differences is so profound, it is tempting, as in the twentieth century, to keep trying to seek a cure by focusing only on those groups and individuals who are already facing established problems because of their disadvantaged position. The lure of high-profile needs, with the promise of short-term, measurable changes in health status has a political appeal, too.

The real challenge, however, is to maintain a preventive focus in mainstream services, focusing on the activities that will provide a small immediate, but significant long-term, contribution towards ameliorating health inequalities. In the end, the ordinary, everyday preventive work of mainstream, rather than specialised, public health workers was selected as the focus for this section. Increasingly, the evidence points towards the importance of the early years of life in setting the pattern of health in the adult years; social and emotional support for parents, and the development of coping ability and parenting skills are significant ways of reducing later health inequalities (Acheson 1998).

In the first chapter of this section, Appleton and Clemerson-Trew go further, explaining why child protection should be viewed as a major public health issue. They explain the continuum of need and why this is an issue of concern not only for health visitors and school nurses, but for all nurses working in the community. While this stance may be considered contentious by some, it is consistent with a growing international recognition of the level of harm from this cause. Child abuse is recognised by the World Health Organization (WHO) as a major public health problem that impairs the health and welfare of children and adolescents (Djeddah et al 2000). Prevention requires involvement across a range of levels, including the child, parents, whole family, community and society as a whole (WHO 1999).

In Chapter 10, Dalziel explains ways of engaging the community as a whole in identifying and dealing with the difficulties they perceive as existing for themselves, whether their main issues are focused on child health, housing, transport or anything else. The key message from this chapter is that the priority needs must be defined by those who experience them. A major purpose of the community development philosophy is to promote local empowerment, not dependence on service providers; it is not an approach to be used only by a small proportion of public health workers, but is a key approach and philosophy that should underpin the work carried out by them all. This is not always an easy way of working, particularly if there is political opposition to working without previously defined objectives and aims, set by health service managers or government. However, it is an approach that is very much in tune with recent policy statements, that emphasise the importance of listening to lay views, working *with* communities rather than *for* them (Department of Health 1999a,b, Scottish Executive Health Department 2000).

The Scottish National Health plan is the first major UK policy document to focus strongly on breastfeeding, setting a target of 50 per cent of all mothers brestfeeding at six weeks by 2005 (Scottish Executive Health Department 2000). Again, this is a key public health target, given the enormous impact that breastfeeding (or not) has on the future health of both mother and child. Sally Kendall sets out the evidence in Chapter 11, explaining not only why this is such an important aspect of our national health, but also why it cannot be promoted solely by focusing on individuals who have made a private decision to breastfeed. Instead, a cultural change across society is needed to enable women to choose breastfeeding as the most obvious, natural and straightforward way to feed their infants; this pushes the issue firmly into the public arena.

Finally, public health begins where this book ends: with the family. In his independent review of inequalities in health, Acheson (1998) recommended a strengthening of the emotional and social support offered to families with young children, specifically suggesting that the health visiting role should be strengthened. Paradoxically, as the extent of evidence mounts that home visiting is a very effective mechanism for reducing health inequalities and for preventing a whole a range of health and social problems (Ciliska et al 1999, Elkan et al 2000), so there has been mounting pressure to reduce this form of service delivery. As Bidmead shows in Chapter 12, however, home visiting by rote is not recommended, nor is it the only way of achieving parenting support. Again, the focus is on the needs of the whole population of parents, with groups, parent education, the promotion of coping skills, community and individual development all contributing to the well-being of families, for the good of the public health.

This book could have been twice as long and still had major omissions and readers may well wish to seek more information about the many issues that are not covered. Overall, the book aims to demystify and explain the contribution that can be made by grass roots practitioners to the public health whilst supplying some of the key background research and information about policies needed for practice. Hopefully, therefore, it will suffice for some and whet the appetite for others who wish to develop deeper knowledge about specialist areas of practice or to think of becoming a public health specialist in future.

REFERENCES

Acheson D 1998 Independent inquiry into inequalities in health. The Stationery Office, London

Ciliska D, Mastrilli P, Ploeg J, Hayward S, Brunton G, Underwood J 1999 The effectiveness of home visiting as a delivery strategy for public health nursing intervention to clients in prenatal and postnatal period: a systematic review. Effective Public Health Practice Project for the Public Health Branch, Ontario Ministry of Health, Ontario

Department of Health 1999a Saving Lives: Our Healthier Nation (Cmnd 4386). The Stationery Office, London

Department of Health 1999b Making a Difference: strengthening the nursing, health visiting and midwifery contribution to health and healthcare. Department of Health, London

Djeddah C, Facchin P, Ranzanto C, Romer C 2000 Child abuse: current problems and key public health challenges. Social Science and Medicine 51:905–915

Elkan R, Kendrick D, Hewitt M, Robinson J J A, Tolley K, Blair M, Dewey M, Williams D, Brummell K 2000 The effectiveness of domiciliary visiting: a systematic review of international studies and a selective review of the British literature. Health Technology Assessment 4:13

Scottish Executive Health Department 2000 Our National Health: A plan for action, a plan for change. The Stationery Office, Edinburgh

World Health Organization 1999 Report of the Consultation on child abuse. World Health Organization, Geneva

RESOURCE

Network for innovation in health visiting and school nursing, at the Centre for Innovation in Primary Care, Walsh Court, 10 Bell's Square, Sheffield S1 2FY; email hvsn-network@innovate.org.uk, or go to www.innovate.org.uk.

9 Child protection as a public health issue

Jane Appleton & Jill Clemerson-Trew

KEY ISSUES

- Describing children 'in need' in relation to public health.
- The children in need continuum.
- Child health promotion and the identification of children in need.
- The roles and potential interventions of community health care nurses within the children in need continuum.
- The identification of children in need of protection.

INTRODUCTION

In order to fully promote and advance children's rights within society, it is of fundamental importance that the identification of 'children in need' and the protection of children from abuse are recognised as public health issues. Surprisingly, the work which community nurses undertake to identify needs and protect children is often unacknowledged as public health activity. This chapter will demonstrate how, in current health and social care practice, work with 'children in need' and 'children in need of protection' is increasingly being viewed in this way.

The chapter will initially begin by exploring definitions of 'children in need' and definitions of 'public health'. Although these definitions do not have obvious links, the authors will demonstrate that the identification of children in need, through services that are developed from sound public health principles, is of paramount importance for the well-being of all children in our society. The phrases 'child(ren) in need' and 'child protection' will be used throughout the chapter as these encompass the more recent, broad concept of protecting children, rather than the narrower historical one, usually associated with child abuse. Themes will be developed through the chapter which will illustrate the public health basis of child protection work. These themes will be examined within the context of contemporary community nursing practice.

DEFINITIONS

Defining children in need and child protection

The difficulty in defining child abuse is highlighted by the Department of Health (1995) in 'Messages from Research'. There are many definitions of child abuse

BOX 9.1	Children Act (1989) definitions of 'children in need' and 'significant harm'

A child will be 'in need' (Part III Sect 17(10) p 13) if:

- '...he is unlikely to achieve or maintain, or have the opportunity of achieving or maintaining a reasonable standard of health or development without the provision for him of services by the local authority',
- '...his health or development is likely to be significantly impaired, or further impaired without the provision of such services,' or
- '...he is disabled'.

'Significant harm' (Part IV Sect 31(9) pp 27–28) is defined as:

- '..."harm" means ill-treatment or the impairment of health or development',
- '..."development" means physical, intellectual, emotional, social, or behavioural development',
- '..."health" means physical or mental health',
- '..."ill-treatment" includes sexual abuse and forms of ill-treatment which are not physical'

and the relative nature of this concept is accentuated in Meadow's (1993 p 1) classic definition, where, 'a child is considered to be abused if he or she is treated by an adult in a way that is unacceptable in a given culture at a given time'. The Children Act (1989) defined child protection in terms of 'children in need' and 'significant harm' (see Box 9.1).

When a child protection conference is convened:

'... the conference should consider the following question when determining whether to register a child:

- Is the child at continuing risk of significant harm?

The test should be that either:

- The child can be shown to have suffered ill-treatment or impairment of health or development as a result of physical, emotional, or sexual abuse or neglect, and professional judgement is that further ill-treatment or impairment are likely; *or*
- Professional judgement, substantiated by the findings of enquiries in this individual case or by research evidence, is that the child is likely to suffer ill-treatment or the impairment of health or development as a result of physical, emotional, or sexual abuse or neglect.' (Department of Health 1999b Sect 5(64) p 55).

Over the last twelve years various theories and models for child protection work have been debated and the 'integrated' model is now widely accepted. This child protection model takes an eclectic viewpoint by combining the individual, social, environmental and interactive models, and supports the view that child abuse and neglect is multifactoral; it also recognises the potential complexity of family life. This model has been described by Browne (1995) and encompasses four elements that mitigate for or against the child's present situation. These include:

1. The range of differing relationships and potential disputes between care-givers which may impact on the children.
2. The relationships with and between the children, including the size and spacing of the family, attachments to and expectations of the child(ren).
3. 'Stress generated by the child, for example, an unwanted child' (Browne 1995 p 53), one who is difficult to discipline, demanding or temperamental, or a child who is often ill or has physical or learning disabilities.
4. Environmental and sociological stresses, such as housing issues, social isolation, unemployment, and 'threats to the care-givers authority, values and self-esteem' (Browne 1995 p 53).

'Working Together to Safeguard Children' (Department of Health 1999b Sect 2.17 p 7) recognises that 'there are no absolute criteria on which to rely when judging what constitutes significant harm'. It also suggests sources of stress for children and families based on research, these include social exclusion, domestic violence, mental illness of a parent or carer and drug and alcohol misuse (Department of Health 1999b Sect 2.20–2.24 p 9).

Defining public health

It is not appropriate to offer here detailed definitions and discussion on what constitutes public health as this is being covered elsewhere in this book. However, is it interesting to consider the commonalities between some key definitions of public health and the focus of 'children in need' and 'children in need of protection', as described above. Acheson (1988) defines public health as 'the science and art of preventing disease, prolonging life and promoting health through the organised efforts of society'. The Royal College of Nursing has described public health as:

'A collective view of the health needs and health care of a population rather than an emphasis on an individual perspective. A central component of this collective approach is an emphasis on partnership at all stages and levels of the public health process. This means partnership with communities and clients within them, as well as partnerships across and between professional groups. Team work is an essential prerequisite to effective public health work'. (Royal College of Nursing 1994 p1)

Definitions: discussion

Although the above definitions and models do not have obvious similarities, there are links or parallels that can be drawn between them. Indeed since the mid-1990s there has been a change of focus for much of the work that in the late 1980s and early 1990s would have been considered to be child protection work. Since the publication of 'Messages from Research' (Department of Health 1995) and the subsequent 're-focusing debate' it is widely accepted that child protection must be viewed as a broad concept which includes all elements of 'children in need' and 'significant harm'. This also encompasses the need to preventatively identify children and their families who need professional input and support. Interagency forums and Area Child Protection Committees are largely in agreement that initial responses to referrals should be seen as 'children in need' cases, while the child protection focus is retained for the more serious or chronic cases (Department of Health 1995, 1999b, Thorpe & Bilson 1998).

The structural and organisational efforts of society and communities to support positive outcomes for children and provide advice and guidance for parents must be based on whole-population approaches. Such collective approaches are required, at least initially, to ensure those children who are in need (and their families) are reached and offered services. These approaches to service provision fit closely with the public health concepts as defined above and the expanding public health agenda being proposed in 'Our Healthier Nation' (Department of Health 1998a). Government policy is increasingly recognising the importance of supporting children and their families, while emphasising the need for families and local communities to work more closely together to improve the health outcomes of society.

There are additional key themes in public health working to identify children who may be in need and children who are in need of protection. These include partnership with both children and their parents and between professionals and their agencies to ensure the needs of these children are met (Department of Health 1995, 1999b, 1999c). This theme of partnership fits closely to the definition of public health offered by the Royal College of Nursing (1994), with its emphasis on multidisciplinary activities and professionals working openly together and with families. Indeed 'Working Together to Safeguard Children' (Department of Health 1999b p 75) has outlined 15 basic principles for partnership working between professionals' and families to promote 'best possible outcomes for children'. A further theme is that of 'equity of access', which is a cornerstone of public health work and supported by the professions who provide universal services for children and their families (Burke 1998). Similarly, the concepts of the 'organised efforts of society' which Acheson (1988) describes are reflected in two ways. First, there is a reliance on the community to identify children and families in need of professional support, and secondly they are reflected in the systems set up by individual agencies to ensure children are growing, developing and being educated appropriately.

DESCRIBING 'CHILDREN IN NEED' IN RELATION TO PUBLIC HEALTH

'Child(ren) in need' must be defined as a public health issue using concepts of public health intervention that are principally societal and not those that focus solely on the individual. This is essential so that potentially vulnerable children can be identified at an early stage in the 'children in need' continuum and receive the services and support that they and their families need to maximise the health and well-being of the child and family and potentially to prevent child abuse. The government consultation document 'Supporting Families' (Home Office 1998) reiterated the need for children's interests to be viewed as paramount in our society. It can be argued that there are three reasons why 'children in need' must be viewed as a public health concept:

1. The 'child(ren) in need' continuum.
2. The world view
3. Childhood outcomes.

The 'child(ren) in need' continuum

It is only recently that the idea of 'children in need' has been conceptualised as a continuum. This viewpoint has emerged from 'Messages from Research' (Department of Health 1995), and the 'refocussing debate' which followed the publication of this influential document has confirmed that professionals relate to this viewpoint. The 'refocussing debate' has centred around the need to identify areas in which more interagency work can be undertaken preventatively with 'children in need' rather than waiting until children are 'in need of protection'. It has also highlighted the dilemmas in practice between working preventatively with children in need of services as opposed to children in need of protection. The research evidence presented in this document suggests that the focus on child protection investigation does not result in support to children and families in many cases. In practice there are very good systems in place for the assessment and inquiry into child protection concerns. Yet research demonstrates that much time and energy from social workers is put into this aspect of practice, rather than intervening and working preventatively at an early stage to prevent a higher level of family breakdown (Thorpe & Bilson 1998). This clearly has implications for community health workers.

'Working Together to Safeguard Children' (Department of Health 1999b) emphasises the need for 'initial' and 'core' assessments to consider the welfare needs of children. These assessments are the response to a referral whether or not significant harm is likely to have occurred or to continue. This guidance encourages social services to make assessments with other agencies to prevent further breakdown of the child's situation.

Figure 9.1 illustrates the 'child(ren) in need' continuum and the range of family-centred interventions which community nurses might undertake with families. In the UK, 'children in need' identification is addressed through public health values and concepts, principally universal access to professionals through child health promotion programmes (Hall 1996), which include the total population and ensure follow-up of families who do not initially take up the service. Individual work with a child and family would only take place once a health need has been identified, and this individual focus is not reached unless the whole population has access to child health promotion review services. The Child Health Promotion Programme implemented by health authorities, primary care groups/trusts and community trusts ensures that regular contacts are offered by members of the primary health care team to families with young children. This provides the gateway to health needs assessment and increased levels of preventative intervention by health service personnel (Appleton & Clemerson 1999). This enables professionals to reach all children and identify those who, with their families, are potentially in need of advice, support and guidance, including those children who are potentially vulnerable to abuse. Thus a broad picture of child protection emerges, which encompasses a spectrum ranging from protection from abuse, to protection from disease (immunisation), protection from harm (accidents in the roads and home) through to

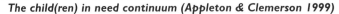

| FIGURE 9.1 | *The child(ren) in need continuum (Appleton & Clemerson 1999)* |

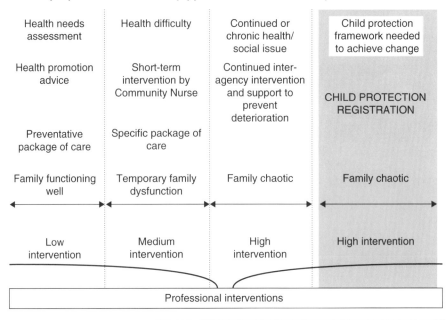

maximising children's potential by stimulation, play and education. It should encourage supported, responsible parenting leading to children reaching their maximum potential socially, emotionally and educationally.

At one end of the continuum (low professional intervention) a parent might seek professional guidance or reassurance which would constitute the beginning of base-line preventative work. For example, a mother seeking advice on a feeding difficulty. This may lead to the professional suggesting ways of managing a difficulty and supporting a change in parenting pattern or referring children in need and their families for specialist assessment and input. Further along the child protection continuum, at the medium intervention level, programmes promoting the development of parenting skills may be offered through family centres or child guidance. Still further along, day or respite care for children might be offered and the provision of services for 'children looked after' (Children Act 1989 Part III Sect 22(1) p 17). At the other end of the continuum, the high level of intervention will include children who are the subject of child protection registration and the minority of cases which culminate in court proceedings (Department of Health 1995). It is important to recognise that multidisciplinary and multiagency assessment and care planning could occur at any point along the continuum. In child protection work this shift from child abuse to concepts on a continuum is analogous to the 'individual vs community discussion' in public health.

The world view

The second reason for viewing 'children in need' as a public health issue is the global recognition or world view of the need for broad concepts of child protection systems and interventions to prevent child exploitation and abuse. Child protection and child abuse does not discriminate against sex, age, social class, community or country, which is illustrated by the international interest in this area and the existence of organisations such as the International Society for the Prevention of Child Abuse and Neglect (ISPCAN). This international society was founded in 1976 with the aim of 'prevent(ing) cruelty to children in every nation, whether cruelty is in the form of abuse, neglect, or exploitation, whether it is in the family or in the society' (ISPCAN 1996 p 4). There are also a number of initiatives to emphasise children's rights, such as the adoption in many countries of the United Nations Convention of the Rights of the Child which was ratified by the UK Government in December 1991. This policy document has led to the increasing development of child-friendly and child-focused policies at a national level in many countries. Progress towards implementing the UN Convention varies from some countries where children are viewed as an integral part of society, to the other extreme where children are still exploited as slave labour and other children are left to live on the streets. Other international organisations promoting children's issues and supported by world governments include the World Health Organization and UNICEF. Clearly it is accepted that child protection issues can and do occur in all cultures and countries across the globe and across all social groups.

Childhood outcomes

The third and perhaps most important argument for viewing 'children in need' as a public health issue is the impact of unidentified or unresolved children in need issues or child abuse on the individual and society. Indeed it is only recently that the government has acknowledged the impact on the public's health of wider influences such as poverty, unemployment, homelessness and social exclusion (Department of Health 1998a). Farrington (1995 p 100) provides evidence of the correlation between problems in child rearing and 'consequent childhood behaviour problems, later delinquency and criminality'. He also highlights the possible long-term mental health and behavioural problems associated with childhood physical abuse or neglect.

Research evidence suggests that there may be a correlation between adult mental health problems, a history of abuse in their past and the subsequent ability to parent successfully and positively rear children (Gibbons et al 1995). Child abuse can result in poor self-esteem or an inability to make social relationships. As a worst-case scenario this may lead to childhood delinquency, offending behaviour, substance misuse and later delinquency, violence and imprisonment. Bifulco and Moran (1998) have illustrated through in-depth interviews with over 800 women, that childhood abuse and neglect can increase the probability of women suffering depression in adult life. Their research evidence also demonstrates how such negative childhood experiences can result in low self-esteem for women and abusive relationships in their adult life. This supports the findings of Mullen et al (1996), who studied the long-term impact of childhood physical, emotional and sexual abuse in a group of women and found that a history of any form of abuse was associated with increased risk of mental health problems, interpersonal problems and sexual difficulties.

A study by Glaser and Prior (1997) indicated links between parental attributes and outcomes for children's emotional health. These parental attributes were mental illness, domestic violence and alcohol or drug misuse, which appeared to impair parenting and affect children's emotional and social development. These researchers raised questions about the appropriateness of professionals' early responses to concerns about children's emotional health. Rather than immediately using formal child protection procedures in the investigation and assessment of suspected emotional abuse, they suggest using alternative strategies, where a multidisciplinary approach is taken and preventative work with the child and family in the form of planned interventions undertaken over a time-limited period.

> 'This process does, however, depend on the parents' recognition of the concerns about the child, and their willingness to become involved and work with professionals towards change' (Glaser & Prior 1997 p 27).

Reder and Duncan (1999) suggest that a further effect of childhood distress can be seen in family life-cycles, particularly at times of transition such as birth, death or loss of a job. Unresolved child in need or child protection issues might affect an adult so their ability to adjust to changes may be prolonged, or result in psychological symptoms or relationship struggles.

'Messages from Research' (Department of Health 1995) has described the long-term ill-effect for children of living in a low-warmth/high-criticism environment as far more damaging than a single incident of over-chastisement. Indeed Smith et al (1995) have estimated that as many as 350 000 children in any one year may be living in this kind of low-warmth/high-criticism environment. Roberts (1996) and Hagell (1998) have also reported the negative impact of children growing up in such uncaring surroundings. Roberts (1996) describes how absence of family support interventions during childhood may result in high levels of aggression and risk-taking behaviour in adulthood. However, it is important to highlight that, in spite of adversity or adverse backgrounds, people can and do rise above past abuse, poverty, loss and relationship difficulties to become mature and balanced individuals (Bifulco & Moran 1998).

In this section the authors have outlined three arguments to explain why work with children in need must be viewed as public health practice. First, the 'children in need' continuum demonstrates that children in need and child protection should be regarded as broad concepts. Secondly, there are initiatives across the world to work with children, who in the context of their culture can be regarded as being 'in need of protection'. Finally, there is evidence which links the failure to address the needs of children to a negative outcome in terms of their social and emotional development and their ability to form positive social relationships.

CHILD PROTECTION STATISTICS

Since 1988 the Department of Health has collated child protection statistics on an annual basis on the numbers of children registered on Local Authority Child Protection Registers, and those subsequently de-registered. Prior to this time no national statistics were maintained (Corby 1990). The most recently available statistics demonstrate that the protection of children is a significant public health issue affecting many children in society.

> 'At 31 March 1999 there were 31 900 children and young people on child protection registers in England. This figure represents [a rate of] 28 children in every 10 000', in the population aged less than 18 years' (Department of Health 1999a).

These statistics are based on the responses from all local authorities with social services responsibilities. However, it is worth pointing out that caution needs to be maintained when interpreting these child protection statistics as they are not a record of all child abuse (Department of Health 1997a). As Corby (1990 p 305) has stated child protection statistics reflect only 'the tip of the iceberg', as 'they do not show the true extent of violence and ill-treatment towards children in our society'. The statistics 'refer only to abuse which is officially recognised' (Corby 1990 p 305).

Another example of the extent of serious injury and death to children is the number of Part 8 reviews carried out by Area Child Protection Committees (ACPCs). Such reviews are conducted, 'when a child dies, and abuse or neglect are known or suspected to be a factor in the death' (Department of Health 1999b p 87). Part 8 reviews examine the involvement of agencies and professionals with the child and family to establish, 'whether there are any lessons to be learned about the ways in which [the agencies] work together to safeguard children' (Department of Health 1999b p 87). Reder and Duncan (1999 p 22) commenting on 'Part 8' notification statistics provided by the Department of Health, report that out of 120 child deaths for the year ending March 1995, '54 were the result of non-accidental injuries', or required further investigation. These researchers also describe the inherent difficulties in estimating child abuse fatalities because of, 'problems of definition, recognition, misdiagnosis and data collection' (Reder & Duncan 1999 p 2). They put forward three arguments for why 'Part 8' reviews do not provide an accurate indicator of non-accidental injury. Reder and Duncan (1999 pp 22–23) state: '"Child abuse" is not a precise diagnosis and parameters for concluding whether maltreatment caused or contributed to a death are ambiguous. It is possible that pathologists and coroners are cautious about recording a death as being the result of non-accidental injuries. Second, criteria for setting up the reviews leave room for flexibility and local circumstances may lead one APCP to review a particular case, which, if it occurred elsewhere, would not be considered necessary. Third, the quality of the information available may not allow a reviewer to form an opinion as to the likely contribution of maltreatment to the child's death.'

Furthermore, the child homicide figures illustrated in Table 9.1 from the Office of National Statistics would be disputed as a gross underestimation of child deaths at the hand of their carers, by organisations purporting to represent children's best interests (Wyre 1998).

The central problem seems to be that accurate figures are not currently recorded for fatal child abuse. Indeed the National Society for the Prevention of Cruelty to Children (NSPCC) in what is described as 'a very conservative estimate' of child homicide, suggests that, 'each week at least one child dies following abuse and neglect' (NSPCC 2000). This organisation is continuing to push for more accurate and reliable official figures. The NSPCC is currently compiling a factfile of the various official government statistics relating to children

TABLE 9.1	Numbers of child deaths (children under 16 years -of -age) through 'child battering and other maltreatment' in England and Wales (Office for National Statistics 1997 Crown copyright material is reproduced with the permission of the Controller of The Stationery Office)

Year	Total Numbers	Boys	Girls
1997	5	4	1
1996	13	8	5
1995	5	4	1
1994	6	2	4

TABLE 9.2	Children looked after by local authorities at 31 March in England (Department of Health 1999a; Crown copyright material is reproduced with the permission of the Controller of The Stationery Office)

	1994	1995	1996	1997	1998	1999
Total	49 300	49 500	50 500	51 000	53 300	55 300
Age groups						
Under 1 year	1400	1600	1600	1700	1800	2200
1–4 years	6500	6700	7300	8100	8700	9200
5–9 years	10 300	10 100	10 500	10 800	11 800	12 500
10–15 years	21 300	21 600	21 600	21 400	22 000	22 400
16 and over	9800	9400	9400	9000	9000	9000

and child protection into a single publication, which it intends to update on an annual basis to review child protection trends. Indeed Wilczynski (1994) and Creighton (1995) also maintain that the official homicide statistics grossly underestimate the actual incidence of fatal child abuse. Furthermore, recent controversial research indicates that the cause of some child deaths, registered by coroners as sudden infant death syndrome (SIDS), may in fact be undiscovered child homicide (Meadow 1999).

The statistics for children looked after by local authorities also provide an indicator of the numbers of children in need. Children looked after include, '(i) children who are accommodated under a voluntary agreement with their parents, (ii) children who are the subject of a care order and (iii) children who are compulsorily accommodated. This included children on remand and those subject to short term emergency orders or the protection of the child' (Department of Health 1997b p 9). In England on 31 March 1999, it was estimated that 53 300 children were being looked after by local authorities (Department of Health 1999a). Table 9.2 illustrates the numbers of children looked after by local authorities since March 1994. It also illustrates the increasing numbers of children looked after by local authorities. 'At 31 March 1999, 4% more [children were looked after] than a year earlier ... representing 49 per 10 000 children under 18' (Department of Health 1999a). Parents may, while recognising the needs of their children and themselves, agree to the use of support by a foster family to augment their parenting ability and/or energies.

Indeed at 31 March 1996, 20 300 (40%) children accommodated by local authorities were placed, with the agreement of their parents, under Section 20 of the Children Act 1989 (Department of Health 1997b). Such placements may be time-limited to cover a period of family or parental stress.

Clearly the above statistics do not offer a complete picture of the numbers of children in need, however, they do go some way towards demonstrating that 'children in need of protection' is a significant public health issue affecting the child population.

CHILD HEALTH PROMOTION AND THE IDENTIFICATION OF CHILDREN IN NEED

Before considering the responsibilities of community nurses in children in need work it is vital to outline the nature of universal services available to all children and families. Children and their families are offered the child health promotion programme (Hall 1996), which is implemented in all provider settings in the United Kingdom by primary health care teams, through the work of GPs, practice nurses and the health visiting and school nursing services. Indeed 'Making a Difference' (Department of Health 1999d) has reiterated the family-centred public health role of many community nurses working with children and young families. The child health promotion programme consists of a planned programme of contacts with the child and parent(s) to review the child's health and development. The ethos of this programme includes a recognition of the vital and 'central role of parents, and the importance of parent "empowerment"' (Hall 1996 p 17), which again reflects a public health approach. It is the vehicle through which health professionals have contact with children and families and undertake both child and family health needs assessment.

As highlighted earlier, child health promotion work forms the basis for assessment and targeted work which is the basis of the child(ren) in need continuum. Figure 9.2 illustrates a public health framework for protecting children in local communities. It highlights the variety of services available to children and their families, ranging from universal services to those specifically for 'children in need' and 'children in need of protection'. It is this universal contact with all children in our communities that guarantees 'equity of access' (Burke 1998) to child health promotion services.

Currently, some disciplines within community nursing provide a universal service to the whole child population in the UK; these are midwifery, health visiting, school nursing and practice nursing. These community nursing disciplines who have a public health role will undoubtedly have more contact with children and families than others, yet it is important to point out that all community nurses have an important potential role in the recognition of children in need and child protection issues.

In 1994 the UKCC (United Kingdom Central Council 1994) adopted four principles, that were initially developed for health visiting practice, as required learning outcomes for community nurse education. Despite a subsequent review which then removed these principles (UKCC 1998), the authors strongly believe that the four principles do continue to provide a substantial framework for delivering public health interventions. Clearly, each community nursing disci-

FIGURE 9.2   *The Public Health Framework in Child Protection*

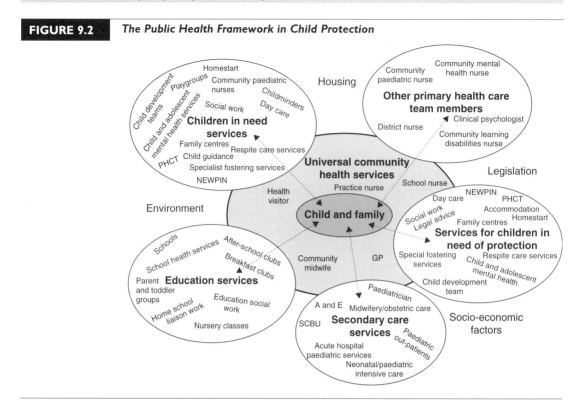

pline has a different focus of practice in relation to child protection. However, all have similar responsibilities in the identification and referral of child(ren) in need of protection. Table 9.3 illustrates the roles and potential interventions of all community health care nurses within the 'child(ren) in need' continuum. This table demonstrates that all disciplines of community nurses, not just those directly associated with children and their families, have a potentially important public health role in the identification of 'children in need' and 'children in need of protection'.

Increased health interventions by community nurses

Midwives, health visitors, practice nurses and school nurses are the main groups of community nurses who will implement the Child Health Promotion Programme and therefore have contact with all children and their parents. This means that they are potentially in a unique position to identify families experiencing stress (Appleton 1996). Community nurses are able to identify those parents who may be in need of advice, support and guidance, including those children who are potentially 'in need' or 'in need of protection'. All health authorities, primary care groups/trusts and community trusts should have clear policies and procedures for employees in suspected or actual child protection cases, as this is a Department of Health requirement (Department of Health and Social Security 1999b). In addition, most community nurses will have access to practice guidelines and protocols, as well as

TABLE 9.3 The roles and potential interventions of community health care nurses within 'the children in need' continuum

Principles	Health Visitor	School Nurse	Community Mental Health Nurse	Community Paediatric Nurse	District Nurse	Practice Nurse	Midwife	Community Learning Disability Nurse
Search for health needs	Contact with each family in order to identify health needs and parenting difficulties. This contact may be on an individual basis or through community groups	Review of each school child's record at school entry in order to identify health needs, particularly emotional and social health	Through work with parents with mental health difficulties, identifying the effects of these on family dynamics and children's emotional health	Contact with families with sick children cared for at home and the recognition of the changes in family dynamics and support systems	Contact with children through their grandparents, parents/carers or direct contact with sick children. Identifying the effects of ill-health in the family on the child	Contact with pre-school children through the immunisation programme. Identification of parenting support needs	Contact with antenatal and postnatal parents. Identify negative attitudes to parenting and concerns around parent/baby dynamics	Contact with children of clients with learning disabilities. Identifying the effect of the learning disability on family dynamics and parenting skills
Stimulation of awareness of health needs	Raise issues surrounding children and family health and parenting needs with the individual family	Raise issues surrounding children's health needs with the individual child and potentially their family	Encouraging parents to recognise the effects of their mental health difficulties on the child	Enabling the family to be aware of the normal processes of emotional adaptation to having a sick child	Encourage the family to be aware of the emotional needs of the child in relation to ill-health in a close family member	Raising issues with the parent surrounding the need for parenting support	Raising issues with the parent surrounding the need for adjustment to being parents and skills support	Consistently work with clients to ensure their awareness of the need to enhance parenting abilities
Facilitation of health-enhancing activities	Providing a planned programme of care, e.g. behaviour modification programme for an identified health need	Providing a planned programme of care for a child's health need in partnership with the family, e.g. nutrition or self-esteem	Encourage self-awareness in parents and the need to recognise and reward positive behaviour in the child. Liaison with HV and SN	Encouraging the family to adapt their coping mechanisms for living with a sick child at home. Liaison with HV and SN	Making use of strategies and adapting coping mechanisms to meet the emotional needs of the family. Liaison with HV and SN	Advise contact with HV, GP and SN and liaise with these professionals	Encouraging self-awareness skills and teaching practical baby care skills. Liaison with HV, GP and paediatrician	Provide detailed and practical programmes of care which will teach and reinforce parenting abilities. Liaison with HV and GP
Influence on policies affecting health	Influencing local children's services and child protection policies and practice development	School population health initiatives often involving parents	Representing and campaigning on behalf of the client group	Representing the support needs of families with sick children locally	Representing the support needs of a family with a sick member	Influencing the development of primary health care team child protection practice	Influencing the development of preventative child protection practice between midwifery and primary health care services	Representing the rights of this client group and their children in the development of child-care services.

focused training and clinical supervision, which will aid in the identification of families who may be experiencing stress or vulnerability. Furthermore, community nurses should be referring to the 'Framework' recently outlined by the Department of Health (2000) for assessing children in need and their families. This document offers a core foundation for a systematic approach to assessing children and families needs, while emphasising the need to safeguard and promote children's welfare. It incorporates three key areas (Department of Health 2000 p 17):

- Developmental needs of children
- Capacity of parents or caregivers to respond appropriately to those needs
- Impact of wider family and environmental factors on parenting capacity and the child.

The following sections will explore and illustrate the levels of family-based interventions that community nurses may undertake with children in need.

Low professional intervention

An important emphasis in community nurse education is a focus on the development of effective interpersonal and assessment skills. This enables practitioners to develop a flexible approach with families and to understand the broad range of family circumstances and backgrounds. The working relationship formed with families plays a significant role in influencing the preventive public health work in the community. Society recognises that parenting is not easy and that all parents need advice, support and sources of knowledge and all parents learn skills as they parent (Home Office 1998).

The possession of well developed assessment skills is a fundamental area of responsibility for all community nurses in order that children's and their parents' health needs can be competently identified. Through the Child Health Promotion Programme a parent would be offered health promotional advice and would have the opportunity to ask for specific guidance on an expressed health need (Ewles & Simnett 1995). Indeed, Gould (1998) would argue that it is the working relationship formed with individuals which informs preventive public health work. It is essential that the advice given by the community nurse is delivered in a sensitive and acceptable way, in the context of a professional caring and befriending relationship. This type of health promotional advice is invariably related to the age and developmental stage of the child and may include a focus on the parents' health need. It is often included in a protocol that covers the Child Health Promotion Programme, for example, advice given by a practice nurse both before and following administration of a baby's immunisation.

Medium professional intervention

In view of their role in implementing the Child Health Promotion Programme midwives, health visitors and school nurses are in a unique position to identify the necessity for a health need assessment and the requirement to undertake short-term preventative work with families experiencing stress. Following an initial or targeted child and family health assessment the community nurse may identify one or more health needs that need short-term, targeted intervention with individual families or school children. For example, a parent might seek professional guidance or reassurance from a midwife or health visitor and this may lead to the professional suggesting ways of managing a difficulty and supporting a change in parenting pattern. In addition, the community nurse might enable the parents to join a suitable peer group which would meet their support needs. A school health service example might be when a child has been bullied and the school nurse is working with the teacher and parents to increase the child's self-esteem and ability to socialise appropriately with his/her peers.

Community mental health nurses are available to advise and assist health visitors and community midwives in the assessment of mothers who appear to be emotionally low or depressed in the early weeks and months following a baby's birth. This may result in a period of short-term support and counselling for the mother, and possibly her partner, from one of the community nurses. Close liaison with other members of the primary health care team, e.g. the GP and clinical psychologist, would be an essential element of practice. Such joint assessment, support and interprofessional supervision by members of the primary health care team is a core element of public health working.

An illustration of the type of short-term targeted intervention undertaken by a health visitor could be management of a child's sleep problem. As part of the Child Health Promotion Programme preventative advice on the establishment of a child's sleep pattern will normally have been given at the 8-month contact. If the parents then raise further concerns about difficulties in their child's sleep pattern at the 18-month–2-year contact, the health visitor would offer a targeted care plan to the parents which is likely to consist of 3–4 home visits. At the first visit the health visitor would explore and assess sleeping routines and agree a sleep-management programme. Subsequent visits would evaluate with the parents the success of the agreed programme, assessing any subtle changes to the child's routine and encouraging and praising where there has been obvious improvement.

The above shows some examples of the type of short-term preventive work which has been particularly highlighted for its importance by the Report of the National Commission of Inquiry into the Prevention of Child Abuse (National Society for the Prevention of Cruelty to Children 1996). However, when a professional such as a health visitor holds a caseload of 350–450 families and school nurses cover a population of 2500 school-aged children, realistically their increased interventions with families can only be short-term and targeted. There cannot be an expectation by the individual health professional or other agencies that health visitors and school nurses can work intensively over a considerable period of time with a child or family. However, there are currently government moves to promote positive parenting and family friendly initiatives within the Department of Health and Home Office policy, which will impact on community nursing practice, for example 'Sure Start' initiatives and the green paper 'Supporting Families' (Home Office 1998). Health visitors have been cited as key health professionals in preventative work with families who might experience parenting stresses.

In the long term, the health visitor will have ongoing contact with the family to evaluate and reassess the care plan and family's circumstances and their care plan may change to focus on enabling the mother and children to engage with local support networks. For example, a local mother and toddler group. Any ongoing support for parenting skills could be met by referral to a family centre. The worth of such tangible, albeit short-term, support from an approachable and caring health professional is often underrated. The bottom line is, it's about parents being valued, believed and not condemned, and somebody saying to them 'well done'.

High professional intervention

High intervention cases will involve working jointly with another agency or another section of the health service. A key feature of this level of working is that the professional who identifies the need for this level of intervention will remain proactively engaged with the family. This will include ongoing work and the monitoring of progress with the other agencies or professional group who are involved. It is not a case of referring the family and being able to withdraw after a short period of support. Box 9.2 offers a case history example of high-intervention work.

BOX 9.2   *High-intervention work case history*

The family has three children aged five, three and fifteen months and the mother is six months pregnant. Mother's first partner left when she was pregnant with her second child and she met her present partner soon after the birth of that baby. Both the mother and her partner have stormy relationships with their families and have spent periods in care as children when their parents were going through difficult times. The five-year-old is not in school regularly, is difficult to manage in class, has a poor concentration span and appears to have difficulty in coordination. The class teacher and the school's head have met the mother once to discuss this but she has now failed to attend two arranged meetings. The school nurse has carried out school-entry screening of vision, hearing and growth and because of the school's concerns has referred for a specialist school medical.

The three-year-old is shy and very quiet with delayed speech; she has a place in the local day nursery and has had appointments arranged with the speech therapist. She has not been taken to the day nursery regularly and is in danger of losing the place, and has failed to attend her last appointment with the speech therapist. The fifteen-month-old baby girl gained weight erratically between the ages of four and ten months and the heath visitor wondered if she was being fed regularly. Mother has been to the GP to confirm her pregnancy and was booked in to see the midwife at the next antenatal session. As she had diabetes of pregnancy with her last baby her health assessment is particularly important, however she has not attended any appointments.

The family seemed initially to cope well but as successive children have come along a pattern of lurching from crisis to crisis has developed. They regularly seek financial support from social services and have difficulty paying the rent and the debts from the last time they were nearly evicted.

BOX 9.2	*Cont'd*

Following assessment, the identification of health needs and the agreement of care plans, the family has already had considerable offers of support for the issues relating to each of the children and have not been able to consistently take up that support. The pattern of their difficulty in coping is affecting the children. The school teachers, the school nurse and the health visitor are concerned that the parents need to be confronted with the effects on the children and offered a comprehensive care programme including support for their parenting skills.

The health visitor has tried to work with the family, as agreed with them in a care plan, to enable them to take up the services that would support their parenting, with increasingly little success. She has offered to work with them on stimulating and playing with the children and on the programme outlined by the speech therapist. The midwife has tried to visit at home, as well as inviting the mother to clinics, however contact has not yet been established. The health visitor and school teacher/head teacher make a joint 'child in need' referral to social services suggesting a meeting to share information about their professional assessments and to agree a multiagency approach to the family that would aim to result in their cooperation with a support package. This package or plan would include some of the issues and plans that the single agencies have been working on. Its strength comes from the joint approach to the family by the agencies and the negotiation with the parents about the seriousness of the needs of the children and the support on offer for them to change.

There is usually a time-lag between referral to social services and a meeting with the family to agree a care plan. Social services having received the referral have the responsibility of collating the assessment data from all the professionals who have been working with the family to varying degrees of success. During this time, the midwife and school health service would continue to try to establish contact, while the health visitor would be the most appropriate person to support the family while reiterating the need for change and that professionals are there to help.

In the above case history, if the family refuse to cooperate or just continue to avoid contacts and appointments, then the agencies would need to discuss whether the children were suffering continuing risk of significant harm and whether child protection procedures were needed.

Work with families whose parenting difficulties or vulnerabilities are long-lasting or chronic in nature is often perceived by health and other professionals as particularly difficult and challenging. Although an individual practitioner may not have very many families who need this level of intervention, the workload is widely acknowledged as being high and sometimes stressful (Appleton 1996).

These examples have been offered as an illustration of the range of increased interventions that can be offered to children and families where there is an identified health need. They are family-based interventions along the 'child(ren) in need' continuum, which the authors have demonstrated is a fundamental element of public health community nursing practice.

THE IDENTIFICATION OF CHILDREN IN NEED OF PROTECTION

The identification of children in need of protection flows from single agency work with 'children in need' and their families. Where single agency 'children in need' work has not resulted in improvement for the children there will be a need to discuss the child and family's situation with an agency which has statutory responsibility under The Children Act (1989). The Act identifies social services as the agency statutorily responsible for carrying out assessments of 'children in need' and 'children in need of protection'. The above case history example (Box 9.2) illustrates how health professionals regularly identify the need for social work intervention and support in such families. However, research evidence indicates that until recently social work intervention has often only been accessible if a referral is couched as a child protection issue (Gibbons et al 1995, Hallett 1995). It is important to clarify at this point that the majority of cases fall within 'child(ren) in need' referral criteria and only in chronic or very severe cases will a child protection investigation be needed.

'Messages from Research' (Department of Health 1995) suggests that the best course of action to meet the needs of the majority of children and their families is a 'child in need' inquiry. As already outlined, although social services are the responsible statutory agency for such inquiries, many professionals who are in contact with the family will have undertaken a recent needs assessment and can provide that information for social services. Following this initial assessment a meeting is held between the professionals and the family, the focus of which should be the parent's perception of the child(ren)'s needs and what would enable those needs to be met. This meeting should result in a plan that is agreed between all parties to address the child(ren)'s and parent's needs. This form of joint working has been outlined as part of the refocusing debate and falls within children in need legislation in The Children Act (1989 Sect 17). The recently published 'Working Together to Safeguard Children' (Department of Health 1999b) guidance reiterates the need for social services coordination of multiagency children in need assessments that result in welfare support for the child and family. The joint agency care plan agreed with the parents should include practical steps that the parents agree to carry out to achieve change in their parenting with the support of appropriate professionals. Some activities may be jointly undertaken, for example a family centre worker and speech therapist might work with the parents on a child's language development. The extended family may also be included in the care plan, for example to give regular breaks for the parents.

After a relatively short period of intensive work with a family on a joint agency 'children in need' care plan, it will be clear whether the family are able and willing to change, with support, the patterns that resulted in the original concerns for the children. The reasons for a lack of improvement are usually multifactorial and may be due to the family's inability to change or due to their avoidance of professionals who are offering support and intervention. Other reasons might include situations where a family or parents do not agree with the professionals' assessment and do not perceive the need to change their parenting patterns and behaviours. It is important to recognise that a minority of parents may not be able to put their children's needs before their own and this is usually due to other influences in their lives such as the use of drugs or alcohol, mental health difficulties or being in a relationship that makes a parent very vulnerable (Glaser & Prior 1997). In these cases it will be of vital importance to formally consider whether the children are 'at risk of significant harm'. This will usually be addressed through child protection procedures, including a social services investigation and a child protection conference.

If the child protection conference decides to place children on the child protection register the resulting child protection plan may not differ significantly to the 'children in need' care plan that may have preceded it. This reflects that the changes needed for the physical, emotional and social health of the child(ren) and family are not different, but that the context of the work is more formal and potentially 'serious'. It is only after this progression from 'children in need' work through child protection procedures that professionals can demonstrate that a court case for the protection of the children should be considered. A court case will only be appropriate when the preventative 'children in need' work and the child protection plan have not resulted in major improvements for the children and their family. In the majority of cases, the identification of 'children in need of protection' flows from 'children in need' work. The assessment of risk and subsequent framework for work with the family will usually be related to the omissions or commissions of parents and their ability or willingness to change. It is therefore apparent that contributions by health professionals working with children 'in need' or 'in need of protection' should be a progression from normal working practices within a framework of good quality needs-based clinical practice.

CONCLUSION

There is a continuing debate within community nursing about the extent to which services generally, and not only in terms of 'child(ren) in need', should be targeted at the level of the individual or the community. The authors have argued that child protection work based on the principles of public health must adopt a combination of both whole-population and individual approaches. In order to view 'child protection' as a public health concept, practitioners will need to be familiar with the 'child(ren) in need' continuum and the concepts of universality and targeted services. Universal services will be necessary at an initial contact or assessment level to identify the 'needs' of a given population, which can then be targeted and met through group and community work or individual interventions, such as support to parents. 'Child(ren) in need' can only be targeted by ensuring universal contact with all children in our communities.

In addition, community practitioners will need to be knowledgeable about the legislative and multiagency practice issues surrounding the very different concepts of children 'in need' and 'in need of protection'. The chapter has described how the Child Health Promotion Programme is the universal service offered to all families with children. This review programme ensures contacts at key child developmental stages and provides the gateway to family health needs assessment from which targeted family-based interventions may ensue. The authors feel strongly that it must be in children's best interests for society to ensure that effective steps are taken to identify the needs of children, as research evidence indicates that a failure to address these needs may lead to negative outcomes in terms of a child's social development, emotional growth and ability to form positive social relationships. Throughout the chapter the authors have therefore illustrated that it is these two concepts, that of a universal initial contact service and the 'children in need' continuum, which underpin both effective professional practice and provide the foundation for all public health work with children and their families

DISCUSSION QUESTIONS

- Discuss how the concept of the 'children in need continuum' would benefit multidisciplinary and multiagency work.
- Discuss how in your professional practice the child health promotion programme will lead to the identification of children in need.
- Looking at Figure 9.2, list the contact names for each service in your practice area.
- Using case examples from group members, discuss the assessments that would be available from health professionals to forward with a referral of a child and their family to social services.

ACKNOWLEDGEMENT

Ideas for this chapter developed from an article first published in Community Practitioner (1999) 72(5):134–136.

FURTHER READING

Clarke M L 2000 Out of the wilderness and into the fold: the school nurse and child protection. Child Abuse Review 9(5):364–374

Department of Health 2000 Assessing Children in Need and their Families: Practice Guidance. The Stationery Office, London

Department of Health, Department of Education, Home Office 2000 Framework for the Assessment of Children in Need and their Families. The Stationery Office, London

REFERENCES

Acheson D 1988 Public Health in England. HMSO, London.

Appleton J V 1996 Working with vulnerable families: a health visiting perspective. Journal of Advanced Nursing 23:912–918

Appleton J & Clemerson J 1999 Family-based interventions with children in need. Community Practioner 72 (5):134-136

Bifulco A & Moran P 1998 Wednesday's Child. Routledge, London

Browne K 1995 Child abuse: defining, understanding and intervening. In: Wilson K & James A (eds) The Child Protection Handbook. Baillière Tindall, London

Burke W 1998 Letter to Members of the RCN Health Visitor Forum. Royal College of Nursing, London

Corby B 1990 Making use of child protection statistics. Children and Society 4(3):304–314

Creighton S J 1995 Fatal child abuse – How preventable is it? Child Abuse Review 4:318–328

Department of Health 1989 An Introduction to the Children Act 1989. HMSO, London

Department of Health/Dartington Social Research Unit 1995 Child Protection: Messages from Research. HMSO, London

Department of Health 1997a Statistics of Children and Young People on Child Protection Registers. Year Ending 31 March 1997, England. Government Statistical Service, London

Department of Health 1997b Children Looked After by Local Authorities. Year Ending 31 March 1996, England. Government Statistical Service, London

Department of Health 1998a Our Healthier Nation: a contract for health (Cmnd 3852). The Stationery Office, London

Department of Health 1998b Health and Personal Social Service Statistics 1998. The Stationery Office, London Web site at http://www.doh.gov.uk/HPSSS/INDEX.HTM

Department of Health 1999a Health and Personal Social Service Statistics 1999. The Stationery Office, London Web site at http://www.doh.gov.uk/HPSSS/INDEX.HTM

Department of Health 1999b Working Together to Safeguard Children: A guide for inter-agency working to safeguard and promote the welfare of children. Department of Health, London

Department of Health 1999c Framework for the Assessment of Children in Need and their Families. Consultation Draft. Department of Health, London

Department of Health 1999d Making a Difference: strengthening the nursing, midwifery and health visiting contribution to health and health care. Department of Health, London

Department of Health 2000 Framework for the Assessment of Children in Need and their Families. The Stationery Office, London

Ewles L & Simnett I 1995 Promoting Health: A Practical Guide, 3rd edn. Scutari Press, London

Farrington D 1995 Intensive health visiting and the prevention of juvenile crime. Health Visitor 68(3):100–102

Gibbons J, Conroy S & Bell C 1995 Operating the Child Protection System: A Study of Child Protection Practices in English Local Authorities. HMSO, London

Glaser D & Prior V 1997 Is the term child protection applicable to emotional abuse? Child Abuse Review 6:315–329

Gould E 1998 All for one and one for all. Nursing Times 94(1):32–33

Hagell A 1998 Dangerous Care: reviewing the risks to children from their carers. Policy Studies Institute, University of Westminster, London

Hall D M B 1996 Health for all Children. Report of the Third Joint Working Party on Child Health Surveillance. Oxford University Press, Oxford

Hallett C 1995 Interagency Coordination in Child Protection. HMSO, London

Home Office 1998 Supporting Families: a consultation document. The Stationery Office, London

International Society for the Prevention of Child Abuse and Neglect 1996 Eleventh International Congress on Child Abuse and Neglect. Conference Programme. International Society for Prevention of Child Abuse and Neglect, Dublin

Meadow R (ed) 1993 ABC of Child Abuse, 2nd edn. BMJ Publishing Group, London

Meadow R 1999 Unnatural sudden infant death. Archives of Disease in Childhood 80:7–14

Mullen P E, Martin J L, Anderson J C, Romans S E & Herbison G P 1996 The long term impact of the physical, emotional, and sexual abuse of children: a community study. Child Abuse and Neglect 20(1):7–21

National Society for the Prevention of Cruelty to Children 1996 Report of the National Commission of Inquiry into the Prevention of Child Abuse. Childhood Matters. Volume 1: The Report. The Stationery Office, London

National Society for the Prevention of Cruelty to Children 2000 About the NSPCC – Some Key facts. NSPCC, London Web site at http://www.nspcc.org.uk/aboutus/

Office for National Statistics 1997 Statistics for child battering and other maltreatment. In: Mortality Statistics Cause England and Wales (Series DH2, No. 24). Office for National Statistics, London

Reder P & Duncan S 1999 Lost Innocents. A Follow-up Study of Fatal Child Abuse. Routledge, London

Roberts I 1996 Family support and the health of children. Children and Society 10:217–224

Royal College of Nursing 1994 Public Health: Nursing Rises to the Challenge. Royal College of Nursing, London

Smith M, Bee P, Heverin A & Nobes G 1995b Parental control within the family: the nature and extent of parental violence to children. In: Department of Health/Dartington Social Research Unit (eds) Child Protection Messages from Research. HMSO, London

Thorpe D & Bilson A 1998 From protection to concern: child protection careers without apologies. Children and Society 12:373–386

United Kingdom Central Council 1994 The Future of Professional Practice – the Council's standards for education and practice following registration. UKCC, London

United Kingdom Central Council 1998 Standards for Specialist Education and Practice. UKCC, London

Wilczynski A 1994 The incidence of child homicide: how accurate are the official statistics? Journal of Clinical Forensic Medicine 1:61–66

Wyre R 1998 Understanding the perpetrator. Paper presented at the 'Protecting the Child in Need' Conference. Institute of Education, London, 10 December

10 Community development as a public health function

Yvonne Dalziel

KEY ISSUES

- The origins and influences on community development.
- Exploration of the key concepts of community development in health.
- Refocusing health visiting to a model of community development practice
- The development of methods appropriate to community development ethics.
- Application of community development process to key areas of health visiting practice.

INTRODUCTION

It is generally agreed that poor health and poverty are inextricably linked and that ill-health will not be solved by medicine, but by more effective public health measures and socioeconomic change. An equitable and accessible food supply, tackling crime, responding differently to mental health issues and housing and environmental needs and to the building of social capacity are some of the issues which, if addressed, would have a long-term impact on community health.

This chapter suggests that the ideology and methods of community development offer nurses involved in public health work an approach to address the inequalities in health which underpin many of the health problems in our communities. It will briefly explore the historical context of community development and the radical influences on the community health movement in the 1960s and 1970s that are arguably still pertinent to the implementation of a public health nursing strategy today.

The outline of a model of community development that focuses on child health will suggest how the application of the methods to one area of nursing activity can have an impact on the health of the wider community. Finally, the chapter suggests that if community development is to become the mainstream approach, nurses will need strong leadership, changes in the nurse education curriculum, and the development of structures and policies to support them in thinking and doing differently.

COMMUNITY DEVELOPMENT: ORIGINS AND INFLUENCES

Although community development is now gaining recognition as an approach to health, the methods and thinking that constitute community development are not new. Jones (1990) suggests that it was used by colonial governments to, 'ensure the governability and modernisation of their empires' (Jones 1990 p 32). It was more recent events, however, that nurtured its growth and its value as an approach to addressing health issues.

According to Jones (1990), community development and health work has evolved over the last ten years, incorporating a number of different influences which have built onto a basic community development model. The growing movement in health occurring in the last few decades has used community development as an ideological and practical framework to bring about change in how health as a concept is regarded. Previously used as a method in community work to address housing and social policy needs, the first health projects using community development principles did not appear in the UK until the late 1970s. The emergence of social movements of the late 1960s and 1970s, like the women's movement, civil rights, black power and the self-help movement, were key influences in supporting the growth of the approach.

A social movement is defined as: 'collectively acting with some continuity to promote change in the society or group to which it is a part' (Turner & Killian in Schiller & Levin 1983 p 1344). The social movements of this time grew from the disaffection of people who felt marginal to and excluded from decision-making processes. It was a reaction to the dominant male, white middle-class systems and the attitudes that discriminated against women, black people and the poor. The movements demanded justice, freedom, democracy and the end of discrimination. Underpinning their emergence was a belief system that held the primacy of individual experience as the basis of knowledge and expertise. The primary challenge of both the women's health movement, (which grew out of the women's liberation movement) and the self-help movement was to demystify health knowledge and take its ownership away from the male-dominated medical profession, which so jealously guarded it as its own. As a consequence they developed an anti-professional view of health and the causes of ill-health and encouraged individuals to become experts in their own bodies. They encouraged people to view what they knew, derived from their own experiences, as being as important as the theoretical knowledge that had evolved conceptually and been filtered through a dominant male medical ideology. In consciousness-raising and self-help health groups, women began to see how this latter view of themselves was reinforced by their contact with the medical profession and that it adversely affected their health and their access to health services.

The Black Report (Townsend & Davidson 1982) indicated that the groups for whom the social movements had, potentially, the greatest impact were those who are socially and economically disadvantaged, who are more likely to experience poorer health and have shorter lives than more affluent people. The community development ethos will bring into the awareness of nurses that these groups of people and others who feel socially excluded from mainstream society, e.g. homeless, disabled, etc, have knowledge and experience about their own lives that when harnessed can strengthen and sustain their communities.

The right of people to participate in health decisions is enshrined in the Alma-Ata Declaration of 1977 (World Health Organization 1978). It states that, 'the people have a right and a duty to participate individually and collectively in the planning and implementation of their care'. The desire for a public health movement to tackle health problems resulted in 1981 in the WHO policy 'Health For All by the year 2000'. Central to the attainment of its targets is the development of primary care and the concepts of participation, collaboration and equity that were central to the Alma-Ata Declaration.

The dominance of the medical model in public health thinking and its focus on epidemiology and medicine has left an ontological deficit in what nurses working in public health know about the poorest communities; what they need to promote health and to build the social capacity of their neighbourhoods and communities. Nurse involvement in public health work, through activities like community-based needs assessment and public involvement in primary care planning and delivery of services, would legitimate the community development approach and support the move away from the clinical model based on individual transactions to a social contract with entire communities (Ashton & Seymour 1988). To fit the new agenda of addressing social as well as individual change in health, community nursing practice requires change in its approach to health as a concept and to the methods and the activities of its daily practice.

The key tenets of a community development approach – collective action, self-determination, democracy and promotion of self-confidence – are central to any policy to tackle inequalities in health. So what is community development, how does it fit into public health work and what activities might health visitors engage in to bring about change?

ELEMENTS OF COMMUNITY DEVELOPMENT

A community development approach is a useful way to move from exclusion to inclusion in the decision-making process for marginal groups, and the principles of the approach could form an essential ideology for groups of nurses. The approach is concerned with the notion of shared power between health professionals and lay people and the move from dependency to involvement. The concepts which underpin this approach are about equal access to resources, promoting democracy and involvement in decision-making about health, taking action to bring about change, sharing power and working in partnership with communities.

Underlying each is the concept of shared authority. This means that each person takes equal responsibility for the decision-making and each is accountable for the outcomes. Although conceptually different, each element of community development is related to and has an impact on the others. For example, when individuals are involved as equal partners and their knowledge affirmed, skills used and opinions heard, they feel more in control and are then more able to begin to form alliances with others to bring about the changes they desire. A brief outline of each of the different elements will demonstrate this.

Equity

Although very closely connected and often confused as one concept, equity and equality are not the same thing. People all have the right to equal access to available health services for the maintenance and promotion of health but, to be fair, people do not all need to be treated in the same way. Instead, those who stand to benefit the most and whose needs are the greatest are given priority: this is 'equity'. In a culture of scarce resources, this may mean unequal distribution, even taking away from the most well-off to give extra services to the most needy. All too often, what happens is the opposite; those most in need have the worst or fewest services. Inequalities in health care are not only about the provision of services but also how those services are delivered. Addressing inequalities means challenging practices that discriminate against individuals on whatever basis – poverty, race, disability, language, sexuality or age – in the provision of essentials for health. It also involves examining the provision, quality, uptake, accessibility and availability to those who have the greatest need.

Empowerment

This is also discussed at length in Chapter 7. Rappaport defines empowerment as 'the process by which people, organisations and communities gain mastery over their lives' (Rappaport et al 1984 p 3). The empowerment process involves building individual and collective confidence and raising the esteem of individuals and communities through valuing their knowledge and experience and supporting them to be part of the decision-making process. Kiefer (1983) views empowerment as attainment of what he calls 'participatory competence'. Beigal (1984) views empowerment as both capacity and equity; capacity being use of power to solve problems and equity referring to getting one's fair share of resources. Empowerment skills include problem-solving, assertiveness and confidence-building strategies.

Participation

The concept of participation is about supporting the people who are affected by decisions to have some influence over their outcome, and for nurses it is an important approach to the attainment of health. Perceptions of power affects participation. Steve Lukes (1978) suggests that there are different levels of power; the visible manifestations of power, the unseen but tangible manifestations of power, and internalised powerlessness. People on the margins of society experiencing this third level of powerlessness become passive and dependent. Believing themselves unable to influence events and decisions affecting their lives, they consciously exclude themselves from opportunities to be part of the process of decision-making. People who experience internal powerlessness are often those who do not attend for clinic appointments, come to parentcraft classes or attend their children's school evenings. They don't believe their involvement can make a difference to their lives.

Keifer (1983) suggests that participatory competence is a life-long achievement and includes three aspects:

1. Development of a more positive self-concept or sense of self-competence
2. Construction of more critical or analytical understanding of surrounding social and political environment, and
3. Cultivation of individual and collective resources for social and political action.

Consultation, rather than participation, happens when decisions have already been made and there is little likelihood of any change but the public is still asked

| BOX 10.1 | *Levels of participation or involvement (adapted from Taylor et al 1997)* |

1. **Information giving** – details of services, decision-making structures, helplines, media slots, etc.
2. **Gathering information** – views on existing services, needs assessment, concerns about services, focus groups, community meetings.
3. **Consultation** – asking for comment on formulated plans or proposals.
4. **Involvement in policy development and decision-making** – getting users directly involved with management to develop training and quality standards for professional staff.
5. **Joint working** – equal basis to develop projects, services, information packs, local forum, community health projects.
6. **Community or user control** – involvement in planning and delivering services.

to comment about a proposal. This is a poor substitute for real participation and being part of the planning process. There are six different levels of participation or involvement from information-giving to user-control (Box 10.1).

Nurses can support their communities to be involved in any of these different levels. Involving people as part of the decision-making process is beneficial not only to the people living in communities but to the service providers. Giving users a voice in what they need avoids mismatch of services and may in the long run be more economical.

Partnership and alliances

A key concept in the community development process is partnership and the building of alliances. Alliance is defined as partnership for action; a virtual organisation that is created by the interaction between partner agencies and sectors (Duffy 1996). The purpose of agencies working together and with local people is to develop common priorities and strategies on issues and policies that affect health. Partnerships for health work involve a wider spectrum than that usually associated with the health sector. For example, a health alliance would involve nurses working in partnership with agencies such as environmental health, education, social work, voluntary organisations, health projects, work places and local industries. Funnell et al (1995) identify five key features of alliance building (Box 10.2).

The culture of fundholding in primary care has left a legacy of isolation and actively not working with others, that may linger for some time. Fundholding did not support partnership and alliances with other practitioners, let alone other agencies or the community in which the practice was located. General practitioners were encouraged to believe that they owned their nurses and often referred to community staff as 'my health visitor' or 'my district nurse'. Working from within general practice, with its small-business focus and therefore some competition with other practices, nurses were often prevented from

| BOX 10.2 | *Features of alliance building (Funnell et al 1995)* |

- Commitment to the shared goals of the alliance
- Community involvement in all alliance activities – community representatives must have the necessary training and skills to participate equally
- Communication where partners share relevant information and commit to simplicity, openness and honesty
- Joint working with equal ownership and appropriate input from each partner
- Accountability
- Evaluation is built into alliance work and results are used constructively

working with their colleagues in neighbouring areas because they might be giving benefit to patients from another practice. This is contrary to new thinking about health and public involvement and fragments community work. Nurses need to defend their right to work with geographical, as opposed to practice, populations and to be part of the move to shift resources away from practices to communities. The benefits of community partnerships to nurses in relation to pooling information, knowledge, experience, skills and resources are too important to the promotion of health to be lost to medical politics. Joint working can be more efficient and effective and can widen and deepen the impact of health initiatives. In return, nurses must be willing to share knowledge and power with each other and other agencies and, importantly, the community and to be involved in supporting community involvement.

Collective action

The author's and other experienced community development worker's experience suggests that the knowledge of what constitutes community development in primary care is very incomplete. Many health visitors maintain that they have been working in community development for years and need learn nothing new. They believe that running groups, giving input into a women's group or working with mother and toddler groups is community development. Small group work is an important method in community development and is to be encouraged, but it is not the whole story.

What is missing from primary care is the action part of community development. Concepts like partnership or equity are very palatable, empowerment is what many feel they are doing already, but collective action is more scary because it is about the transfer of power and control.

Collective action occurs when people act together to bring about changes in their circumstances that they identify need to be changed. The women's health movement and radical groups of the 1960s and '1970s are examples of collective action. Today self-help groups formed around a variety of issues and pressure groups, like disability coalitions or environmental groups, use collective action to bring about change. When community development is working well, the evidence of this is in visible collective action. Health visitors working with groups where they make the tea or put away the toys because that is what

BOX 10.3	*Labonte's (1998) framework for community development*
	1. The adoption of a model of positive health
	2. An analytical model of health determinants
	3. Community development as a theory of social change
	4. A model of community development practice
	5. An accountability framework
	6. Development of methods appropriate to community development ethics

the participants want, need to ask themselves what they are doing. Rather than supporting dependency and passivity they can ask themselves how they could support social action in their neighbourhood to bring about changes in confidence and self-esteem.

REFOCUSING HEALTH VISITING

Health visitors have been supporting a range of families, not just vulnerable families, for years and are increasingly being viewed, with other community nurses and school nurses, as an untapped resource for promoting wider community health. They are the ideal practitioners to take forward the new agendas in health described in the recent government document 'Towards a Healthier Scotland' (Scottish Office 1999). They are in the community, have easy access to large numbers of families and individuals, develop the kind of relationships that engender trust, and importantly, the principles of health visiting support them to work for policy change and to support collective action for health.

Labonte (1998) maintains that community development offers the best means by which health authorities can begin to tackle the determinants of health. The model he offers would provide public health nurses with a methodological and philosophical framework (Box 10.3).

A model of positive health

The WHO definition of health is well-used but, arguably, its concern with promoting health rather than illness is rarely fully understood or operationalised. A change in how health as a concept is viewed would switch community nursing activities from an illness and disease prevention focus to an emphasis on promoting health and well-being. Labonte's model of positive health views health as being more about the quality of our emotional and social situations than about our experience of disease or disability. This model includes elements like:

- Feeling vital and full of energy
- Having a sense of purpose in life
- Experiencing a connectedness to 'community'

- Being able to do things one enjoys
- Having good social relationships
- Experiencing a sense of control over one's life and living conditions.

A model of positive health would move the focus primarily away from a disease and illness-prevention model to one that supports the development of social capital in communities. In child health, the switch would be from screening activities such as hearing tests and vision testing, to focusing on the life circumstances in which children live. With this approach a sense of meaning, promoting self-confidence and the family's relationship to the wider community, would be viewed as being as important as an individual child's development.

An analytical model of health determinants

It is thought that inequality in health has psychological as well as physical effects. An understanding of how unequal access to resources may adversely affect health are not clearly understood but Wilkinson (1994, 1996) argues that the psychological effects of poverty and limited access to resources creates chronic anxiety. He says, 'the deep divisions in our society are both a reflection and a cause of financial and human waste on a scale we cannot afford'. He maintains that there is evidence to suggest that the national infant mortality rises if the rich get richer while the real incomes of the poor remain constant. An analytical model would view housing, a clean and nourishing environment, access to food and appropriate services as essentials for health, and determinants that needs assessment would incorporate as standard.

Community development as a theory of social change

Community development is an approach to health that, 'encompasses a commitment to a holistic approach to health; one which recognises the central importance of social support and social networks'. A community way of working attempts to, 'facilitate individual and collective action around common needs and concerns identified by the community itself and not imposed from outside' (Beattie 1990). The emphasis is on working collaboratively to address equity and support democracy and the participation of the community in issues that affect their lives, and taking collective action to offer a more empowering and positive health promotion message (Box 10.4).

A model of community development practice

Labonte's (1998) model of community development outlines a range of social organisations and relationships necessary for the promotion of health. The activities associated with the development of these relationships could form the core activities for community nurses to engage in tackling the key determinants of health, e.g. housing, poverty and environment. Labonte describes them as 'strategic spheres', that rely on their interrelatedness and dependency on one another, for change to occur.

| BOX 10.4 | *Principles and values of community development (from Voluntary Activity Unit 1996)* |

- Combating social exclusion, poverty and disadvantage
- Antidiscriminatory action in relation to race, age, disability, gender and sexual orientation
- Commitment to community-led, collective, democratic processes of action, empowerment and participation
- Preventive action
- Commitment to partnerships between common interest groups, governments and citizens
- Public issue and public policy focus
- Range of activities from self-help services to campaigning for action

Support of individuals

Community nurses are already engaged in the support of individuals but community development emphasises individual support as an essential component of the strategic approach to social change. Personal support would include basic support, empathy and affirming trust, advocacy, counselling, education and crisis-intervention, as well as referral to other agencies or community groups. Where this approach deviates from mainstream community nursing is in the belief that promoting confidence by enabling the development of new skills and opportunities is not enough on its own. Support must take place within a framework which views personal support as an important component of social or collective action to bring about social change.

Development of support groups

Concepts of democracy, participation and empowerment are central to a community development approach. Local democracy means everyone having a say in what is right for them and for their community, creating structures to encourage participation and involvement, working together to improve the community and influence local policy and enabling people to take effective action. Here the individual support which is an essential part of health visiting core work is extended, to encourage people to come together to improve social support and increase social networks. It is believed that this process builds support for personal change, overcomes learned helplessness and creates the ground for social action to occur.

The process of involvement is an empowering action in itself. The author's experience of helping a women's group set up a food cooperative in their neighbourhood demonstrated that health gain for the volunteers was not limited only to an increased intake of fruit and vegetables, but to the increase in self-esteem resulting from involvement. Being part of the project supported the concept of health outlined by Labonte (1998); increased sense of purpose and a sense of being connected to the community. Activities to facilitate participation, which can often be difficult for groups that feel themselves to be marginalised, are like those in social support, e.g. confidence-building, raising awareness of health issues, increasing access to information through making documents and literature available and developing strategies. This could be part of mainstream public health nursing practice.

Community organising

Community development is about bringing people together to deal with the issues and needs in their area that they define as problematic. It is about working from expressed needs, helping create structures where individuals are not powerless and where there is a commitment to include people who feel excluded because of poverty, disadvantage and isolation. Public health nursing activity would help communities to organise to take effective action through developing support groups, working with people to plan things and to identify issues for action. One of the difficulties of the community development approach is the involvement of individuals who are under-represented in the democratic process. Community nurses, using their contacts and the nature of the relationships they develop, could play an important part in reaching such individuals and encouraging them to become involved in local action on community-defined needs.

Community nurses also have an important role in strengthening communities and helping them develop resources. Social capital (see Chapter 7) is often referred to as 'social glue' and is claimed to impact on health in a number of ways, e.g. by increasing life-expectancy and decreasing infant mortality. Loosely, it means developing social trust, reciprocity and mutual support between neighbours and creating services in the community that are relevant and support empowerment among their users. Social capital is also demonstrated by involvement in civic activities, e.g. voting, going to church and participation in local events.

Alliance-building, political action

Community development methods and concepts support a view that empowered communities should work in partnership with local authorities, local businesses and health professionals to bring about change. They are all key stakeholders in the promotion of health. As argued earlier, improvements in public health are more dependent on changes in social and economic policy than medicine, and so the involvement of agencies like housing, police and education working collaboratively with local communities in the promotion of health is essential.

An accountability framework

Accountability is similar to evaluation, although it is broader in meaning. Labonte (1998) makes the point that accountability is often more of an ethical or moral nature than legal. Public health nurses would have what he calls a 'dual accountability tension', in that health authorities employ them and so they have accountability to their employers, but in working alongside the community as equal partners they would also have accountability to them. The conflict that can arise for workers when local people are challenging their employing authority about services they want is not the problem that Labonte suggests it might be, if current policy about involvement and working from the needs of local people is adhered to.

Development of methods appropriate to community development ethics

In order to enhance and support community development ways of working it is essential that public health nurses be aware of and can use methods of working and evaluating community development that uphold the values of the approach. The Voluntary Activity Unit (1996) offer the following suggestions in relation to evaluation, that are equally valid for undertaking other community development initiatives:

- Work with communities must be negotiated to ensure that the criteria and methods used are sanctioned by the constituencies on whose behalf they act.
- Communities are encouraged to ask a series of questions about evaluation such as, 'what will be evaluated and by whom?', 'what perspective will be used to identify success or failure?', 'What methods will be used?', 'What happens to the products of evaluation, who will have access to it and for what purposes?'.
- Evaluation should be regarded as a learning process for communities and the other agencies involved and so there must be a commitment to involvement of them as evaluators. The process is then always based on partnership and collaboration rather than on a lone researcher.
- Evaluation should be regarded an empowering process that increases community and personal knowledge, raises self-esteem and confidence and allows for community control.
- Recognition that qualitative data is as valid as quantitative information is important. As motivation for action often springs from the quality of personal and community life, indicators and measures must reflect lived experience and give commitment to the voice of people not usually asked for their views.
- Resources should be made available to allow real participation, e.g. training, crèche or sitter support or translation facilities.
- Value should be given to the process as well as to task goals, e.g. getting people together or involved is acknowledged as an outcome of a piece of community work.

Working with a community development approach will not only involve a change in practice for community nurses and the need to enhance skills such as group work, but will radically change the relationships nurses have with the people with whom they are involved. No longer working *for* patients or clients but working *with* them, acknowledging the value of local expertise and knowledge and being able to support the emergence of leaders from within the community to take things forward.

COMMUNITY DEVELOPMENT ACTIVITY IN NURSING

Underpinning the community development approach are a set of activities designed to mobilise neighbourhoods or communities of interest to harness their own skills and resources to provide action for change. These activities are encompassed within the community development process. In many ways the community development process parallels Labonte's (1998) model of community development practice discussed earlier. There are four distinct elements in the process: reflection, analysis, developing strategies and taking action. One element has an impact on the other, which leads onto the next and so on in a continuous cycle. Several discrete stages of activities support the elements; some may overlap, some happen simultaneously and, like Labonte's model, although they are difficult to separate they are all, nevertheless, integral to the process.

Craig (1998) offers a model of public health practice for nurses that this section builds on to outline the community development process and its accompanying activities.

Networking or 'just hanging about'

This involves visiting mother and toddler groups, women's groups, the local cafe and talking to people, to find out who the key individuals are in a community. The purpose is to build-up a picture of the neighbourhood, the culture and the values of the local people, what their needs are and where their interests and energy lie in addressing them.

Identifying supports in the community

Developing from 'hanging about' and still part of networking is the next stage. Here the public health nurse moves onto encouraging people to become involved in addressing local health needs. They may need support to do this, e.g. awareness-raising sessions to help people focus on issues of health and to clarify what health means to them. People may also need help to organise themselves to progress to the action stage. This may mean the group becoming constituted and seeking charitable status. Groups often need to be formalised in this way to obtain funding and, although often initially resisted, it can be a very good process for a group. It helps them clarify their aims and objectives and begin to learn about how organisations operate, even one as small as theirs, and that there are different roles and tasks to be undertaken.

Needs assessment and identifying issues

It will be important for the public health nurse to be working closely with local people to identify main concerns, identifying what needs to be done and developing support to do it. This can be achieved by running a health day in the community centre or doing community profiles or needs assessment.

It was discussed earlier how people who perceive themselves as excluded from society due to poverty, colour, class or homelessness find it difficult to participate due to feelings of powerlessness – often called apathy or indifference by professionals. Public health nurses could help marginalised communities like people who are homeless or vulnerable families with children on the 'At-Risk' register be part of activities like community profiling and needs assessment by involving them in the process. That involvement would, according to Burton and Harrison (1997), produce some important benefits:

- Providing information from people's lived experience. This may produce the impetus for action in the community.

- Enabling new structures to develop as a framework evolves for allocation of tasks. Groups of people getting together to undertake pieces of work can together create new opportunities for further action.

- Enabling people to increase their knowledge about their community. The process of asking questions of neighbours and others creates a wider knowledge of what is in their neighbourhood for those involved in the process.

- Facilitating personal development and the acquisition of new skills. Training is usually necessary for those involved in asking the questions and analysing and disseminating the data.

- Creations of more effective services by feeding the information back up through the system. This helps health authorities commission services that are more meaningful to community need.

- More democratic health service through public involvement at all levels. Often at this stage it is not possible to undertake a formal needs assessment, due to lack of resources, funding and personnel, or it may not be appropriate because the needs are apparent.

Testing ideas on informal networks

Instead of formal needs assessment, groups may decide to take action on what they perceive are their immediate health difficulties and then through a variety of methods check this out with the larger community. These can include:

- Informal contact
- Holding training days
- Small surveys
- Discussion groups
- Running a seminar or conference in the community.

Nurses at this stage in the process will be shaping, collecting and getting support for ideas, setting up support groups, offering opportunities for volunteering, training and supporting participation.

Bringing together key individuals to develop strategies

This next stage in the process involves clarifying opportunities for change and developing strategies. One group the author worked with identified a lack of trained crèche workers to care for their children while they were engaged in committee meetings as an issue. With key workers, locally, they decided to seek funding and to offer a training course for local people wanting to work in crèches. Another area identified for action was the lack of shops locally selling quality affordable fruit and vegetables. After holding a public seminar and asking other projects involved in food work to speak about setting up a fruit and vegetable cooperative, the group decided to take action collectively and set up such a cooperative for themselves.

Taking action with the community

This next stage, supporting the action of the community around their defined needs, is a key one for a public health nurse working with a community development approach. Activities at this time will focus on supporting communities to seek funding to initiate new ventures or to develop existing projects, and building alliances between the community and the people who can help them. This may mean setting up evaluation or monitoring systems for projects and community activities and supporting their growth and development. These activities will be underpinned by sharing information, joint working and networking.

One of the outcomes of the community development process must be to influence policy. However, policy change need not be huge change. The creation of new structures, however small, can impact on policy. The courses for crèche workers referred to earlier were so successful that other agencies asked to employ the workers and soon the availability of training began to alter crèche policy in the area. Community education workers eventually undertook to organise and fund the training and to compile a register of trained workers. After the establishment of the food cooperative, volunteers started working with other agencies and eventually community centres locally began to reduce the sales of sweets and to offer fruit instead to youth and children's groups. The community cafe widened the variety of food for sale and tried to reduce the amount of fried food they offered. Playgroups and nursery schools implemented a healthy-eating policy and local primary schools supplied fruit in tuck shops. The local GP fundholders even provided core funding to sustain the food cooperative.

To bring about major change that will impact on the lives of the most discriminated against people in our society requires that local people have access to the existing decision-making structures like health boards, city councils and government, so that their voices can be heard. Influencing policy is a key principle of health visiting but is one that nurses have shied away from in the past. There may be several reasons for this; the structures for nurses to feed into policy have not existed, it is regarded as 'too political', but it may be also that nursing as a low-status profession is implicated in the lack of action by nurses. Like the low-status groups they work with (women and children, the poor and older people) nurses do not readily avail themselves of the active participation in the democratic process that may bring about change. Like these groups, this may also be a manifestation of their internalised powerlessness (Lukes 1978). If nurses are to be involved in other people's empowering process there may need to be a place in nurse training to focus on the 'participatory competence' of nurses, to prepare them to be able to engage in this.

The impact of community development work can be considerable. The crèche training provided employment for local women, offered new skills and knowledge and improved childcare in crèches. The establishment of the food cooperative impacted on food costs, created a new community focus, and led onto new training courses. It also initiated the development of new groups and community activities. It is clear from this brief example of food work and childcare that nurses working alongside local people in this way can have a considerable impact on public health issues through influencing policy locally, to bring about structural changes. However, in the future, public health nursing will not only be about undertaking different activities but also applying different methods to existing practice.

BRINGING COMMUNITY DEVELOPMENT INTO HEALTH VISITING PRACTICE

Health visitor workloads are currently defined by caseloads in most cases. A caseload of under-five's will by definition restrict health visitors to spending time developing a relationship with individuals primarily, being available when they have a crisis, visiting them at home, seeing them in the clinic, giving advice and counsel and generally overseeing the development of the children. This individualistic model of care feeds the ego and the sense of being important and vital to others. It encourages health visitors to know the answers and creates dependence, on the part of the patients, for their knowledge and skills. The current individualistic culture and medical model structure of the GP practice, coupled with the statutory obligation to fulfil certain responsibilities for individual families, further supports this dependence and renders casework as a core activity very powerful. It was shown earlier from the small study of health visitors trained in community development methods (Dalziel 1997) that given a choice between community development work or responding to caseload demands the caseload was given priority every time. This was because of external client demand and pressure from GPs and nurse managers to maintain the status quo.

Recent research carried out for Lothian Health (Dalziel & McLachlan 2000) in relation to community development training in primary care found that primary care staff liked the community development way of working and wanted to do more, but felt constrained by caseloads and lack of support within the structures. The research suggested that in order for community development to be integrated into mainstream working it needs:

- Recognition within NHS structures and at all levels of management of the value of this kind of training and the community development way of working
- Consideration of practical support for the training including how practice-based health professionals can be released to attend training
- Funding of posts for dedicated workers to provide on-going advice and support to implement the approach
- Further research to assess the health gains of such activities.

The model for health visitor community development work, with some exceptions, e.g. Stockport, has currently been one health visitor working alone in an area, sometimes part of a team but probably isolated and on the margins within that team because the activities and philosophy of the work were in conflict with those of mainstream colleagues. The lone health visitor working without a caseload is often inadequately supported by management and materially poorly resourced. The introduction of the new government papers on public health have created a sea-change in attitudes to a community development way of working, which suggest that this pattern of working can be changed. The benefits of having a health visitor with a caseload working in a community development way as opposed to a lone community development worker are substantial:

- Ready access to existing communities of interest, i.e. women with young children, older people, antenatal, or to other groups with which health visitors are involved
- General acceptance by other professionals of their role in community health
- Existing knowledge of the area and available services.

CHILD HEALTH AND COMMUNITY DEVELOPMENT

Most areas of health visiting activity are amenable to a community development approach, but child health is good place to start. Child health is at the core of health visiting activity and has a potential impact on community health that may be as yet unappreciated, not least because adherence to the caseload paradigm with its focus on the individual child and individual family blocks health visitors from working in a more population-based way. Paradoxically, the demands of current child care provision keep primary care isolated from the communities they serve.

Health visitors have traditionally jealously guarded their work with the well population and contact with every family and resisted the more community-orientated community development approach. Perhaps they fear it will move them away from their unique role as health professionals with this population. Individual family work is valuable and can be retained within a community development framework, but arguably this focus on individual care and individual contact also prevents any possible social action to solve or discover the community or population problems. What individual visiting reveals are individual symptoms of a wider community stress: bits of a jigsaw that all look the same but are in fact unique and only make sense when fitted together with the other pieces. The individual approach, on its own, can do little to change the life circumstances that contribute to unhealthy lifestyles and illness. Without a population approach, work with families sits outside the new public health agenda.

The changing focus on positive health that values being connected, having a sense of purpose, and has a focus on strengthening communities, makes traditional health visiting activities insufficient for the new agenda. The current activities are located within a personal care strategy and so have a remit for child health which focuses on surveillance, screening and advice to mothers about feeding, weaning, sleeping behaviour, etc. Focus on a positive model of health, as opposed to illness prevention, would create different priorities for action. Although immunisation, weighing, hearing and vision testing and developmental testing are important activities, without the causes and solutions to what is found by surveillance being located within a bigger community picture, they are of little value and need to be replaced by an emphasis on different criteria for health. Instead of the questions health visitors traditionally ask about weight, hearing and developmental progress, they might ask questions that more properly focus on a wider public-health agenda like:

- Has this child access to good food, adequate shelter and a safe environment?
- Is there the potential in this family/community for him to develop supportive, nourishing relationships and a sense of belonging?
- Is there the opportunity for him to be educated and do fulfilling work when he is older?
- Is there freedom from discrimination and harassment?
- Are there accessible relevant health and social-welfare services in the area?

In this agenda, good housing, the abolition of poverty, opportunity for nourishing social relationships and for fulfilling work in the future and a pleasant environment are viewed as essentials for the promotion of health, and of equal status as immunisation and child development.

A community development public health approach would move the emphasis away from an exclusive focus on individual behaviour to participation, collaboration with the local community and some understanding of the social circumstances that create ill-health. Key areas of child health that are amenable to this change include:

- Well-baby clinics
- Child development
- Child protection.

WELL-BABY CLINICS

It could be argued that traditional child health clinics encourage and support a dependency culture where young parents feel pressurised into taking their child to the baby clinic 'to be checked'. This might have overtones of the policing role of health visitors but also perhaps professional input encourages them to feel that what they know about their child is not enough on its own and needs to be confirmed or supported by health visitors. This can be disempowering and deskilling for parents.

Clinics also operate very much on an individualistic model of care with individual advice and support being offered, often in a cultural and social vacuum. Advice and help that lies outwith this prevailing culture will be largely ignored. Child-rearing is an activity embedded in cultural norms and women from the same culture can offer advice and help as part of their natural interaction with young mothers. They are then likely to be more acceptable purveyors of guidance and support than health visitors.

Health visitors and other health professionals often demonstrate contempt for the input of lay women by calling it 'old wives tales' to diminish its value.

A community development approach to public health would use this valuable community resource and incorporate it into a new structure for young parents. The Patchwork community clinic in Edinburgh is a good example of this approach in action.

The Patchwork experience

A group of health visitors in an area of high deprivation in the city were aware that the traditional service they offered to parents was often inadequate and not meeting the complex myriad of need resulting from economic and social disadvantage. After completing the 'Community Development in Primary Care' (Dalziel 1999) training programme run by the author, they decided to work differently.

Following the community development process they ran a series of focus groups to find out what local parents wanted, and then worked with them to achieve action for change. They formed a steering group composed of parents, health visitors and representatives from community education and from the local health project. They then moved the baby clinic from the general practice building to the community centre. This shift from buildings that are medically orientated into the community centre, where the environment fosters social and community activities, immediately created a more equal partnership and reduced the perceived authority of the health visitor. In this model of shared authority, child-rearing is returned to the community, where it rightly belongs. Health visiting activities then centre on working with the child-rearing constituency, lay workers and parents, to find out what needs they have, not necessarily by formal needs assessment but by talking to them, forming support groups or organising child-rearing seminars or exchanges, in which they are equal participants. Parents are part of the decision-making progress and can dictate what happens in Patchwork.

The Patchwork experience encourages new friendships among the women and reduces the isolation that can lead to postnatal depression. It acts as a source of information about what is happening in the community, encourages breastfeeding support groups, and runs parenting groups around issues defined by the parents. These events promote good practice, help parents learn about social relationships and allow them to get support and help for difficulties from each other. Community education workers involved in the initiative encourage parents to produce their own local leaflets on best child health practice and on sources of support and help locally.

The social action resulting from this new structure is currently centred around antenatal education and breastfeeding. The uptake of traditional parentcraft classes run by health visitors and midwives is very poor. One of the Patchwork volunteers was interested in addressing this issue and working with a local midwife is finding out what women who live in this area want from antenatal education and how they can be involved as peer educators. She has also started, with some other women, a breastfeeding support network. Arguably, this will have as much or more impact on local women as the breastfeeding strategies currently devised within cultural and social vacuums by professionals.

Valuing local expertise and knowledge around something as seminal as child-rearing is part of building social capital. The acceptance of lay knowledge and experience alongside professional expertise strengthens partnerships with communities and will ultimately shift patterns of dependency from health professionals and diminish community helplessness.

CHILD DEVELOPMENT

Working alongside parents and lay workers in a community based child-rearing 'clinic' with local parents, it should be possible to organise or facilitate a range of child development activities to help parents be the expert in their child's development. These activities take several forms, e.g. booklets, seminar-type activities or fun events, but local parents would be actively involved in developing information on stages in child development for themselves and other parents.

In this paradigm, new parents are encouraged to monitor their child's progression, reporting when something seems wrong, rather than being dependent on the health visitor to be the judge of what is 'normal'. Arguably, this is what parents, relatives and friends do anyway in their day-to-day contact with a child. Parents could also have open access to other services: child psychology, speech therapy or vision and hearing testing, if they decide that they need it. Shifting the responsibility to the parents to judge child progression, and changing structures to support this reduces dependency, increases knowledge and confidence, and promotes self-esteem.

CHILD PROTECTION

In the preface to her book 'The Case of Mary Bell' (who was convicted of murder when a child of ten years old), Gitta Sereny (1998) says, 'The reason such tragedies happen is that there is still too much ignorance within families about how to live and how to love'.

It is no accident that vulnerable families living in poverty in poor social circumstances are more often involved in child protection issues. Due to the stress of living with multiple difficulties, children of such families are usually exposed to more harm than more affluent families. Overburdened with debt and lack of money, often experiencing psychological and relationship difficulties or mental health problems, many families cannot sustain the support and nourishment necessary for their children's health because of their own needs. The public health agenda would view the development of resources to respond to such parental need, and services to offer relevant support, as the way forward. The work of public health nurses mobilising communities, and supporting the development of local resources like Credit Unions and Welfare Advice, may prevent some of these family relationships breaking down irreparably. Community development concepts applied to child protection issues would view equity in resources and a collective and democratic approach as being more likely to offer the support individuals and communities need than individual home-visiting on its own.

Public health nurses need to be part of the movement to encourage a shift away from an individual blaming and punishment agenda to one of looking at what communities have and what families in difficult circumstances need to support them. It would offer an opportunity for perpetrators and suspected abusers to be involved in support and training programmes, to help them look at their violence and the correct use of their power, but also to harness that knowledge and experience to help others. This is part of building social capital.

CONCLUSION

The chapter is being written at a time when the author's employer, a primary care NHS trust in Scotland, has just adopted community development as the mainstream approach for primary care staff. Although this may seem like a radical move, and in some ways it is, it also fits in with the new way of thinking about public health and health promotion that is the current policy agenda. The trust believes that the use of community development concepts like joint working and partnership with the community, public involvement in primary care services, addressing equity and inequality issues, collective action and an empowering agenda, will provide primary care staff with the thinking and the methods to work differently.

In time, a community development approach will dismantle the current primary care culture and do much to help community nurses undo some of the learning imbued by nurse training. It will challenge the notion that health professionals are the experts in health and that individuals are passive recipients in the process. As this way of working becomes commonplace, the dominant culture of professionally held power and expertise in health will give way to a culture of shared authority between nurses and the community which they serve. Public involvement in primary care planning and delivery, a targeted emphasis on resources to address inequalities in health and joint working with the community will become the core work, and surveillance and policing greatly reduced or eliminated.

The adoption of this approach is far-reaching and offers nurses a set of principles that will move the profession into a new era in its development. It may be the beginning of the separation of nursing from the shadow of medicine and the emergence of community nurses regaining their role as autonomous practitioners largely divorced from the medical model and working as public health promoters building social capacity.

This new paradigm for nursing will see nurses as no longer the 'experts' holding onto health knowledge to retain professional distance and power relations with the people they are supposed to be supporting in health, but working with the notion of achieving shared authority. No longer attached to general practice and constrained by the hierarchical nature of primary care teams, they will be able to work across practice boundaries to shift the energy and resources from medicine and illness and general practice interests to issues that concern the community at large, however they are defined. Nurses will be accountable for their work and its outcomes to their management and defined by their accountability to the communities they serve.

None of this can happen in isolation, but needs to be supported by major structural change within health organisations like primary care trusts, Local health care cooperatives and primary care groups. Integration will only happen when the appropriate culture and structures are in place to support the approach. If the community development approach to public health is to be allowed to have the impact it could, it needs to stop being as a marginal viewed 'add on' to what is perceived as core work. As a way of working it has been less favoured in the past by health visitors because it is slow, and for a while input will be largely invisible. It also involves nurses shedding the dependant, relatively distant, professional relationship fostered by 'caseload as core activity', and adopting a relationship where working alongside people, rather than for them, is preferred. Within the present health visiting framework health visitors may be drawn to fulfilling the caseload remit because it is clearer, more highly valued and, initially, more emotionally rewarding.

Nursing will need leadership at all levels if it is to achieve this major cultural and organisational change. It needs strong informed leadership at a government level, in health boards and authorities, in trusts and at a local level. It will require changes in the nurse education curriculum, post-registration training, a rethink about student placements, and allocation of resources to make the transition. It needs brave nursing management to gather the lone health visitors working with a public health or community development remit, with or without a caseload and probably without peers, and bring them in from the margins to the centre of community nursing, to use their innovation, ideas, skills and knowledge and to make their activities central and not an 'extra' that so-called real nurses have no time to do. The experience and contacts gained by these workers will form the core of the new curriculum of the future and their skills will be used to train and support other nurses.

Community development offers a way of working in public health that could have a profound influence on the shape of nursing, but it needs to be properly funded and supported and the relevant training provided. New structures and the culture that will develop from an adoption of the principles of a community development approach can help primary care to look outside medicine and to view other agencies, like housing, education, environmental health and local businesses, as also having a key role in public health and to welcome their support in partnership.

DISCUSSION QUESTIONS

- Does the autonomy of health visiting benefit or hinder the public health agenda?
- Is surveillance a relevant component of public health/health visiting?
- Who cares for the children – community or professional responsibility?
- Can health visiting risk an analysis of existing power relationships?

FURTHER READING

Craig P & Lindsay G 2000 Nursing for Public Health. Churchill Livingstone, Edinburgh

Jones J 1999 Private Troubles and Public Issues – a community development approach to health. Community Learning

Smithies J, Webster G 1998 Community Involvement in Health. Ashgate Publishing, Aldershot

REFERENCES

Ashton J & Seymour H 1988 The New Public Health. Open University Press, Milton Keynes

Beattie A (ed) 1990 Roots and Branches. Open University Press, Milton Keynes

Beigal D E 1984 Help seeking and receiving in urban ethnic neighbourhoods: strategies for empowerment. In: Rappaport J, Swift C & Hess R (eds) Studies in Empowerment: Steps towards Understanding and Action. Hawthorn Press, New York

Burton P & Harrison L 1997 Identifying Local Health Needs. Policy Press, University of Bristol, Bristol

Craig P 1998 A description of the public role of health visitors. Unpublished MSc thesis. University of Glasgow, Glasgow

Dalziel Y 1997 Community Development in Primary Care, unpublished report. Edinburgh Health Care NHS Trust, Edinburgh

Dalziel Y 1999 Community Development in Primary Care. Lothian Health, Edinburgh

Dalziel Y & McLachlan S 2000 Preliminary Report of the CHART Project. Lothian Health, Edinburgh

Duffy S 1996 Partnerships in Action. Health Education Board, Edinburgh

Funnell R, Oldfield K & Speller V 1995 Towards Healthier Alliances. Health Education Authority, London

Jones J 1990 Community Development and Health Education: Concepts and Philosophy. In: Beattie A (ed) Roots and Branches. Open University Press, Milton Keynes

Kiefer C H 1983 Citizen Empowerment: A developmental perspective. Prevention in Human Services 3(23):9–37

Labonte R 1998 A Community Development Approach to Health Promotion. Health Education Board for Scotland, Edinburgh

Lukes S 1978 Power: a radical view. Macmillan, London

Peckham S, Makdonald J, Taylor P 1996 Primary care and public health – project report phase 1. Public Health Alliance, Birmingham

Rappaport J, Swift C & Hess R (eds) 1984 Studies in Empowerment: Steps towards Understanding and Action. Hawthorn Press, New York

Schiller P L & Levin J S 1983 Is Self-care a social movement? Social Science and Medicine 17:1343–1352

Scottish Office 1999 Towards a Healthier Scotland. HMSO, Edinburgh

Sereny G 1998 Cries Unheard. The Case of Mary Bell. Macmillan, London

Taylor P, Peckham S & Turton P 1997 A public health model of primary care–from concept to reality. Public Health Alliance, Birmingham

Townsend P & Davidson N 1982 Inequalities in Health. Penguin, Harmondsworth

Voluntary Activity Unit 1997 Monitoring and Evaluation of Community Development in Northern Ireland. Department of Health and Social Services, Belfast

Wilkinson R 1994 Divided we fall. British Medical Journal 304: 1113-1114

Wilkinson R 1996 Unhealthy Societies: the Afflictions of Inequality. Routledge, New York

World Health Organization 1978 Alma-Ata 1977, Primary Health Care. World Health Organization, Geneva

11 Breastfeeding and public health

Sally Kendall

KEY ISSUES

- Breastfeeding makes a significant contribution to public health.
- Public health policy focuses on the prevention of disease and does not recognise the contribution to positive health which breastfeeding can provide, particularly in relation to women's own perceptions of the benefits to health.
- The incidence and prevalence of breastfeeding in the UK continues to be low relative to other countries and there are marked variations according to socio-economic group and region.
- There are many factors including cultural barriers and breastfeeding in the workplace which make it difficult for women to breastfeed beyond the first few weeks of life.
- There is great scope for health professionals (especially health visitors and midwives) to promote and support breastfeeding.

INTRODUCTION

Breastfeeding as a public health issue is hardly a new phenomenon. During the nineteenth century, as the industrial revolution really began to have a major effect on the economy in western Europe, infant mortality was at an all-time high. Urban living became a necessity for many in the search for work and poor housing, overcrowding, squalor and the attendant scourges of infestation and infection such as cholera, typhoid and syphilis took their toll on as many as 250 infants per 1000. As Gabrielle Palmer (1993) reliably informs us in her book 'The Politics of Breastfeeding', the movement of industry away from cottages and family-based units in the rural areas and into the urban settings had a serious economic and social outcome for women and their children.

Whereas child-rearing and infant feeding had been a natural part of the daily life of the cottage industrialist, with the move to a capitalist economy where the means of production was centrally based in a factory, women who had to work to survive did not have the flexibility to breastfeed their infants, thereby providing protection from infection as well as essential nutrients, or therefore to manage their own fertility via this method. Breastfeeding as the natural method of feeding therefore became increasingly redundant, as entrepreneurs such as Henri Nestle realised the niche market for artificial feeding and started to produce dried milk powder to replace breastfeeding.

Prior to this time, the only alternative to breastfeeding had been wet-nursing – the practice of hiring another woman to feed your baby. This in itself had been a source of respectable income for many women, who gained both stability and status by breastfeeding the babies of noble women. The vast majority of women, however, fed their own babies and not only was infant mortality *lower* in most areas before the industrial revolution (about 150 per 1000), but women were also able to take advantage of the contraceptive effects of lactation to space their families. Indeed, Palmer (1993) remarks on the fact that noble-women often had much larger families, with miscarriages and stillbirths than working women, as they did not tend to breastfeed their own babies. The daughters of the cottage-industry families would have been brought up not only as skilled helpers in the industry, but as able mothers who would have no difficulty in breastfeeding their own children alongside the hard and often long working day.

Combining work outside the home with child-rearing, within an economy which was driven by capitalism and controlled by patriarchy, deprived women of the power they had had to determine the health and future of their offspring. The only way to maintain some independent means of sustaining themselves and their children was to work in the factories and mills. While breastfeeding continued to be successfully sustained in rural areas, it declined in the urban populations as artificial milks flooded the market and were seen by many women as the only viable alternative. Public health officials such as Dr Reid, (cited by Palmer 1993) who exhorted women to return to natural feeding of their infants, overlooked the fact that most women were powerless to do so, and thus the moral debate over breastfeeding vs artificial feeding was inaugurated. Women who breastfed were either 'harlots or fallen women' who wet-nursed to make a living, or impoverished women of little moral worth. Working women, for whom breastfeeding was impossible, were portrayed as selfish beings who worked to make their own lives better and had little care for their children.

Women in the nineteenth century were thus in a 'Catch 22' situation and the legacy of that continues for women today, where arrangements to breast-feed or express milk in the workplace remain unusual and breastfeeding in public can still cause a moral outcry. Indeed, the influence of westernised economic thought can now be seen to be infiltrating traditional agricultural economies in the developing world. Maher (1995) describes how, in one North African tribe, women have been almost forced into artificial feeding through the transformation from a self-sufficient agriculture to a cash-crop economy. The men command the power in the community through the sale of cash crops in the urban markets and therefore retain the profits. The women can only maintain a degree of power by using some of the wealth to purchase formula milk for their infants, a practice which is undoubtedly reinforced by westernised marketing methods. To breastfeed means to surrender access to the means of survival which the women themselves have played a major part in producing.

In today's western civilisation it would be difficult to ascribe infant mortality rates to the decline and rise again of breastfeeding – there have been so many other major public health and social reforms. However, there are many public health benefits associated with breastfeeding, which will be discussed later in this chapter, and breastfeeding continues to be a political issue demanding considerable structural and economic changes if the possible cost benefits to the public are to be truly realised.

INCIDENCE AND PREVALENCE OF BREASTFEEDING IN THE UK

How popular was breastfeeding in the late 1990s in the UK? Without a doubt there was a significant shift from the 1960s and 1970s, when not only was bottle-feeding seen to be the most efficient and proper way to feed a baby, but also the feminist movement (ironically) probably contributed to women 'liberating' themselves from their bodily functions and perceiving breastfeeding as domi-nation by men which tied them to the home. Surveys of infant feeding are conducted every five years by the Office of National Statistics (ONS) and these provide a rich database of information on infant feeding practices, which reveal differences around the country which may be linked to public health issues.

The most recent survey was conducted in 1995 and published in 1997, with reference to the previous 1990 survey. The ONS randomly selected a sample of over 12 000 women from registrations of births compiled by the General Register Offices of England and Wales, Scotland and Northern Ireland. Of these, a total of 74% responded to an initial questionnaire when their babies were between 6 and 10 weeks old. These were followed up by further questionnaires when the babies were 5 months and 9 months old respectively. The ONS define the incidence of breastfeeding as the proportion of babies who were breastfed initially, even if they were put to the breast only once. Prevalence of breastfeeding is defined as the proportion of babies who were wholly or partially breastfed at specific ages. These definitions have been used since the 1975 survey and are therefore helpful for comparative purposes. However, they do disguise the fact that some babies may only be breastfed for a very short time and, in relation to incidence in particular, these babies are counted in the same way as babies who were exclusively breastfed from the moment of birth.

The health benefits of exclusive breastfeeding for 4 months as recommended by the Committee on Medical Aspects of food (Department of Health 1994) are therefore difficult to extract from the ONS data. However, as Table 11.1 shows, there has been an overall increase in the incidence of breastfeeding since 1990. The obvious issue which these data draw our attention to is one of difference in

TABLE 11.1	*Incidence of breastfeeding by country (1975, 1980, 1985, 1990 and 1995) (Foster et al 1997)*																
	England and Wales					**Scotland**				**Northern Ireland**		**Great Britain**				**United Kingdom**	
	1975	1980	1985	1990	1995	1980	1985	1990	1995	1990	1995	1980	1985	1990	1995	1990	1995
Percentage who breastfed initially	51	67	65	64	68	50	48	50	55	36	45	65	64	63	67	62	66
Base	1544	3755	4671	4942	4598	1718	1895	1981	1863	1497	1476	4224	5223	5413	5018	5533	5181

TABLE 11.2	Prevalence of breastfeeding at ages up to nine months by country (1990 and 1995 United Kingdom) (Foster et al 1997)

Age of baby	England and Wales		Scotland		Northern Ireland		United Kingdom	
	1990	1995	1990	1995	1990	1995	1990	1995
	Percentage breastfeeding at each age							
Birth	64	68	50	55	36	45	62	66
I week	54	58	41	46	29	35	53	56
2 weeks	51	54	39	44	27	32	50	53
6 weeks	39	44	30	36	17	25	39	42
4 months	25	28	20	24	8	12	25	27
6 months	21	22	16	19	5	8	21	21
8 months	15	16	12	14	3	6	–	15
9 months *	12	14	9	13	3	5	11	14
Base	4942	4598	1981	1863	1497	1476	5533	5181

* Based on a reduced number of cases in 1995

the incidence of breastfeeding between the UK its constituent countries. Northern Ireland appears to be particularly low at 45%, compared to Scotland at 55% and England and Wales at 66%. There are regional variations within these figures – for example, the incidence of breastfeeding in London and the South East in 1995 was 82% compared with 61% in the north of England. Although there have been significant increases since 1990, the overall figures do not compare favourably with other European countries. For example, in Italy the incidence at birth was 85.3% and 41.8% at 3 months, based on exclusive breastfeeding (Giovanni et al 1999). Prevalence of breastfeeding would also indicate positive changes since 1990 (see Table 11.2).

However, it is important to note that breastfeeding drops dramatically after 6 weeks and that these figures include babies who are receiving other forms of nourishment as well as breast milk. Again, health benefits over time are difficult to extract unless exclusive breastfeeding is counted and identified as the independent variable. Finally, the ONS measures duration of breastfeeding, which is defined as the length of time a baby is breastfed from initiation to weaning, but again includes other forms of nutrition. The figures suggest that there has been a small increase from 18–21% of babies who continue to receive breast milk at 9 months of age. Unfortunately, data are not systematically collected beyond this period so there is little national evidence of the effects of longer-term breastfeeding. The ONS survey also provides an interpretation of the data which demonstrates significant positive correlations between incidence, prevalence and duration of breastfeeding, and social class and education of the mother. The Acheson Report (Department of Health 1999b) on inequalities in health also identifies the differences in prevalence in breastfeeding among different social groups and calls for policies which can address these differences. These data are critical to the interpretation and understanding of local health needs analyses, as will be expected within primary care groups (Department of Health 1997), as other correlates of health gain are also strongly associated with these variables (e.g. smoking behaviour). To realise the necessary health improvements, account has to be taken by public health analysts and practitioners of the co-variates affecting health behaviour and ultimately public health outcomes. The positive changes in breastfeeding rates should be correlated with other health data and some epidemiologists – notably Howie and colleagues (Wilson et al 1998) – have conducted some rigorous analyses of these possible relationships.

PUBLIC HEALTH BENEFITS OF BREASTFEEDING

The white paper 'Saving Lives: Our Healthier Nation' (Department of Health 1999a) refers to areas for health improvement and outlines proposals for a 'third way' of both managing and preventing ill-health. The document goes a lot further than its predecessor in acknowledging the social and economic causes of ill-health, recognising that there are real inequalities in health. However, while attention is focused on the major health concerns in England (coronary heart disease, cancer, accidents and mental health) the document promotes a modernist rather than a post-modernist approach to health (Kelly et al 1993), that is, the emphasis continues to be on disease and scientific measurement of the causes and changes in disease patterns, rather than a focus on positive health and the factors (both social and biological) which contribute to what Antonovsky (1987) has described as salutogenesis, or the causes of health. There is very little evidence in the document, for example, about the ways in which improving the incidence and prevalence of breastfeeding could have a significant impact on some of these issues.

There is evidence that breastfeeding can be important in preventing breast cancer (e.g. Chilvers 1993) in premenopausal women and breast cancer was responsible for 18% of female mortality from cancer in 1996 (Foster et al 1997). The target set by the government is for *reducing* cancer deaths, not for *increasing* activities such as breastfeeding. It is well-recognised that breastfeeding is the most beneficial method of feeding an infant and yet breastfeeding per se is not given attention in the document. From a post-modernist construction it would be valid not only to consider the medical outcomes of promoting breastfeeding, but also the perceived benefits from women's perspectives. Such indicators of health are significant by their absence in the current white paper and therefore in policy terms will be entirely unevaluated. Nevertheless, it remains the case that breastfeeding is a social and cultural activity as well as a biological phenomenon, which needs to be analysed within all these domains.

Across the world, it has been estimated that over a million babies per year die from unsafe formula-feeding techniques and that babies who are bottle-fed in poor conditions are 25 times more likely to die than breastfed babies (Baby Milk Action 1991). For example, in relation to gastroenteritis, Bauchner et al (1986) found from a review of over 40 studies since 1970, that breastfeeding had a protective effect. Howie et al (1990), in a study of 618 children in Dundee, found that babies who were breastfed for 13 weeks were not only protected from gastroenteritis, but also the benefits lasted for up to one year.

Breastfeeding has also been identified as a protective factor in sudden infant death syndrome (SIDS) (Savage 1992) and shown to be important in protection in the longer-term from diseases such as Crohn's disease (Koletzko et al 1989) and insulin-dependent diabetes (Metcalf & Baum 1992). Clearly, the initiation and continuation of breastfeeding should lead to significant health gains and cost savings within the health services. Most of the evidence on the public health benefits of breastfeeding is predicated on its relationship with the reduction of risk for certain diseases for either baby or mother. For this section of the chapter I will concentrate on two major pieces of research which have demonstrated the health gains to infants prospectively, a systematic review of the health gains to women from breastfeeding and some implications for public health of the benefits of lactational ammenorrhoea. This will be contrasted with some research which explores breastfeeding from womens' perspectives.

HEALTH GAINS FOR INFANTS

As already indicated, there has been much research conducted into the ways in which babies can benefit from breast milk – not all of which is conclusive. However, two published reports of a prospective study conducted in Dundee have found some convincing findings about the public health benefits of breastfeeding for infants. The first of these was published in 1990 (Howie et al 1990) and reported on the relation between breastfeeding and infant illness in the first 2 years of life, with particular reference to gastroenteritis. The study was based on a prospective, observational design of 750 pairs of mothers and infants, of whom 618 were followed up for 24 months after birth. The infants were observed in detail by health visitors at 2 weeks, monthly for 6 months and then 3-monthly up to 24 months. This regularity of surveillance minimised detection bias, as did rigorous definitions of the diseases being observed for, and the ways in which the health visitors were instructed to ask parents questions. Gastrointestinal illness, for example, was defined as vomiting or diarrhoea or both, lasting as a discrete illness for 48 hours or more. The main outcome measure was the prevalence of gastrointestinal disease in infants during the follow-up. Women were categorised for the purposes of the study by their breastfeeding behaviour at 13 weeks as either full breastfeeders ($n = 97$), partial breastfeeders ($n = 130$), early weaners ($n = 180$) or bottle-feeders ($n = 257$). This was a helpful distinction, as several previous studies had not made any attempt to define breastfeeding.

The results showed that there were 50 episodes of gastrointestinal illness among bottle-fed babies compared to two among fully breastfed babies. When these data were adjusted for variables such as social class and parental smoking, it was found that there was a significant difference in the prevalence of gastrointestinal illness at 13 weeks between babies who were either fully or partially breastfed and those who were bottle-fed. There was also evidence that other illnesses were less prevalent among the breastfed babies, for example respiratory illness was also less common. These benefits were observed to persist up to the first year of life, with fewer babies who were breastfed requiring admission to hospital with gastrointestinal illness. The authors point out that nothing in their study undermines the view that babies should be fully breastfed for 4–6 months. However, they do emphasise that some mothers either decide to bottle-feed from the outset or give up breastfeeding prematurely because of the pressures of returning to work. They urge that women should be enabled to breastfeed for a minimum of 3 months through statutory maternity rights and crèche facilities at work. This recommendation is significant in the light of the historical overview at the beginning of this chapter.

Interestingly, the green paper 'Our Healthier Nation' (Department of Health 1998) did refer to the idea of the 'healthy workplace' and enjoined employers to consider a contract for health which included issues such as child-care facilities. It is a matter of some considerable interest that this does not feature strongly in the policy document 'Saving Lives' (Department of Health 1999a), and therefore there is no real policy incentive for employers to consider child-friendly environments which include time out to breastfeed or express milk. It is on such important matters for women that health visitors, midwives and other community nurses should be commenting and lobbying government, using the evidence produced by research such as Howie et al's (1990) to support their arguments.

The importance for public health of Howie et al's (1990) paper lies in its methodological rigour and the significance of its findings, which clearly have implications for cost evaluation also, although the researchers do not carry out this exercise themselves. Eight years after the publication of this work, the researchers published their findings of the 7-year follow-up of the same cohort of infants (Wilson et al 1998). This type of long-term follow-up is fairly unusual as it is costly, but provides strong evidence on the benefits of breastfeeding. In this stage of the study the team analysed the relationship between infant feeding practices and childhood respiratory illness, growth, body composition and blood pressure. Of the original 674 children in the cohort, 545 were available for the study, the mean age of whom was 7.3 years. Outcome measures were prevalence of respiratory illness, height, body mass index, percentage body fat and blood pressure. Parents of the children were asked to complete a questionnaire about childhood illnesses and family history of allergy (545 or 81% of the original cohort) at around the age of seven years, and anthropometric measures including blood pressure, body composition, percentage body fat, skin-fold thickness, weight and body mass index and height were completed by 412 or 61% of the original cohort. The same definitions and data of breastfeeding were used as for the original study. The main findings from this study have important implications for child health as they confirm that exclusively breastfeeding infants up to at least 15 weeks does confer health benefits into later childhood. For example, there is a significant reduction in respiratory illness during the first 7 years of life for exclusively breastfed infants, and exclusive formula-feeding is associated with higher blood pressure (mean difference 3 mmHg systolic blood pressure) at the age of seven. Early introduction of solids is associated with increased weight, percentage body fat and risk of wheezing in childhood.

As the authors point out, the observed effects on body composition and blood pressure of bottle-feeding and early solids may be magnified over time and become important antecedents of adult health. This again is significant in the light of the recent document 'Saving Lives: Our Healthier Nation' (Department of Health 1999a). The target towards reducing coronary heart disease and strokes by 33% in the under 65 age-group by 2002 may well be difficult to achieve, as the cohort group on which the effects will be measured will not be those who benefited from full breastfeeding in their infancy. These will be post-war babies who were victims of child-care practices which favoured rigidly structured feeding regimes and therefore rejected breastfeeding in favour of formula. No reference is made in the document to the potential health gains in later life from exclusive breastfeeding, although the findings from Wilson et al's (1998) study do confirm the advice of the Commission on Medical Aspects of Food (COMA) report (Department of Health, 1994), to continue breastfeeding for up to four months. This advice is also supported by the American Academy of Pediatrics (1997) who advise that 'exclusive breastfeeding is ideal nutrition and sufficient to support optimum growth and development for approximately six months after birth' (para 6 p. 4). It would, therefore, be appropriate for practitioners to utilise the evidence from Wilson et al's (1998) study to support their own arguments to promote, audit and evaluate breastfeeding practice within their own localities.

HEALTH BENEFITS FOR WOMEN

The evaluation of the health benefits of breastfeeding have tended to focus almost exclusively on the health gains for infants and children. However, lactation is a naturally occurring physiological phenomenon which may confer health benefits to those women in whom the natural course of events takes place. Clearly, there are many women who do not lactate either because they have never been pregnant or because they suppress lactation after birth. For those women who are feeding an infant, it is not possible to assign them to an intervention or control group, as the choice to breastfeed has to be personal. Epidemiological studies can therefore only be observational of the different feeding behaviours. Heinig and Dewey (1997) have conducted one of the few rigorous reviews of the health benefits of breastfeeding for women. It provides further evidence of the longer-term public health gains for the adult female population which can be conferred through breastfeeding and should be seen alongside the evidence on health gains for infants and children.

In their review, Heinig and Dewey use Bauchner et al's (1986) standards for including studies in the review. These are listed in Box 11.1

A total of 144 studies were reviewed by the Heinig and Dewey using the standards listed, where at least three out of the four applied. These papers fell into various categories which included recovery from childbirth, maternal postpartum weight-loss, metabolism of lipids and glucose, suppression of fertility, cancer risk (breast, ovarian and endometrial) and bone density. The reader is referred to the original review for a full report on the findings, but for the

BOX 11.1	*Bauchner et al's (1986) standards for studies to be reviewed*

- Avoidance of detection bias through prospective study design and active surveillance of subjects
- Adequate control of confounding variables
- Clearly-defined outcome events
- Clear definition of breastfeeding

purposes of discussing the public health issues related to breastfeeding, this part of the chapter will address those factors which are relevant to the health targets set out by the government. As previously indicated, the targets as set out in the current public health white paper (Department of Health 1999a) do little to inspire the uptake of health-promoting activities such as breastfeeding, as the emphasis is on the reduction of disease. The targets (Department of Health 1999a) which could be affected by increasing the number of women who breastfeed are:

- To reduce (from baseline of 1996) the number of deaths from cancer among people aged under 65 by at least a further fifth (20%) by 2010

- To reduce (from baseline of 1996) the death rate from heart disease and strokes and related illnesses among people under 65 years by at least a further third (33%) by 2010.

As part of the strategy for health, primary care groups are also encouraged to identify local needs and set local targets for health, providing the opportunity for areas of high prevalence of particular diseases or high rates of unemployment, for example, to be targeted in specified ways.

Breastfeeding and cancer

The evidence on cancer and breastfeeding as presented by Heinig and Dewey (1997) does suggest that there may be significant benefits of breastfeeding, which are mainly conferred to pre-menopausal women and are dependent on patterns and duration of breastfeeding. In the case of breast cancer, they reviewed 20 studies all of which were unequivocal in their findings that lactation does not *increase* the risk of breast cancer. The studies were mixed in their conclusions about the risk-reduction for pre- and postmenopausal women, although most suggest that the cumulative duration of breastfeeding is important, especially beyond 9 months. One study suggested that a lifetime total of 24 months or longer of breastfeeding could reduce the incidence of breast cancer by as much as 25% (Newcombe et al 1994). This study involved more than 14 000 pre- and postmenopausal women. A UK study by Chilvers (1993) suggested that there was a lower risk of breast cancer associated with the number of children breastfed for at least 3 months. Heinig and Dewey are careful to point out that it is difficult to make comparisons between the 20 studies, as factors such as tumour type, patterns of breastfeeding behaviour and menopausal status are not always taken into account. They recommend that further studies should be undertaken which control for these variables. However, the evidence appears to be robust enough for organisations such as UNICEF to use it in their promotional material for the Baby Friendly Initiative (UNICEF 1996).

In relation to ovarian and endometrial cancer, the authors remain somewhat cautious in their conclusions, as the few studies which have been conducted in this area do tend to conflict. In a meta-analysis of 12 case-control studies in the USA it was found that breastfeeding for 6 months or more was associated with reduced risk of ovarian cancer (Whittemore 1994). Some studies of ovarian cancer (e.g. Gwinn et al 1990) suggest that it is lactational anovulation which exerts the protective effect against ovarian cancer, as circulating gonadotrophins are reduced and it is these hormones which have been associated with ovarian malignancy. Other studies have shown no relationship between lactation and reduction in ovarian cancer risk (e.g. Cramer et al 1983, Hartge et al 1989).

Breastfeeding provides a theoretical protection against endometrial cancer as the risk of endometrial cancer is said to increase in response to circulating oestrogens unopposed by progesterone. During lactation, oestrogen is reduced more than is progesterone. However, the evidence for this protective effect is conflicting. One study (Brinton et al 1992) found no difference in risk for endometrial cancer among those women who had ever fed and those who had never breastfed, while a study by Rosenblatt and Thomas (1995) found a significant decreasing trend in risk of endometrial cancer with increasing cumulative duration of breastfeeding. Again, one of the factors which may explain the difference in these findings is the extent to which the researchers define the pattern of breastfeeding. For example, 'ever breastfed' is a very different definition to total length of duration of breastfeeding. Neither study appears to report on exclusive breastfeeders.

To conclude on the effect of breastfeeding in reduction of cancer risk, it would seem that there is no reason *not* to encourage breastfeeding, especially of sustained duration, and that it is likely that there is some protection for premenopausal women against the risk of cancer of the breast and possibly ovaries if they breastfeed.

Breastfeeding and heart disease and stroke

In relation to coronary heart disease and strokes, the prospective study by Wilson et al (1998) on children at seven years of age has already been discussed in some detail and shown that breastfeeding for at least 15 weeks does have a potential beneficial effect on blood pressure and body fat in adult life, both of which are risk factors in coronary heart disease and stroke. However, this study is relevant to the breastfed child – does the mother also share any reduction in risk for these diseases? Heinig and Dewey's (1997) review reports on one main study which has investigated cholesterol metabolism and lactation and has some implications for heart disease risk. Raised cholesterol and triglyceride serum levels are recognised risk factors in the development of atherosclerosis and atherothrombosis, leading to coronary events such as angina and heart attack. During pregnancy, serum cholesterol levels rise above that of the pre-pregnancy level but during lactation this is secreted into the milk at a rate similar to that of cholesterol-lowering medication (Kallio et al 1992). It is thought that this is promoted by an enzyme in the mammary gland which is activated by prolactin (Kallio et al 1992). Kallio et al (1992) studied cholesterol metabolism in women who exclusively breastfed their infants for up to 12 months. These researchers found that total cholesterol, low density lipoprotein and triglycerides declined to levels significantly lower than the pre-pregnant state during lactation and returned to normal values after lactation ceased. It is hypothesised that repeated periods of lactation may help to reduce atherosclerotic damage over time, thus reducing the overall risk of coronary heart disease. Heinig and Dewey (1997) recommend that more research be done in this area.

To conclude on women's health in relation to government targets, it seems that there is some evidence to suggest that breastfeeding protects against some cancers and possibly reduces coronary heart disease risk-factors. This is valuable evidence in public health terms but does need further confirmation. It is also important to bear in mind that for many women across the world, especially in developing countries, breastfeeding acts as the only way of spacing families because of lactational anovulation. Spacing of families is known to reduce maternal and infant morbidity and mortality. In the western world, breastfeeding does not have such a significant contraceptive effect because the pattern of breastfeeding does not sustain the hormone levels required to prevent ovulation. For example, night feeding and frequent feeding after the first 2–3 months are reduced by western mothers. In 1988, researchers from around the world met in Italy and stated that:

> 'Breastfeeding provides 98% protection from pregnancy in the first six months postpartum if the mother is fully or nearly fully breastfeeding and has not experienced vaginal bleeding after the 56th day postpartum. Additional contraception is required in lactating women who are partially breastfeeding, who have started menstruating or have been breastfeeding for more than 6 months' (Kennedy et al 1989 p 477).

This was an important statement for women whose only access to contraception is through breastfeeding, as long as women are informed of the need to feed often and frequently during the night. For many traditional communities this is the normal pattern of feeding, but aggressive marketing by formula producers has resulted in changes in these patterns, with the subsequent loss of the contraceptive effect (Palmer 1993). Maher (1995) comments on communities in west Africa, where feeding up to 3 years of age is the cultural norm and that as a consequence women bear between six and eight children during their fertile lifetime, as opposed to their potential for around 17. This must bring health benefits to both mother and children, as repeated pregnancies and childbirth are in themselves risk-factors for maternal and child mortality. The implications for western women of lactational ammenorhoea have to be viewed cautiously, while breastfeeding practice tends to be up to six feeds a day as opposed to 12 or more feeds among traditional communities.

WOMEN'S PERSPECTIVES ON THE BENEFITS OF BREASTFEEDING

Typically, when women are asked about the benefits of breastfeeding for them, they do not focus on risk-factors for disease. It seems that while social scientists grapple for concepts which can adequately describe and explain health as opposed to disease, women are natural 'post-modernists' in their own explanations of health, well-being and breastfeeding. For example, Hauck and Reinbold (1996) conducted a study to determine the criteria western Australian women used to decide whether breastfeeding was successful. A series of 183 telephone interviews was followed by 19 in-depth interviews with ten unsuccessful and nine successful breastfeeders. Success or failure was a personally defined experience, not necessarily based on conventional notions of duration. The four major categories which emerged from a content analysis of the data were giving, persistence, meeting expectations and accomplishing personal goals. Such criteria are not consistent with medical orthodoxy related to health outcomes, being scientifically immeasurable, but nevertheless are authentic outcomes for the women themselves.

Dignam (1995) explored the concept of intimacy with breastfeeding mothers and associated intimacy with reciprocity, mutual joy, harmony, concern for others, trust and closeness. While none of these characteristics could either be measured or defined as conventional outcomes, they nevertheless could be conceptually associated with theories on mental health. For example, Antonovsky's (1984) theory of the sense of coherence is interesting in the light of the characteristics women associate with breastfeeding. Antonovsky defines a sense of coherence as:

> 'A global orientation that expresses the extent to which one has a pervasive, enduring though dynamic feeling of confidence that one's internal and external environments are predictable and that there is a high probability that things will work out as well as can reasonably be expected' (Antonovsky 1984 p 10).

When we consider characteristics such as harmony and mutual joy, it becomes feasible that, if Antonovsky's theory that the sense of coherence is central to mental well-being holds true, then breastfeeding could contribute to mental health in a positive way. This aspect of breastfeeding should be explored in more detail and valued more highly by the more conventional health analysts. Currently, these aspects of breastfeeding remain 'hidden' behind the cloak of qualitative research, which itself is not highly valued in the medical domain. Of course, a post-modernist would pose the question, 'Why is breastfeeding in the medical domain in the first place?' This is perhaps the most enduring question in the analysis of public health and breastfeeding, as it becomes more evident that the contrast between the private experience of breastfeeding and the epidemiologically defined public health benefits are quite disparate.

WHY DON'T MORE WOMEN BREASTFEED?

Despite all the evidence on the positive benefits for health which breastfeeding can confer, it is clear from the UK evidence on incidence and prevalence (Office of National Statistics 1997) that while about two-thirds of women may breastfeed at birth, this rapidly declines over the first six weeks and beyond and about a third of all babies in the UK never have the opportunity to be nurtured by human milk. The ONS survey identified some of the variables associated with breastfeeding and breastfeeding patterns, these being social class, age of leaving school and region. While it is useful for public health purposes to know that breastfeeding incidence and prevalence decreases among the manual socioeconomic groups, it is also important to understand the explanations for the differences in behaviour towards infant feeding found among various social groupings in the UK. It is equally important to acknowledge that, because women from one socioeconomic group are statistically less likely to breastfeed than women from another, this does not in itself indicate lack of intention or motivation and may be indicative of cultural or social barriers to breastfeeding, rather than an active decision not to breastfeed.

It would seem that if education, class and region are important statistical variables then one explanation underlying these may be culture. Culture here could refer to the infant feeding or social culture within which women exist, or the wider cultural context of the western medicalised environment in which women are expected to breastfeed. It has been argued in a previous paper (Kendall 1995) that practitioners should acknowledge and explore cultural norms and expectations before exhorting women to breastfeed; it is particularly necessary to appreciate that for some families the notion of healthiness is not a priority and neither is it ascribed to behaviours such as breastfeeding which may be regarded as unacceptable or even obscene. For example, Gordon (1998) found in her work in Northern Ireland that the partners of breastfeeding mothers were often of the view that only wayward women did that sort of thing, equating breastfeeding with 'whoring'. Under this type of cultural pressure within a strongly patriarchal society, a woman must probably respect the wishes of her husband before anything else and would not want her family or husband's family to think she was 'loose'.

Professional discourse on this topic often refers to the 'failure' to breastfeed. For example, Wylie and Verber (1994) report on women's breastfeeding behaviour at 28 days postpartum, commenting that 'failing to breastfeed this cohort of babies will inevitably mean increased artificial feeding for the next cohort – we only have one chance to get it right' (p 118). This implies that women are weak and uncaring and somehow failing in their responsibility to nurture their babies appropriately. Clearly, from the evidence already cited, the public health view is that breastfeeding should both be initiated by more women and continued for longer. However, the barriers to breastfeeding may be more societal than individual.

Hoddinott and Pill (1999) conducted a qualitative study among working class women in east London found that the decision to breastfeed was more influenced by 'embodied knowledge', that is having first-hand experience of observing friends and relatives breastfeeding, than theoretical knowledge related to health benefits. The implication of this study is that it is important to find ways of exposing more women to positive experiences of breastfeeding than to provide information about how much healthier their babies will be in the future. A study by Buckell and Thompson (1995) of two contrasting social areas in an outer London borough, found that women in the less affluent area had equally strong intentions to breastfeed as women in an area of higher affluence (house ownership, employment, professional occupations) and that initiation of breastfeeding for both groups was even higher than the national average (82.8% and 85.3% respectively). However, women from the less affluent area were less likely to maintain breastfeeding up to the 3-month point. Given high motivation and initiation, it is disappointing from a public health perspective that the group where other indicators of poor health (e.g. smoking, depression) are also high, that breastfeeding is not continued regularly beyond three months. The study suggests that some of the explanation for this may be that they come from a 'bottle-feeding culture' although this is not explored in any detail. The complexities of the ways in which a bottle-feeding culture is created by the formula milk companies aggressively marketing their products, alongside a social security system which rewards mothers on low income who formula-feed with milk tokens, may have something to contribute to our understanding of the variations between social groups in the UK and infant feeding practices. One hypothesis for tackling the 'bottle-feeding culture' may be to investigate the effects of greater exposure to positive breastfeeding experiences, one being tried in the Lambeth, Southwark and Lewisham health action zone.

The way in which we disseminate information about breastfeeding may also be an important factor, since it is apparent that information alone does not significantly change behaviour. Britton (1998) has discussed the ways in which antenatal information influences women's breastfeeding experiences. From a series of qualitative focus groups with a total of 30 mothers aged between 20 and 39 years, the majority of whom were primigravidae and had breastfed between 5 days and were continuing at the time of the study (up to 20 weeks), Britton found that there were three main sources of influence antenatally. These were the media construction of breastfeeding, professional influence through antenatal classes and information from other women. The participants commented on how the media construction was often falsely rosy in its perspective and did not portray the realities of night-time and the exhaustion associated with a crying baby and sore nipples. Antenatal classes were criticised for putting too much emphasis on labour and the physiological aspects of breastfeeding, rather than the emotional and social aspects. The most supportive and relevant to the needs of this group of women was the information they received from other women who had previously breastfed, including other women in the focus groups. This information is supportive of the idea that if health professionals explored women's concepts of successful breastfeeding, rather than the medically determined outcomes, then their 'success' rate at helping women to breastfeed might be improved. Britton concludes that midwives and health visitors should probably do more to facilitate peer learning and peer support for breastfeeding.

COMMUNITY PRACTITIONERS AND THE PROMOTION OF PUBLIC HEALTH THROUGH BREASTFEEDING

The foregoing discussion has raised the dilemma for the community practitioner of how, having collated the evidence for health improvement through breastfeeding, are culturally and socially acceptable methods of promoting the incidence, prevalence and duration of breastfeeding to be achieved? Is breastfeeding a public health issue or is it simply a matter of personal preference? Should breastfeeding be part of healthy public policy, for example in terms of the workplace, public places, health service policy? There are, embedded in these deliberately rhetorical questions, three levels of public health action to be addressed – the individual/community, the professional sphere and the policy-making process.

Each of these will be addressed in terms of the contribution each level could make separately to improving public health through breastfeeding, and also, it will be concluded, how a concerted action could facilitate a shift from a bottle-feeding to a breastfeeding culture.

THE INDIVIDUAL/COMMUNITY

Britton's (1998) study has raised the question of support for breastfeeding women coming primarily from other experienced breastfeeders, rather than through a professionally led route such as antenatal classes. This is not a novel idea and studies have been conducted to review the effectiveness of mother-to-mother programmes. I would argue that if the evidence from a range of qualitative studies on breastfeeding is analysed concurrently, then a theoretical position emerges which proposes that women gain more support for breast-feeding from other women than they do from health professionals because other experienced breastfeeders promote the outcomes as defined by women, rather than medically-determined outcomes. These outcomes could be significant for the mental well-being of both mother and baby, which have been largely over-looked in the medical literature. For example, Locklin (1995) focused on 17 low-income, culturally-diverse women in a qualitative study which involved peer counsellors to support breastfeeding. Through the constant comparative analytic approach, five themes emerged from her data which indicated the empowering effect which this type of support had on the breastfeeding experience. The five themes were:

- Making the discovery
- Seeking a connection
- Comforting each other
- Becoming empowered, and
- Telling the world.

As suggested in relation to Dignam's (1995) study, these themes are highly suggestive of the sense of coherence Antonovsky (1984) has described.

In Tarkka and Paunonen's (1996) study of social support to 200 new mothers, they found that the support they received least of in hospital was emotional support. Locklin's study would suggest that this could be provided through the peer support system and this would also support Britton's (1998) conclusions. A study in Glasgow was reported by Gribble (1996). At that time, the breastfeeding rate in the Easterhouse district of Glasgow was 12%, one of the lowest in Europe. A 'breastfeeding helper' scheme was set up and organised by midwives, as it was understood that the culturally embedded and negative attitudes towards breastfeeding on the estate would be more likely to respond to local women who 'spoke their language' than to health professionals. The six trained helpers involved found that they were able to encourage other women to breastfeed, or at least to give it serious consideration, and that an additional bonus was that their own self-esteem and self-confidence increased, enabling them to become spokeswomen on behalf of breastfeeding in the community. The outcomes on breastfeeding rates were unreported, but these qualitative effects of peer support are relevant to public health initiatives.

One of the recent initiatives of the Department of Health in England has been to set up health action zones (HAZ) (Department of Health 1998) in specified areas of the country where health indicators such as housing tenure, unemploy-ment, ethnic mix, population trends, and morbidity and mortality rates are suggestive of inequalities in health compared with more affluent areas. The HAZs provide the opportunity for health authorities and primary care groups to work in partnership with other agencies to analyse the health needs of the population and to target the HAZ in response to this. The HAZs are currently in the process of developing their strategies and undergoing evaluation.

One example of an HAZ is in the Lambeth, Southwark and Lewisham health authority. One part of their initiative is to conduct an outcome-based evaluation of the effectiveness of mother-to-mother support for breastfeeding. This will involve collaboration with general practice and training of midwives and health visitors to work with community mothers in this way. Most previous research has been of a qualitative nature, so the results of this trial will have important implications for the way in which community-based intelligence can influence child and maternal health (Rowe & Sikorski 2001). It is to be hoped that such a large-scale outcome-based study will draw on the client-determined outcomes as a measure of effectiveness, as well as the conventional public health outcomes.

THE PROFESSIONAL SPHERE

The professional scope for contributing to public health through the promotion of breastfeeding centres around the way in which professional groups can be trained to improve their support of breastfeeding families and the effectiveness of professional advice and support. It has already been noted that Britton (1998) implied that the women in her study found that the information received in antenatal classes was over-medicalised and did little to prepare them for the experience of breastfeeding.

It is not unusual to find examples of women in the literature who give up breastfeeding either because professional support was indifferent or because advice was conflicting from different professional groups. Approaches to assess the level of professional attitude, knowledge and skill in relation to breastfeeding have been reported, as well as studies on effectiveness of professional advice and training initiatives. One of the methodological problems for all of these studies is the difficulty in demonstrating long-term changes in breastfeeding rates, partly because randomised controlled trials are ethically difficult to design and also because long-term observational studies, like the Wilson et al (1998) study discussed above, are very costly to run. Evidence of effectiveness of professional intervention programmes has therefore to be based on short-term indicators such as client satisfaction or audit of professional activity.

Patton et al (1996) reported on a correlational study carried out in the USA, which looked at nurses' attitudes and behaviours towards breastfeeding in relation to their support of breastfeeding. The study relied on nurses self-reports and did not attempt to link this with mothers views. A 19-item questionnaire was administered to which 230 obstetric nurses responded. While 64% of the sample would recommend or actively encourage breastfeeding, the researchers found that this was closely correlated with their personal experience of breastfeeding and their educational level. The main barriers to promoting breastfeeding were lack of knowledge and the shortened length of hospital stay. A further factor was the time-consuming nature of breastfeeding support. It might be assumed that those nurses who had had positive experiences of breastfeeding themselves would view the time factor more favourably and see this as a resource-effective activity, although the researchers do not comment on this possible association.

Another study in the USA (Freed et al 1995) investigated physicians' breastfeeding knowledge and experience. They used a national random sample of 3115 residents and 1920 practising physicians in paediatrics, obstetrics and family medicine. Again a questionnaire was administered with a similar response rate of 68%. All groups demonstrated significant knowledge deficits in breastfeeding – for example, less than 50% of residents chose the appropriate clinical management of breast abscess or breastfed jaundiced infant. More than 30% of practising physicians chose the incorrect advice for mothers with low milk supply. Low milk supply is one of the recurring factors which are perceived by mothers to be a reason to stop breastfeeding; lack of medical knowledge in this area perhaps accounts for why many women do give up between birth and 6 weeks. Over 50% of the physicians thought they had not had enough preparation during residency for counselling breastfeeding women. Interestingly, as with the nurses in Patton's (1996) study, the greatest predictor of physician's self-confidence in breastfeeding counselling was personal or spousal breastfeeding experience.

An audit conducted in northern Birmingham (Robertson & Goddard, 1997) also found that most of their client respondents did not feel adequately prepared for the 'how to' of breastfeeding, although 73% had decided before 28 weeks of pregnancy that they wished to breastfeed. While 50% initially breastfed, by 6 months only 17% continued to do so. The audit results from the professional group, like the American studies, were strongly suggestive that while professionals were widely involved in giving breastfeeding advice, they did not have adequate training. The UK study does not provide a complete picture of the data, and they do not address the issue of the personal experience of professionals, it is therefore difficult to draw direct comparisons, especially in the light of the fact that none of these three studies provide a proper definition of breastfeeding. The implications of these three studies are relevant to the approach which might be taken to promoting breastfeeding through professional support – not only is it important to ensure that professionals have an evidence-based knowledge about breastfeeding, but also to draw on the peer support concept in the context of professional support, as it would seem that the likelihood of giving confident and appropriate advice is enhanced if the professional has a positive personal experience of breastfeeding and is able to draw upon those client-determined outcomes referred to earlier, such as mutual joy and closeness, as a result of their own experience.

PUBLIC HEALTH AND BREASTFEEDING POLICY

The orthodox approaches to public health described above rely heavily on an individualist model of public health, in which women are assigned a responsibility to do what is best for their infants. They retain a taint of the victim-blaming culture of right wing 1980s thinking, where women who do not breast-feed 'bring their problems on themselves and their babies'. Thus, eczema, asthma, gastroenteritis, otitis media, and even sudden infant death can be blamed on the formula-feeding mother. The new public health (Ashton & Seymour 1990) would argue for a more structuralist approach, in which policies addressing the complexities of culture, social variation, multiagency involvement and consumer involvement are developed. There is some evidence that such policies are beginning to emerge in the UK – the example given above of the health action zones (Department of Health 1998) is a recent initiative which is responsive to structural issues related to inequality in health, as well as conceptual issues around health promotion and health improvement such as consumer involvement. Healthy public policy integrates concepts of health, environment, economics, social milieu and work, so that people can expect to be as safe and well as possible in all aspects of their lives. In the UK, Acheson (Department of Health 1999b) reported on inequalities in health and highlighted the need to improve the health of women and children through nutrition. It particularly refers to much of the evidence cited here on the benefits of breastfeeding and states:

> 'We recommend policies which increase the prevalence of breastfeeding' (para 22.1 p 71).

The integration of public policy to meet this recommendation is vital and the full and proper evaluation of initiatives such as health action zones central to the future success and survival of such policy.

Some interesting initiatives are emerging, although as with other matters discussed, most are unevaluated in the traditional sense. For example, women around the world have been campaigning for the right to breastfeed at work. At the beginning of this chapter, I referred to how women have historically been driven into working away from the home, and the inherent difficulties of maintaining breastfeeding in an environment which may be male-dominated, lacks childcare facilities and expresses negative attitudes towards breastfeeding, especially longer-term. In 1993, a campaign in Australia tried to address some of these problems by introducing the 'Mother-friendly workplace initiative', in association with world breastfeeding week (World Association for Breastfeeding Action 1993). The campaign was predicated on the Innocenti Declaration signed by 30 governments (including the UK) in 1990, which states that:

> 'All women should be enabled to practise exclusive breastfeeding and all infants should be fed exclusively on breast milk from birth to four to six months of age'.

The Declaration calls on all governments by 1995 to 'enact imaginative legislation protecting the breastfeeding rights of working women'. The Australian initiative can be seen as an example of healthy public policy in the making because of the way in which it integrates the physical and emotional health benefits to infants and mothers with employment, environmental and economic benefits. For example, it was argued in the document that breastfeeding women are less likely to be absent from work, as their children are healthier and the morale of the women is better since they feel more able to meet their family responsibilities. This, the argument continues, leads to higher productivity. Breastfeeding is environmentally friendly leading to only biodegradable waste and as more women breastfeed at work this would probably have the effect of the workplace becoming a cleaner and safer place for everyone to work in. Economically, as more women breastfeed there would be savings on the health-service budget. The initiative also provides a strategy for employers to provide a workplace environment which supports breastfeeding women. The strategy is built on three tenets – time, space/proximity and support. Time refers to paid maternity leave, as well as time out at work to breastfeed, including flexible working hours. Space and proximity refers to childcare facilities that are based in or near the workplace, comfortable and private facilities for breastfeeding or expressing and a clean work environment that is safe from hazardous waste or chemicals.

Support should be in terms of:

- Ensuring women are aware of their maternity rights
- Full job security
- Ensuring a positive attitude towards breastfeeding at work, and
- Encouraging women to establish their own support networks.

Considering the positive benefits this strategy could bring to the work environment, it is interesting to reflect on the extent to which employers in the UK have adopted it.

Britten (1996) reported on some workplace initiatives which have developed in the UK, largely as result of individual pressure rather than integrated policy. She explores a number of case studies within the context of Health and Safety legislation (Health and Safety Executive 1994), which gives some guidance to employers on the rights of expectant and new mothers at work, but Britten argues is a long way from the 'imaginative legislation' agreed in the Innocenti Declaration. Nevertheless, the case studies do provide examples of the way in which employers could address some of the issues inherent in the healthy workplace initiative proposed by the Department of Health (1998), although this is not prominent in the subsequent white paper. For example, one employer negotiated with Liz that her return to work could be on a flexible basis while she was breastfeeding, she was allowed time-out to express milk and storage arrangements were available in the staff kitchen. Morag had to negotiate with her personnel department to provide expressing facilities which were eventually found in the occupational health department. She had informal agreement to take time-out to express. Davina's return to work was more difficult. Her request to take time-out to breastfeed her 4-month-old baby was turned down by a committee. Davina had to make arrangements to leave her son with her mother and then to take a 25 minute walk there during her break to feed him. It was Davina's health visitor who lobbied the committee on her behalf and eventually the decision was overturned by a minority vote. This case study provides a good example of the way in which practitioners can support and raise awareness of policy within the existing legislative framework. The three case studies described go some way towards meeting the strategic objectives of the 1993 Australian initiative – time, space/proximity and support. However, it is clear that there is still great deal more to be done which could contribute to the development of healthy public policy.

CONCLUSION

This chapter has taken the theme of breastfeeding and public health as its focus. The underlying thesis of the discussion has been the way in which the orthodox discourse on public health interacts with a 'post-modern' agenda of health improvement. Breastfeeding represents an aspect of public health which impacts on traditional public health issues such as morbidity and mortality, but also raises questions about public perceptions of health and health outcomes.

There is ample evidence that breastfeeding is an effective way of reducing risk of disease among infants and mothers. A small percentage of that evidence has been discussed here. The Office of National Statistics (1997) data, which demonstrates an increasing trend in breastfeeding is encouraging, but the continuing variations in breastfeeding across regions and social classes remains a concern. There are still many women in the UK who choose either not to breastfeed or give up in the very early weeks, despite all the health benefits it can bring. Synthesis of trends within the evidence would seem to suggest that recognition of client-determined outcomes might be one way of addressing the reluctance to breastfeed among some groups of women. This can possibly be achieved through drawing on the recent public health strategy (Department of Health 1999a) to develop new ways of enabling women to breastfeed. This should include using mother-to-mother support programmes, introducing practitioner training programmes which challenge beliefs and attitudes as well as improving knowledge and by development of healthy public policy, such as employment conditions which enable women to continue to breastfeed.

The primary care groups and the health improvement programmes (Department of Health 1997) will provide an organisational framework for assessing local health need, developing approaches which contribute towards health improvement and, integral to this, quality improvement techniques such as teamwork and clinical audit, which will monitor and evaluate the effectiveness of interventions. Community practitioners, especially health visitors and midwives, must ensure that they are making a constructive and well-argued contribution to the needs of breastfeeding women in their population, so that the public health benefits can be realised at all levels.

DISCUSSION QUESTIONS

1. Do women in the 21st century have a choice about breastfeeding?
2. How would you advise a woman who was undecided about breastfeeding?
3. What are the issues facing women from low income/low socioeconomic groups in relation to breastfeeding?
4. What are the issues in society which we need to address to improve breastfeeding rates?
5. Do health professionals have a public health responsibility to promote breastfeeding?

FURTHER READING

Heinig M & Dewey K 1997 Health effects of breastfeeding for mothers: a critical review. Nutrition Research Review 10:35–56
This review brings together much of the research into breastfeeding which has findings that support the health of women. The research is wide-ranging and critically analysed, providing both a clear view of the evidence available and the strength of this evidence. The authors have also published a second review on the health effects of breastfeeding for infants.

Hoddinott P & Pill R 1999 Qualitative study of decisions about infant feeding among women in the east end of London. British Medical Journal 318:30–34
This paper provides an interesting insight into women's decisions about breast-feeding. It is of particular relevance as the study was conducted in an inner-city

area. It is also a good example of how qualitative research can demonstrate sound evidence through a systematic approach.

Maher V (ed) 1992 The Anthropology of Breastfeeding. Berg, Oxford
This text draws on the expertise of a collection of anthropologists who have studied breastfeeding in a variety of cultural settings. It not only provides rich descriptions of cultural variation and practice, but enables the reader to think critically about the ways in which we approach breastfeeding in the UK context.

Palmer G 1993 The Politics of Breastfeeding. Pandora Press, London
This text details much of the historical context of breastfeeding. It also provides a critical and important insight into the politics which have disabled women from breastfeeding globally and how this affects health, the environment and global economy.

REFERENCES

American Academy of Pediatrics 1997 Breastfeeding and the use of human milk. Pediatrics 100(6):1035–1039

Antonovsky A 1984 The sense of coherence as a determinant of health. Advances 1:37–50

Antonovsky A 1987 Unravelling the mystery of health: how people manage stress and stay well. Jossey Bass, San Fransisco

Ashton J & Seymour H 1990 The new public health. Open University Press, Milton Keynes

Baby Milk Action 1991 The best start in life (informational poster). Baby Milk Action, Cambridge

Bauchner H, Leventhal J & Shapiro E 1986 Studies of breastfeeding and infections: How good is the evidence? Journal of the American Medical Association 256:887–892

Brinton L, Berman M, Mortel R, Twiggs L, Barret R, Wilbanks G, Lannom L & Hoover R 1992 Reproductive, menstrual and medical risk factors for endometrial cancer: results from case control study. American Journal of Obstetrics and Gynecology 167:1317–1325

Britten J 1996 Employers and Breastfeeding. New Generation March: 26–27

Britton C 1998 The Influence of ante-natal information on breastfeeding experiences. British Journal of Midwifery 6(5):312–315

Buckell M & Thompson R 1995 A comparative breastfeeding study in two contrasting areas. Health Visitor 68(2):63–65

Chilvers C 1993 Breastfeeding and risk of breast cancer in young women. British Medical Journal 307:17–20

Cramer D, Hutchinson G, Welch W, Scully R & Ryan K 1983 Determinants of ovarian cancer risk. Journal of the National Cancer Institute 71:711–716

Department of Health 1994 Weaning and the Weaning Diet. Report of the Committee on Medical Aspects of Food Policy. HMSO, London

Department of Health 1997 The New NHS – Modern and Dependable. The Stationery Office, London

Department of Health 1998 Our Healthier Nation. The Stationery Office, London

Department of Health 1999a Saving lives: Our Healthier Nation. The Stationery Office, London

Department of Health 1999b Independent Inquiry into Inequalities in Health (Sir Donald Acheson, Chair). The Stationery Office, London

Dignam D 1995 Understanding intimacy as experienced by breastfeeding women. Health Care for Women International 16(5):477–485

Foster K, Lader D & Cheeseborough S 1997 Infant Feeding 1995. Office for National Statistics, London

Freed G, Clark S, Sorenson J, Lohr J, Celafo R & Curtis P 1995 National assessment of physician's breastfeeding knowledge, attitudes, training and experience. Journal of the American Medical Association 273(6):472–476

Giovanni M, Banderali G, Agestoni C, Silano M, Radaelli G & Riva E 1999 Epidemiology of breastfeeding in Italy. Acta Paediatrica Supplement 88(430):19–22

Gordon M 1998 Empowerment and breastfeeding. In: Kendall S (ed) Health and Empowerment: research and practice. Arnold, London

Gribble J 1996 An alternative approach. New Generation March: 12–13

Gwinn M, Lee N, Rhodes P, Layde P & Rubin G 1990 Pregnancy, breastfeeding and oral contraceptives and the risk of epithelial ovarian cancer. Journal of Clinical Epidemiology 43:559–568

Hartge P, Schiffman M, Hoover R, McGowan L, Lesher L & Norris H 1989 A case-control study of epithelial ovarian cancer. American Journal of Obstetrics and Gynecology 161:10–16

Hauck Y & Reinbold J 1996 Criteria for successful breastfeeding: mother's perceptions. Journal of the Australian College of Midwives 9(1):21–27

Health and Safety Executive 1994 New and Expectant mothers at work – a guide for employers (HS(G) 122). HMSO, London

Heinig M & Dewey K 1997 Health effects of breastfeeding for mothers: a critical review. Nutrition Research Review 10:35–56

Hoddinott P & Pill R 1999 Qualitative study of decisions about infant feeding among women in the east end of London. British Medical Journal 318:30–34

Howie P, Forsyth J, Ogston S, Clark A & du Florey C 1990 Protective effect of breastfeeding against infection. British Medical Journal 300:11–16

Kallio M, Simes M, Perheentupa J, Salmenpera L & Miettinen T 1992 Serum cholesterol and lipo-protein concentrations in mothers during and after prolonged exclusive lactation. Metabolism 41:1327–1330

Kelly M, Davies J & Charlton B 1993 Healthy cities: a modern problem or a post-modern solution? In: Kelly M et al (eds) Healthy Cities: Research and Practice. Routledge, London

Kendall S 1995 Cross cultural aspects and breastfeeding promotion. Health Visitor 68(11):450–451

Kennedy K, Rivera R & NcNeilly A 1989 Consensus statement on the use of breastfeeding as a family planning method. Contraception 39:477–496

Kolezko S, Sherman P, Corey M et al 1989 Role of infant feeding practices in development of Crohn's disease in childhood. British Medical Journal 298:1617–1618

Locklin M 1995 Telling the world: low income women and their breastfeeding experiences. Journal of Human Lactation 11(4):285–291

Maher V (ed) 1995 The Anthropology of Breastfeeding. Berg, Oxford

Metcalf M & Baum J 1992 Family characteristics and insulin dependent diabetes. Archives of Disease in Childhood 67(6):731–736

Newcombe P, Storer B, Longnecker M, Mittendorf R, Greenberg E, Clapp R, Burke K, Willett W & MacMahon B 1994 Lactation and a reduced risk of pre-menopausal breast cancer. New England Journal of Medicine 330:81–87

Palmer G 1993 The Politics of Breastfeeding. Pandora Press, London

Patton C, Beaman M, Csar N & Lewinski C 1996 Nurses' attitudes and behaviours that promote breastfeeding. Journal of Human Lactation 12(2):111–115

Robertson C & Goddard D 1997 Monitoring the quality of breastfeeding advice. Health Visitor 70(11):422–424

Rosenblatt K & Thomas D 1995 Prolonged lactation and endometrial cancer. WHO collaborative study of neoplasia and steroid contraceptives. International Journal of Epidemiology 24:499–503

Rowe J & Sikorski J 2001 Mother to mother support for breastfeeding. Project Information Sheet 18. Lambeth, Southwark and Lewisham Health Action Zone Quarterly Report, January

Savage F 1992 Breastfeeding – SIDS. Midwifery Digest of Research 2(1):3–5

Tarkka M & Paunonen M 1996 Social support provided by nurses to recent mothers on a maternity ward. Journal of Advanced Nursing 23(6):1202–1206

UNICEF 1996 The Baby Friendly Initiative. UK Committee for UNICEF, London

Whittemore A 1994 Characteristics relating to ovarian cancer risk: implications for prevention and detection. Gynecologic Oncology 55:515–519

Wilson A, Forsyth J, Greene S, Irvine L, Hau C & Howie P 1998 Relation of infant diet to childhood health: seven year follow up of cohort of children in Dundee infant feeding study. British Medical Journal 316:21–25

World Alliance for Breastfeeding Action 1993 Women, work and breastfeeding. World Alliance for Breastfeeding Action, Penang

Wylie J & Verber I 1994 Why women fail to breastfeed: a prospective study from booking to 28 days post-partum. Journal of Human Nutrition and Dietetics 7:115–121

12 Family support as a public health issue

Christine Bidmead

KEY ISSUES

- Is family support a 'public health' issue?
- If it is, how is that support to be provided and who should provide it?
- What is the effect of emerging government policies on the role of professional health workers?
- What are the implications for practice for health visitors, school nurses and midwives?

INTRODUCTION

Public health may be defined as, 'the science and art of preventing disease, prolonging life and promoting health through organised efforts of society' (Acheson 1998). Health visitors have a long history of working with families and have always seen their work as having a public health focus.

In its preamble, the UN Convention on the Rights of the Child (UNICEF 1990) asserts that:

> The family, as the fundamental group in society and the natural environment for the growth and well-being of all its members, particularly children, should be afforded the necessary protection and assistance so that it can fully assume its responsibilities within the community.'

Article 18.2 goes on:

> 'For the purpose of guaranteeing and promoting the rights set forth in the present Convention, States Parties shall render appropriate assistance to parents and legal guardians in the performance of their child-rearing responsibilities and shall ensure the development of institutions, facilities and services for the care of children.'

'Well-being' as applied here is surely health in its widest sense. The idea that raising children is a joint venture between the state and parents recognises that all citizens bear a responsibility for children. The state, therefore, has a duty to provide assistance to parents, acknowledging the need for social support to enhance the opportunities for all children (Pugh et al 1994). Family support is necessary for family health and is, therefore, a public health issue and one which the government has a duty to encourage.

In this chapter we will look in detail at:

- Why family support is necessary for family health
- Family health as a public health issue
- New policies which enhance the health visitor's public health role
- The practicalities of incorporating policy into practice.

In conclusion it will be noted that the role of the health visitor is one that evolves from a focus on the health needs of individual families, to take on the wider dimensions of the health needs of the community in which the health visitor works.

IS FAMILY SUPPORT NECESSARY FOR FAMILY HEALTH?

'Bright Futures', a report by the Mental Health Foundation published in June 1999, emphasises the importance of wider supportive networks in the community. It shows that in spite of really adverse circumstances some children go on to do surprisingly well. The report, therefore, looks at what can be done to increase the resilience of all children. It identifies qualities that research has shown increase children's resilience to adverse circumstances. The factors, as shown in Box 12.1, presuppose parents who are capable of providing the right kind of nurturing environment for their children. This may not be possible through no fault of their own. If they live on a run-down estate with poor housing, no leisure facilities, no work, and an inability to form secure relationships with their children, then those children will be at greater risk of mental and physical health problems later in life, and at greater risk of falling into juvenile crime.

In spite of the positive stance taken in 'Bright Futures' it is still those who are worst off in our society who suffer the worst health (Acheson 1998). Inequalities in health persist. However, the report by Sir Donald Acheson again

BOX 12.1	*Qualities that increase children's resilience to adverse circumstances (Mental Health Foundation 1999)*
	■ Secure attachment to a parent figure
	■ A balance of affection and supervision
	■ Has developed good communication skills
	■ Has a positive attitude
	■ Has learned to problem-solve
	■ Can reflect and learn
	■ Absence of severe discord in the family
	■ Wider supportive networks in the community
	■ Good housing
	■ Good leisure facilities
	■ Support for education

emphasises the strengthening effect of social and community support, which can sustain health in otherwise adverse circumstances.

Research has shown that social support is health-promoting (Oakley et al 1994). Oakley also points out that there is a large body of research that demonstrates that both chronic and acute stress are associated with poor physical and mental health outcomes. Those who live under stressful circumstances with little income, poor housing, and a lack of supportive relationships are more at risk from adverse life-events. In her research she shows how stressful life-events impact more heavily on women's lives and that this has implications for the higher incidence of psychological morbidity. Experiencing stress increases health services use. It would seem that mothers are looking to the health service for support, but that until now service providers have not seen meeting these needs as their role.

FAMILY SUPPORT FOR FAMILIES FROM ETHNIC MINORITIES

The Moyenda Project was a three-year piece of work offered to African-Caribbean and Asian families in London, to explore their needs for family support (Evans & Grant 1995). Although the focus of the report is on social services provision of support, it has strong messages for public health workers. It found that African-Caribbean and Asian parents are under additional stresses and pressure that white families do not face. There are pressures associated with racial discrimination and prejudice with which they have to contend, and the difficulties of living in a white culture against their own lifestyle, customs and languages (see Box 12.2). The report showed that these people had little faith in support agencies to help them. What was needed was:

'A more culturally comfortable group where the effects of racism could be discussed more easily and only then could parents feel that the group

BOX 12.2	*Example from practice*

Shiva was a young Tamil woman recently arrived in this country from Sri Lanka. She was pregnant and did not speak English. The health visitor for the homeless made the Tamil Refugee centre aware of her arrival. She visited her temporary accommodation with a link worker to provide interpretation.

Shiva was very lonely for other Tamil women. This was her first pregnancy and she missed her mother and family back in Sri Lanka. At the refugee centre she became part of a mothers group where she could talk to other women in her own language and from her own culture. She soon made friends and attended English classes at the local college with other Tamil women.

Finding and establishing herself within her own culture was important to enable her and give her the confidence to make the necessary links to begin to integrate into her new environment and culture. She needed a safe base from which to explore.

was a safe place to discuss more everyday concerns of parenting' (cited by Siddall 1995).

The project workers found that white professionals were fearful of acknowledging differences and were in danger of taking a 'colour-blind' approach for fear of being labelled racist. A 'colour-blind' approach may be defined as deciding that, as services are available to all, there is no need to acknowledge the differences of culture and ethnicity which effect the take-up or access to those services. Not acknowledging difference and positively discriminating in favour of ethnic minority groups may, therefore, said to be taking a 'colour-blind' approach.

FAMILY HEALTH AS A PUBLIC HEALTH ISSUE

Early intervention

It is important that parents in particular receive the help and support that they need. The effect of early childhood experience of the skills of handling difficult situations, maintaining self-esteem and the ability to care for oneself, is clearly documented. Attachment theory and its effect on the ability to make successful relationships in later life also has a demonstrable effect on the risk of disease and also the ability to heal (Ministerial Group on the Family 1998). Juvenile crime and delinquency and adult crime and violence are also clearly linked to early home-life and patterns of parenting (Farrington 1995).

Russek and Schwartz (1997) showed, in a study obtained from undergraduates at Harvard University, that perceptions of parental caring predict the health status in mid-life. In the early 1950s initial ratings of parental caring were obtained from a sample of healthy Harvard undergraduate men. During the 35-year follow-up investigation detailed medical and psychological histories and medical records were obtained. The results showed that in mid-life those suffering from illnesses such as coronary artery disease, hypertension, duodenal ulcer and alcoholism, had perceived their parents to have a significantly lower rate of parental caring items (i.e. loving, just, fair, hardworking, clever, strong) while they were in college. 'This effect was independent of the subject's age, family history of illness, smoking behaviour, the death and/or divorce of parents, and the marital history of subjects' (Russek & Schwartz 1997 p 144).

Furthermore, 87% of subjects who rated both their mothers and fathers as low in parental caring had diagnosed diseases in mid-life, whereas only 25% of subjects who rated both their mother and fathers high in parental caring had diagnosed diseases in mid-life. They concluded that:

'Since parents are usually the most meaningful source of social support for much of early life, the perception of parental caring, and parental loving itself, may have important regulatory and predictive effects on biological and psychological health and illness' (Russek & Shwartz 1997 p 144).

If social support enables parents to care for their children in a loving environment, then there will be clear benefits for the health of the whole of our society. Early intervention with family support is clearly indicated for family health and the public health role of the health visitor becomes of paramount importance.

Research has shown how distressing it is for children to experience the breakdown of their parents' relationship (Cockett & Tripp 1994). Studies also show that married people are happier and healthier when compared collectively to their single counterparts and that they tend to stay together longer than do cohabitees (Breen et al 1998).

There is now a considerable movement to encourage health visitors, midwives and community nurses to offer support for relationships when problems first start to occur (One plus One 1998). That this contributes to the health of children and parents cannot now be disputed. The 'Brief Encounters' counselling offered by health visitors has proved highly effective and acceptable to new parents and enabled one in five couples to be identified and given help, compared with one in twenty in the control clinics. The findings of the British Social Attitudes Survey (1992) showed that only 2% of married people would turn to a marriage counsellor if they had a problem. They were much more likely to approach a family member or friend for support. They also turn to health care professionals with whom they have more contact at times of increased stress. This being so, One plus One, an organisation concerned to support relationships, set up its 'Brief Encounters' training to help to enhance the skills and confidence of health visitors and GPs to detect the early signs of distress caused by relationship problems, so that they could respond constructively even when time was limited.

There is much evidence to suggest that physical problems such as reduced foetal growth, low birth weight and weight at one year are linked with health problems in early and late childhood. They are also linked with the risk of cardiovascular diseases later on in life (Acheson 1998).

BOX 12.3	*Example from Practice (Leith 1997)*

Jacqui is the mother of 18-month-old Georgia who has been expelled from her childminder for being too naughty. Jacqui is distraught at her daughter's behaviour but struggles on in spite of feeling totally inadequate to the task of parenting a child that she described as a cross between Rambo and John McEnroe.

At two-and-a-half, Georgia was causing problems in nursery and Jacqui and Georgia were referred to the Child Guidance Service. She attended appointments for two years with little improvement in Georgia's behaviour. At four Georgia was threatened with expulsion from the nursery. Jacqui felt isolated, depressed and unable to cope. She believed that she was a bad parent and did not know where to turn for support. Desperate, she contacted her health visitor who told her about the parenting programme being run at the health centre.

Jacqui jumped at the chance to attend. Over the seven weeks she learned some practical techniques for managing Georgia's behaviour in a positive way. She found sympathy, support and understanding from the other parents in the group and began to realise that she was not such a bad mother after all. Slowly her confidence grew. Georgia's behaviour began to improve a little and Jacqui felt incredible relief. When the seven weeks came to an end she had made new friends who continued to support each other over the coming months and years.

Jacqui is a manager with a supportive housing scheme and has used her new-found parenting skills to help young teenage parents in her work.

Barker (1998) showed that child abuse and child neglect can also have adverse outcomes in later life and the effects of maternal postnatal depression on childhood development are well-documented (Murray 1997).

Cowley (1999) cites examples from the USA that show how effective multifaceted home-visiting programmes can be in improving the range of damaging factors, including low birth weight and damaging and hostile home environments. A 15-year follow-up shows continued good results overall.

The evidence seems to be that to take preventative steps to improve health overall we must tackle the health of the family, and in order to do this we must create what Quinn (1997) calls a 'supportive parent-friendly society' (see Box 12.3). Michael Quinn is founder of the Family Caring Trust, which provides resources for parenting programmes in the community and encourages parent leadership and peer support. He defines a 'Parent-friendly community' as:

- 'A place where parents are valued and supported in their task and are not taken for granted nor made to feel guilty.
- A place where there are structured opportunities to explore with their peers what they and their children need and to be updated and coached on skills in an environment where they feel safe, not patronised.
- A place where those with potential are encouraged and trained to support other parents'.

In order to create these supportive communities a community development approach is necessary (Box 12.4).

BOX 12.4	*Principles of community development (Luck & Jesson 1996)*

- Adopts a broad-based social not medical definition of health
- Takes a positive view of health (i.e. does not focus on illness)
- Seeks to be preventative rather than curative
- Challenges and seeks to influence public policy
- Derives its mandate from users not providers
- Uses a collective approach through work with groups and individuals normally excluded from resource and service-planning
- Places emphasis on participation, confidence-building and defining own health needs
- Is free of bureaucratic structures and professional constraints
- Is open to new ways of working, crossing professional boundaries, bringing people and organisations together
- Aims to reduce inequalities in health which derive from socioeconomic factors and unequal access to healthcare services by challenging medical, institutional, racist or sexist or ageist assumptions

NEW GOVERNMENT POLICIES

Health visitors have been particularly hampered by the focus on the medical model of health. It is not a 'health model' at all but an illness model. Working preventatively with community groups, helping them to define their own health needs, has proved particularly difficult in some areas of the country as we shall see later in this chapter. However, current government policies look set to support this role of health visitors and school nurses.

In November 1996 the Labour Party was preparing its manifesto for the election the following year. As part of that process it published two precursors of the green paper 'Supporting Families'. They were 'Parenting' and 'Early Excellence: a head start for every child' (Labour Party Public Information Service 1996a, 1996b). It was clear from these that the Labour Party had identified the health visitor as crucial to their plans.

Health visitors were heartened to hear that their pivotal role with families giving advice on parenting, early childhood development and support in the immediate postnatal period was at last recognised at the highest level by the then shadow education and employment secretary. Their highly respected profession was acknowledged as able to empower parents to access relevant information and support from other local voluntary and statutory agencies (Labour Party Public Information Service 1996).

These papers launched jointly with the shadow home secretary showed a coordinated approach across health, education and the home office, even in opposition. It foreshadowed the 'joined-up' working that we have all heard so much about since the election in 1997. This is particularly true for 'Sure Start', which is a government interdepartmental initiative.

So support for families was very much to the forefront of Labour policies. In particular there was support for parenting programmes. These, they said, should be given a higher priority by schools, local authorities and voluntary bodies. The national helpline for parents was proposed and more help for parents at key points in the life-cycle, i.e. childbirth, beginning school and adolescence.

The role of health visitors was also seen as crucial in looking at how the NHS could do more to provide parents with more information about help available (Labour Party Public Information Service 1996a).

Now the Labour Party are in government and we have seen just how far-reaching their policies are in the green and white papers so far produced. The role of the health visitor and school nurse is of paramount importance to the implementation of their plans to support families, reduce health inequalities and meet new targets for public health.

In the new NHS, community nurses are given places on primary care group boards so that their voices may be heard when services are being commissioned, local priorities are being identified for health improvement programmes, and user involvement and interagency working are being encouraged. Primary care groups encourage general practitioners to take a public health perspective of their community, and nurses, voices must be heard, supporting the new government strategies that promote family support as a public health issue. It is to be hoped that the unfortunate unequal representation of seven general practitioners to two nurses, that is the formation of most primary care group boards, does not reduce that voice to a mere whisper!

BOX 12.5	*Supporting Families, Chapter I (Ministerial Group on the Family 1998) 'Better Services and Support for Parents' outlines new initiatives:*

- The National Family and Parenting Institute to provide guidance to government on family policy and develop more and better parenting support
- A National Parenting Helpline to be developed by Parentline to offer advice to parents and carers and refer people to local sources of help
- A new enhanced role for health visitors, embracing the whole well-being of parents and children as well as their physical health
- Sure Start, a new £540 million initiative to help children in their early years to grow up with the skills they need to make the most of school
- Helping parents help their children learn, through family literacy and mentoring schemes
- Introduce education for parenthood in the school curriculum
- Help grandparents and older people offer more support to families
- Improve the rules for adoption

Now the Government has given us policies that fully support the roles of health visitors and school nurses it may be helpful to look at these policies in some detail.

'Supporting Families'

This green consultation paper (Ministerial Group on the Family 1998) was the first paper to speak of an 'enhanced role' for the health visitor. Many health visitors read it and thought, 'but this is what I do', while many others may have read it and thought, 'but this is what I have always wanted to do!'. In it, the Government also outlined its plans for the 'Sure Start' programme.

The document was divided into five chapters. The first chapter, summarised in Box 12.5, was perhaps the most significant in terms of its relevance to health visiting and we shall examine this in more detail.

The new enhanced role for health visitors (see Box 12.5) did not seem so new to many in the profession who felt that they had always embraced a holistic approach to the care of parents and children. However, at least the role and the potential of health visitors was acknowledged as providing a service that was universal, non-judgemental, and non-stigmatising.

The Community Practitioners and Health Visitors' Association (CPHVA), in its response to this Government consultation document, redefined the family as:

'A complex set of relationships encompassing biological, emotional, social, economic and civic ties. It is dynamic and changes over time and spans a number of generations' (CPHVA 1999 p 1).

The CPHVA then went on to declare that the 'Supporting Families' paper recognised many elements important to the CPHVA definition of the family. These included:

- The responsibility of the state to vulnerable families who face serious problems
- The recognition that grandparents are key family members
- The value placed on all varieties of parental relationships
- The importance of work policies that make it easier for families to balance home and work.

The Association felt that the rights of children were underplayed in the document and that insufficient note was taken of the fact that we live in a culturally diverse society.

> 'There is a need to identify best practice in ethnic minority communities and to weave those practices into policy at every level' (CPHVA 1999 p 2).

The setting up of a National Family and Parenting Institute feels like a step in the right direction, as it has the potential to encourage a stronger national focus on the family. However, it is not clear whether the Institute will form and be the voice of 'experts', or whether it will be an advocate for parents and families, giving them a voice to be heard. If it is to be successful there needs to be an emphasis on true partnership working with statutory and voluntary agencies.

Among health visitors it was the 'enhanced role of the health visitor' that called for the greatest amount of comment. There is the very real problem of resources. During the last government's term of office there were cuts in the health visiting and school nursing services coupled with the effects of an ageing workforce.

- The number of full-time equivalent Health Visitors in England dropped from 10 680 to 10 070 between 1988 and 1998, having reached an all-time low of 9680 in 1994 (Department of Health 1999c).
- 14% of health visitors are under 40 years old, while 43% are over 50 years old.
- 19% of health visitors intend to leave the profession in the next two years. 77% of that group intend to leave due to planned or early retirement (CPHVA 1998).

It is obvious that urgent action needs to be taken, not only to train more health visitors, but to retain those already in employment. There is also an urgent need to review the education and training of health visitors to ensure that the core training contains skills such as those provided by 'One plus One', described on p 265. This will be particularly necessary given the role envisaged in 'Supporting Families' for health visitors and midwives for supporting couples in their relationship when they have a new baby. Subsequent chapters (Box 12.6) in the 'Supporting Families' document deal with differing themes.

Perhaps one of the most significant initiatives to be announced in this document was 'Sure Start'. The Chancellor's comprehensive spending review in 1998 announced £540 million to be made available over a three-year period to fund local projects delivered by partnerships working across agencies. The aim is to target those in greatest need and to bring providers closer together to provide a seamless service. Sixty 'trailblazer' areas in England were announced in February 1999 (Department of Education and Employment 1999b). They were chosen from across the country because they:

BOX 12.6	*'Supporting Families' chapters*

- Chapter 2 'Better Financial Support for Families' outlines reformation of the tax and benefit system to ensure families get the help they need
- Chapter 3 'Helping Families Balance Work and Home' outlines the government plans to support those with family commitments who wish to work, by creating the best environment to balance work and home
- Chapter 4 'Strengthening Marriage' outlines proposals to protect the interests of children by strengthening marriage and reducing the risks of family breakdown
- Chapter 5 'Better Support for Serious Family Problems' outlines what needs to be done to tackle serious problems in family life, including domestic violence and school-age pregnancy

- Could demonstrate need
- Had existing good practice on which to build
- Gave a good spread around the country
- Gave a good spread of types of area, i.e. rural and urban
- Link with other government initiatives to tackle areas of deprivation.

The aim is to promote the physical, intellectual, emotional and social well-being of children of 0–4 years, to ensure that they are ready to thrive when they get to school. 'Sure Start' will add value to and reconfigure services to parents and children in the area, creating an entirely new service based squarely on the needs of parents and children. Parents and children themselves will work in partnership with providers of services and voluntary agencies to ensure that it is their needs that are being met and not the needs of service providers. It is an exciting initiative that has the potential to change the way services work across the country. When it was first announced, only 5% of children were expected to benefit. However, in July 2000, a further £315 million for the initiative was announced, so that the expanded Sure Start scheme will reach a third of children under 4 years old in England by 2004. Sure Start programmes are also available in Wales, Scotland and Northern Ireland. The fact that families living in these areas will benefit will serve as an example of what can be achieved, and holds out hope for the future of these services generally.

MAKING A DIFFERENCE: STRENGTHENING THE NURSING, MIDWIFERY AND HEALTH VISITING CONTRIBUTION TO HEALTH AND HEALTH CARE

The 'Making a difference' strategy for nursing, midwifery and health visiting, published by the Department of Health in July 1999 encourages health visitors to develop a:

'Family-centred public health role, working with individuals, families and communities to improve health and to tackle health inequalities' (Department of Health 1999b p 61).

This approach is not new to health visiting. 'Making it Happen' (Department of Health 1995), the report of the Standing Nursing and Midwifery Advisory Committee (SNMAC), made little impact at the time due to the politics of the last government. However it now seems to be coming into its own with policies to underpin and support it. In this report (Department of Health 1995 para 4.5 p 20) we read:

> 'The SNMAC states that the unique orientation to health promotion, in terms of meeting both individual and community need, makes health visitors public health workers in the entirety of their role. Their focus on families with children is extendable to other targeted groups in the population, to meet agreed health needs in the wider community.'

What was happening in practice was that there was an unnecessary focus on counting contacts with clients, for the needs of providers of services. 'Korner statistics' became the yardstick for measuring activity, leading to the conclusion that the more contacts a health visitor made the more effective she was as a practitioner. Some health visitors have had dictated to them the number of contacts they are to have a month, irrespective of the clients' needs. The quality of the contact was not considered important. This in turn has led to an over-emphasis on individual one-to-one work at the expense of more group-based, community-orientated interventions.

Health visitors have been hampered in their role by adherence to the medical model of care. GP fundholding made it much more difficult for health visitors to provide the kind of support parents needed due to the need to take a more population-wide approach. Practice populations do not always live in communities (see Box 12.7). They are often widely spread over a large catchment area. In this example we can see how previous policies have hampered a full implementation and use of a health visitors skills in her wider public health role. To be fair, this sort of practice did not occur everywhere.

In some community trusts, GP-attached health visitors were contracted for ten per cent of their working hours to enable a wider public health perspective to be taken. There were also practices that valued the work of health visitors, reduced their caseloads and enabled them to be more effective in

BOX 12.7	*Example from practice*

A health visitor working attached to a GP fundholding practice identified a need for parenting support within the rural community. The health visitor, who had qualified in 1979, saw this as part of her wider role and initiated a group that would include not only the practice population but other parents who would belong to another practice. The group was run in the local school hall thus opening it up to the wider community.

Naturally, at the weekly practice team meeting she conveyed this to the rest of the team. The senior GP partner asked what steps would be taken to ensure that only the practice patients attended. On finding out that the group was intended for the wider community the health visitor was discouraged from advertising the group too widely in case she ended up working with non-practice-registered clients.

BOX 12.8	*Results of modernising the health visiting role (Department of Health 1999a para 11.17)*

- Parents will receive improved support including parenting education, health advice and information
- Individuals and families will be able to have a tailored family health plan, agreed in partnership with the health visitor, to address their parenting and health needs
- A team led by a health visitor, including nurses, nursery nurses, and community workers, will meet the health needs of families and communities
- Health visitors will initiate and develop programmes of outreach, based on the experiences of organisations such as Homestart, Newpin and 'community mothers', where local parents use their experience to support others
- Neighbourhoods or special groups such as homeless people, within a practice or primary care group, will have their needs identified by health visitors, who will lead public health practice and agree local health plans
- Local communities will be helped to identify and address their own health needs, for example accident prevention for older people

their service delivery. Meanwhile, their colleagues down the road struggled with ever-burgeoning caseloads and service delivery was far from equitable.

What we saw developing was a patchwork of good and not-so-good practice, with many health visitors longing to be able to give a quality service to meet the varying needs of their clients. Health needs assessment is now something that all primary care groups are expected to carry out, in partnership with the local community and other agencies (see Chapter 6). It is a basic skill of health visitors and community nurses. Health visitors know the needs of the communities in which they work and are well placed to give voice to their findings in the commissioning of new locally-sensitive services.

'Saving Lives: Our Healthier Nation' (Department of Health 1999a) and 'Making a Difference' (Department of Health 1999b), the new nursing strategy which underpins the public health document, say they will modernise the role of the health visitor. The roles of the midwives and school nurses are also to be expanded and enhanced to include family support (Box 12.8).

We are told that a team led by the health visitor will provide a range of health improvement activities (Box 12.9).

Many health visitors have been able to develop their role beyond the traditional boundaries before this government gave them such resounding support, but many were not able to do so. Some skills have been lost and there will be a need for retraining and new training in group-work skills and relationship skills. With 27% of health visitors due to retire within the next four years there will have to be a considerable recruitment campaign to the profession (Turner 1999). However, it is heartening to read that according to the English National Board the number of health visitors in training has increased more than 12% in the last three years (Community Practitioner 1999).

The word 'support' appears five times in the health improvement activities (Box 12.9), so it is quite clearly considered to be a role to be developed by

---

BOX 12.9 | *Health improvement activities (Department of Health 1999a para 11.8)*

- Child health programmes
- Parenting support and education including support to Sure Start, parenting groups and home visits
- Developing support networks in communities, for example tackling social isolation of older people
- Support and advice for breastfeeding mothers and women at risk of postnatal depression
- Health promotion programmes to target cancer, coronary heart disease and stroke accidents, and mental health
- Advice on family relationships and support to vulnerable children and their families

---

BOX 12.10 | *Public health role for midwives (Department of Health 1999a para 11.23)*

- Targeting vulnerable groups through, for example, pregnancy clubs for single mothers or link workers for black and ethnic minority groups
- Providing preconceptual counselling for prospective parents, targeting smoking cessation, alcohol intake and diet to reduce the risk of low birth-weight and premature babies
- Working with health visitors and others on postnatal depression, breastfeeding and best practice to avoid sudden infant death syndrome

---

health professionals. To provide effective support, health visitors need to be able to give families time and in order to do this they need smaller caseloads and to be able to facilitate group-work initiatives and community development approaches to build up social support in the community.

The nursing strategy (Department of Health 1999b) underpins the enhanced role of the health visitor, calling on the profession to work in new ways across traditional boundaries with other professionals and voluntary organisations, to develop a family-centred public health role. It envisages the health visitor as a leader, leading teams of nursery nurses, nurses and other community workers. Much of the frustration felt in the profession over recent years is waning, as the new mandate from the new government initiatives give a clear message to health visitors to take family support work forward.

'Saving Lives' (Department of Health 1999a) also looks at the role of midwives in relation to public health (Box 12.10). Midwives also have a role in supporting expectant mothers and families with very young children. It says that they are uniquely placed to improve health and tackle inequality through innovative services provided to women and their babies at home and in hospital.

It is interesting to note that, in 'Making a Difference' (Department of Health 1999b), midwives are seen as working in partnership with health visitors and school nurses to help to ensure that young people are well-informed about healthy lifestyle choices, contraception, sexual health, relationships and the

---

BOX 12.11 | *Example from practice*

In a large girls' comprehensive school in North London the school nurse worked with teachers, health visitors, midwives, dietician and priest to provide a day for year ten girls focusing on relationships and parenthood. Topics covered included:

- Relationships
- Contraception
- Pre-conceptual health and diet
- Healthy pregnancy and birth
- Parenting skills
- Single parenthood.

The day was well-evaluated by the girls and another day planned for the following year.

BOX 12.12 | *A public health role for school nursing (Department of Health 1999a para 11.20)*

- School nurses need to be developed and supported to enable them to:
- Lead teams
- Assess the health needs of individuals and school communities and agree individual and school health plans
- Develop multidisciplinary partnerships with teachers, general practitioners, health visitors and child and adolescent mental health professionals to deliver agreed health plans

---

responsibilities associated with pregnancy and childbirth (see Box 12.11). Midwives, health visitors, school nurses and community nurses are teams for family health and support at different stages of the life-cycle. In many areas, however, the midwifery service is aligned to the acute trust services and not a part of the services provided by the community trust. This makes for complications in liaising within what should be the family-focused team. Now would be a good time to reconfigure services and integrate teams into primary care groups or primary care trusts so that team-working could be further developed.

'Saving Lives' (Department of Health 1999a) also identifies school nurses as public health practitioners. It sees the potential to develop their role (Box 12.12) within other government initiatives, such as tackling teenage pregnancy. As we can see from Box 12.11, it was the school nurse who was the team leader for this piece of work within a school. She drew together the professionals concerned and helped them to work together to use each other's expertise to form a day that was beneficial to a whole year-group within a school setting.

The public health role of school nurses is further expanded in 'Making a Difference' (Department of Health 1999b). It says that they should draw on their nursing knowledge and pastoral care experience to support policies such as the healthy schools initiative. They are identified as the profession

BOX 12.13	*Health improvement activities of the school nursing team (Department of Health 1999a para 11.21)*

- Immunisation and vaccination programmes
- Supporting and advising teachers and other school staff on a range of child health issues
- Supporting children with special medical needs
- Supporting and counselling to promote positive mental health in young people
- Contributing to personal health and social education and to citizenship training
- Identifying social care needs, including the need for protection from abuse
- Advising on relationships and sex education by building on their clinical experience and pastoral role
- Liaising between schools, primary care groups and special services in meeting the health and social care needs of children
- Contributing to the identification of children's special educational needs
- Working alongside health visitors to promote parenting

BOX 12.14	*Example from practice*

In North London a health visitor was facilitating parenting groups which were greatly appreciated by the parents. School nurses were very interested in the work and the health visitor invited the school nurse to sit in on the next course that she ran. The school nurse then took the information from the health visitor to the head teacher of the local primary school. After discussions between staff, the school nurse and health visitor, a parenting group was established in the school run by the health visitor and school nurse. The course was run for parents of nursery, reception and year 1 pupils

Training sessions were then set up for school nurses and health visitors in the facilitation of the parenting programmes which were led by the health visitor. This will enable the work to be more widely disseminated within the services.

to help young people make healthy lifestyle choices, to reduce risk-taking behaviour and to focus on issues such as teenage parenthood. They should work in teams to provide integrated programmes of support and health promotion. Box 12.13 lists the health improvement activities of the school nursing team.

It is interesting to note that school nurses are seen as working alongside health visitors to promote parenting. This is perhaps an area for 'transdisciplinary' working. The skill from one group could be learned by another and transferred to a different setting (Box 12.14).

There are many examples of collaborative working in practice, not only between disciplines but also between agencies. Box 12.15 demonstrates just one example.

'Our Healthier Nation' and 'Making a Difference' put midwives, health visitors and school nurses firmly at the centre of services for families with children.

BOX 12.15	*Example from practice*

The local Parents Centre knew the parenting work being done by the health visitor. Although the main thrust of this voluntary organisation's work was in supporting families with children with special needs, they were keen to support families more widely.

The manager of the centre and the health visitor worked collaboratively to run a course locally. The centre used its resources and contacts to advertise the course widely through schools and the health visitor co-facilitated the group and provided volunteer crèche workers who were parents who had taken part in previous courses.

PRACTICALITIES OF INCORPORATING POLICY INTO PRACTICE

It is my belief that the public health perspective of health visitors evolves from their focus on individual families. It is from working one-to-one with families in a neighbourhood that the health visitor gains an insight into the problems that occur generally in that population. It is a maturing of practice that draws a health visitor from concerns with a particular family to concern for a whole community.

Having met the same problem in differing guises, the health visitor is led to question how this comes to be, or to look for likely causes. Sharing this information with the community can be vital to empowering that community to take action and help itself.

There are two steps that the health visitor takes to building up a supportive community that is able to take care of itself:

1. Working with the individual client in partnership, to help them gain control over their lives and their situation. To help them in developing their own expertise.
2. Supporting these empowered individuals to help their peers do the same. One of the ways that the health visitor can do this is by cooperating with and affirming networks that parents are open to.

Encouraging growth and independence of communities is part of the health visitor role. Let us look for a moment at an example from practice (Box 12.16) and reflect upon its meaning in this context.

What is illustrated in the relationship between Linda and Jo (Box 12.16) is the approach health professionals can take with their clients and the wider community. Just as Linda had to let go of Jo and allow him to explore his surroundings in order to develop, so as health professionals we have to let go of our clients and allow them to take responsibility for their own decisions. Just as Jo got it wrong sometimes and fell over and bumped his head so the decisions parents make will not always be the ones health visitors would have chosen for them, but they will be their own decisions. The same is true of communities. Interestingly, Linda came to take part in a group of parents with sleeping difficulties and was able to share her success. This gave her a sense of achievement

BOX 12.16	*Example from practice*

Linda brought her son Jo to the sleep clinic. He was 6 months old, and woke frequently at night for feeds. More worrying was the fact that he was not rolling over yet and his muscle tone seemed rather flaccid.

Linda was a devoted mother and never let her son want for anything. She gave him her undying attention day and night. Linda was exhausted and was longing for a night's sleep. Linda attended the sleep clinic weekly for a month.

At first Linda would hold Jo on her lap and never put him down on the floor to play with the toys. As the health visitor worked through a sleep plan with Linda things began to change. Linda was able to put Jo on the floor and let him explore his surroundings. Linda began to allow Jo to separate from her and become more independent. As he learned that he could fall asleep on his own he also learned that he could reach his toys by himself by rolling over. Linda began to be able to tolerate Jo's frustration and sometimes crying when he could not reach what he wanted. As she learned to let go and let Jo learn for himself, he not only slept through the night but started to sit up and roll over. What was really important for Linda was learning to separate from Jo, letting him explore his surroundings and find things out for himself.

and accomplishment and improved her self-confidence and self-esteem. It also helped other parents with the same difficulties to believe in themselves to overcome their problems.

Health visitors and nursery nurses working in North London where Linda lived had noted that many of the problems that parents came to them with were around sleeping difficulties. A survey of the health visitors found that they were giving varying levels of support and found it difficult to give the continuing support to parents that was necessary.

Following a meeting of the health visitors at the health centre it was agreed that one health visitor should use one morning a week to run a sleep clinic to help parents with these problems. It was organised to cover a particular geographical patch rather than one particular GP practice. Clients were seen as families where possible, with an appointment system running weekly. All families seen in the clinic also met as a group once a month to share experiences and for mutual support. This way friendships are also made and parents go on supporting each other and are not dependent on the health visitor for support. The health visitor is very much the initiator of the activity and is there should she be needed. It is the parents themselves, however, who do the work with their children and for each other.

The health visitor works in partnership with the parents. Working in partnership means acknowledging them as the 'experts' in the care of their own children. They are the ones who know their own children best. Once they know this and are in control of their own situation they grow in self-confidence and their sense of self-worth is enhanced. What the example from practice in Box 12.17 shows is how working with an individual can benefit the health of the whole community. I use the word 'health' here in its widest possible sense, meaning not only physical health but social and emotional health and well-being.

BOX 12.17	*Example from practice*

Sharon is a young mother of 24 years. She has a son, Rory, who is 2 years old. Sharon has been experiencing difficulties with Rory's behaviour, particularly since she has become pregnant again. She feels tired most of the time and is short-tempered with Rory. She is well supported by her mother who lives nearby. Her husband is in work but seems uninvolved in childcare. The health visitor suggested that Sharon come to the parenting group at the health centre where she could get some tips on managing Rory's behaviour.

The health visitor facilitating the group is concerned about Sharon in the group as she seems quite shy and finds it difficult to speak personally in front of the others. The facilitator suggests to one of the more outgoing members of the group that she could help to draw Sharon out a bit more. This works well and the two become firm friends. Sharon is able to make good use of the group and her self-confidence begins to grow. The seven-week parenting course soon comes to an end but a 'parent assertiveness' programme lasting eight weeks follows two weeks later.

The parents enjoy this and it is of great benefit to everyone taking part. They are committed to each other and to the work they are doing in their families. They have enjoyed it and benefited so much that they want to give something back to help others in the community. Some of them go on to become crèche workers, so that other parents can attend the group. Three or four of them, including Sharon, continue to meet with the health visitor to prepare them to become parenting-group facilitators.

Sharon, with one of the other parents from the course, co-facilitates a programme with the health visitor. Sharon shows a warm, sociable and outgoing personality and is keen to help others. She introduces friends who are struggling at home with their toddlers to the group and supports their continued attendance. She also brings her mother who will be caring for Rory when Sharon has the baby. Sharon also attends meetings at a local school with the health visitor, to speak to parents of reception children about running a parenting course for them at the school. She also attends a meeting for school nurses and health visitors locally to tell them of the impact of the group on her life.

Sharon did not do well at school. She is someone that the education system failed. She felt disadvantaged. However, recently she has had the confidence to apply to the local Adult Education College and has been accepted on an 'access to social work' course. She feels good about herself because she feels that she can make a useful contribution to society.

The groups have been running for some years now. The one thing that parents agree on when the groups have been evaluated is that just knowing that they are not the only ones who are struggling, and that there are other parents with similar problems, greatly reduces the sense of isolation encountered by so many, and they begin to realise that they can support each other. That support is vital to their health, as we have seen earlier in this chapter.

Parenting groups have become fashionable in today's political climate and not everyone agrees that they are a good thing (Smith 1997). Are they truly about empowerment or about social control? The parents that have taken part in the groups that are quoted here would be quite sure that they were about empowerment, and have found them liberating. They did not take part because they had to but because they were looking for help and support for the problems with which they were faced. Had they not found them useful, or if they had felt that they were being told what to do and were having something imposed on them, they would not have come back, let alone have gone on to facilitate such programmes themselves.

As part of the new Crime and Disorder Act 1998, magistrates have the power to impose parenting orders on parents whose children are guilty of offending. The order compels parents to attend a parenting course. The reasoning behind this is that parents must be made to face up to the responsibility that they bear for their children's behaviour. Utting et al (1993) drew attention to the link between parental supervision, discipline and delinquency. The suggestion was that good parenting might help to prevent the acquisition of a criminal record. It is interesting to note that where these new orders have been imposed, many parents have been very grateful for the help that they have received. There has been some initial reluctance to engage in the work, but when this has been overcome they have been surprised at the improvements they have been able to make in family life. The element of mutual support has been very important, with participants exchanging telephone numbers at the end of the course (Williams 1999 Unpublished Parenting Education and Support Forum conference paper)

It is not always necessary for health visitors to be the initiators of groups. There are very many groups already in existence that parents are open to, e.g. playgroups, mother and toddler groups, schools, nurseries, churches and ethnic minority community groups. It is important to recognise this and to work with them. Not only do they welcome parenting programmes but they may also be open to other initiatives.

As can be seen from the practice example in Box 12.18, sometimes unexpected things happen as a result of the individual work that the health visitor does with a family. It is part of the natural progression of the work of the health visitor that begins with the individual and then broadens perspective to include the whole community.

It is true that, as people grow and develop their skills, they move on. As they come to believe in themselves more and gain in self-confidence, they begin to demand that others have confidence in them as well and take on more demanding roles.

BOX 12.18   *Example from practice*

Mira came to the clinic to attend an appointment with the health visitor for her daughter's two-year development check. Although her daughter was healthy, Mira was having difficulty with her behaviour and did not know where to turn for advice. We talked about the management of Mala's tantrums and of her eating difficulties and behaviour at meal times. Mira was a Tamil woman from Sri Lanka. The family had fled the fighting and all Mira's relatives were back home in Sri Lanka. Mira lived on the thirteenth floor of a tower block and often saw no-one else all day. The health visitor agreed to visit Mira monthly for three months to help her implement a behaviour programme with Mala.

BOX 12.18	*Cont'd*

Each time the health visitor visited Mira had made significant progress with Mala. Soon potty training became an issue and three more visits were agreed. Although Mala and her behaviour were the main thrust of the health visitor's work on these visits, it was evident that Mira was very lonely and in need of adult conversation herself during the day. She made contact with the Tamil Refugee Centre and there found more young mothers from her homeland. This was unfortunately quite a distance from where she lived, so she could not attend often. The health visitor talked with Mira about returning to work or taking up some training opportunities. She was keen to do this but was unsure exactly what she wanted to do.

Some three months later the health visitor received a phone call from Mira who was very pleased with herself as she had managed to get a full-time job at the Tamil Refugee Centre. She had been appointed as the 'Women and Children's Health Worker'. She was keen to set up a support group for Tamil women who were parents. The health visitor met with Mira to discuss how this might be achieved and what areas of health and children's welfare the women might like to learn more about. The health visitor showed Mira the parenting programme and they agreed a six-week programme that included nutrition and dealing with children's behaviour.

The groups were well-attended and the discussions lively. The parenting programme was adapted to the group with some sections left out and everything was done through an interpreter. The hope was that eventually Mira would be able to facilitate these groups for herself with health visitor support. Following the second group Mira was gaining in confidence. All seemed well and it looked likely that Mira would be able to take over the running of the groups. Fortunately for Mira, but unfortunately for the health visitor, as happens so often with people who develop, Mira was offered another job that paid her more money and she left the Tamil Refugee Centre.

When using a community development approach clients are always valued as having something to offer rather than as needing to be 'helped'. The health visitor is well placed to do this work and build up the community to develop its own support network. As a result of three years' work in North London one health visitor working with parenting programmes found that:

■ 56% offered to help run the crèche and 43% wanted to help to co-facilitate a course

■ One parent took the programme to use at work with young teenage parents

■ One parent with a group of five or six others set up a 'Playtime' group to help develop parent's play skills that they had learned on the course

■ Another parent decided to open her home to support other parents and go on meeting after the sessions had finished. This enabled them to care for each other's children sometimes in order to get a much-needed break

- Three of the parents helped to co-facilitate groups
- One of the parents was invited to become a school governor at a local primary school with a poor inspection report, in order to help them develop parenting support within the school.

Three other health visitors and one school nurse were also enabled to facilitate groups in other parts of the locality. If each of these were able to empower clients to support other parents, one could see how quickly a supportive community network could be in place.

Parents are genuinely grateful for the experience of being part of these groups. One such parent wrote:

> 'Because I have gained so much from the groups both as a Mum and now as a co-leader I feel more confident and I know that I am doing the best I can for my children. I feel so much happier and more able to deal with the difficult times. Something that really struck me when taking part in the meetings was that, regardless of whether anyone was married, single, living with a partner or living with their parents, we were all experiencing similar situations with our children, and regardless of our cultural background or the language spoken, we all had a mutual understanding and respect for each other as a parent. I was lucky enough to attend a group and feel now that I would like to pass that experience on.' (Japal 1997)

This work has only been able to develop in this area of North London because a group of health visitors could see that this was what their clients were asking for. It was a genuine response to a local need identified by health visitors working on their caseloads with individual families. Between them, they made a team decision that some of the caseload time needed to be dedicated to this work and with the agreement of management they were enabled to work in the way in which they had identified would be useful.

With the added support of government policies in 'Supporting Families', 'Saving Lives' and 'Making a Difference' (Department of Health 1999a, 1999b, Ministerial Group on the Family 1998), it should now be easier for many other health visitors to work in this way. Out of this work has developed 'Sure Start'. The North London area has been identified as a 'trailblazer' and health visitors are working in partnership with many other community groups, both voluntary and statutory, to take this work forward. In this area the health-visiting service was the initiator of the project. It was the natural development of all that had happened previously. Now the work has developed from working with individual community groups to include a whole range of varied groups and service providers. This has not been an easy process.

All the agencies have to learn to work in partnership with each other and with parents (Bidmead 1999). They have to listen to what parents want and they have to listen to each other. Some agencies are very new to this way of working. Although groups have worked together before on some joint-financed projects, their relationship really resembled that of cohabitees, with little commitment from anyone especially when the funding ran out. What is asked for now is a marriage with real commitment to working together in a completely new way.

We have to be open to working across professional boundaries, to work in true partnership with each other, sharing skills for the benefit of the community.

It is an experiment not entirely without evidence for its effectiveness. It may be true to say that no-one knows whether it will be successful in what it sets out to achieve. It is known, however, that supportive social networks within a local community have a protective effect and can help parents with their parenting (Roberts 1996). This is certainly the experience of many health visitors and why many have worked so hard to continue to make the building-up of social support a part of the way in which they work. Unfortunately, it may be a skill that has been lost for some health visitors who have been bound by the individualistic 'medical model' way of working. It is to be hoped that the opportunities offered to health visiting through Sure Start will not be lost because they are not used to partnership-working with other agencies.

As we saw earlier in the chapter, there is evidence for early intervention in health, education and socially (Cowley 1999). It is just that this way of working has never really been tried here in the UK. It is to be hoped that Sure Start programmes will be well evaluated, so that all may learn the lessons from what we hope will turn out to be a small but very significant step in finding new ways of working together for the benefit of parents and children.

HOW ONE SURE START VISION IS TO BE DELIVERED

One of the drawbacks to partnership working that could also be seen in a positive light is the meetings. Instead of one service deciding that a particular intervention would be a good idea there now has to be consultation. This inevitably means a longer process but it may also mean that your particular service finds out that another organisation is providing something similar and prevents duplication of effort and resources. The Sure Start partnership has had to have such conversations in order to reach agreement on the delivery of the Sure Start services. The partnership board in one area consists of the Parent's centre, which is the lead organisation, the temporary accommodation play project, the Turkish Cypriot Association, The Greek Cypriot Association, The Tamil Refugee Centre, the Somali Education and Cultural Association, English for speakers of other languages unit, Relate, Women's Aid, the women's refuge, Homestart, Trans-age action, libraries, the pre-school support service, the home-school liaison service, social services family support unit, educational psychology, health visiting, midwifery, dieticians, physiotherapy, occupational therapy, speech and language therapy, Childminders' Association and oral health promotion. These organisations represent the partnership working together to draw up the delivery plans. A consultant in public health from the health authority also attends.

This local joined-up working reflects the joined-up working at government level. The Secretary of State for Education and Employment is the responsible cabinet minister, reporting to the Prime Minister. Policy is directed by a steering group chaired by the Minister of State for Public Health and involving ministers from the Department of Health, the Department for Education and Employment, the Department for the Environment, Transport and the Regions, the Department of Social Security, the Department for Culture, Media and Sport and the Treasury. Senior officials from these departments and other key departments attend the steering group as necessary. The new

| BOX 12.19 | *Aims and objectives of Sure Start (Department of Education and Employment 1999b)* |

Aim: To work with parents and children to promote the physical, intellectual and social development of pre-school children – particularly those who are disadvantaged – to ensure that they are ready to thrive when they get to school.

Objectives: Sure Start programmes will work efficiently and effectively to achieve this in areas of significant unmet need by:

- Improving social and emotional development, in particular by supporting early bonding between parents and their children, helping families to function, and through early identification and support of children with emotional and behavioural difficulties
- Improving health, in particular by supporting parents in caring for their children to promote healthy development before and after birth
- Improving the ability to learn, in particular by encouraging stimulating and enjoyable play, improving language skills and through early identification and support of children with learning difficulties
- Strengthening families and communities, in particular by enhancing families' opportunities for involvement in the community and improving the sensitivity of existing services to local needs

cross-departmental team, the Sure Start Unit, is based in the Department for Education and Employment and runs the programme at official level.

This high-level partnership working signals to local groups the ways in which they should also be working across all agencies. Local partnerships must include parents and local community groups. Just how diverse a partnership might be can be seen from the groups included in the partnership example mentioned above.

The plans for the delivery of Sure Start have to be written against specific public service agreement targets. Each planned intervention must relate in some way to the target specified. Each intervention has to then have a quarterly breakdown of what it hopes to achieve in the first year. This is no easy task and the work has to be done in addition to most people's usual job. Health visitors are not used to having to be so specific, but it is a very good discipline to have to be. Monitoring and evaluation procedures also have to be written.

Sure Start has to be responsive to local need and yet is being given very exact targets to achieve by the centrally-based Sure Start Unit (see Box 12.19). How those targets are achieved and are translated into actions is up to each local Sure Start project.

Targets have been set for 2001–2002. All parents in a Sure Start area are to have access to parenting support and information. There must be a 10% reduction in the numbers of children re-registered on the child protection register. Every Sure Start programme must have agreed and implemented, in a culturally sensitive way, ways of identifying, caring for and supporting mothers with postnatal depression. There must be a 5% reduction in the proportion of low birthweight babies. The numbers of children admitted to hospital as an emergency with gastroenteritis, respiratory infection or a severe injury during the first year of life must be reduced by 10%. At least 90% of children are to have normal speech and language development at 18 months and three years. All children are to have access to good-quality play and learning opportunities. 75% of families should report personal evidence of improvement in the quality of services providing family support and every local Sure Start programme is to have parent representation on the partnership board.

If health visitors are not involved in local programmes then it is very uncertain that the above targets could be achieved. Health visitors are the professional health personnel who already work in the community giving parenting support and information. Health visitors work with families where there are child-protection issues and have proven efficacy in working with mothers with postnatal depression (Seeley et al 1996). Health visitors and midwives work with low birth-weight babies and babies with failure to thrive. Health visitors are used to following up accident and emergency admissions to hospital in the first year of life following trauma, respiratory tract infections and gastroenteritis. This is the bread and butter work of health visiting.

Where health visitors are involved in the Sure Start initiative they can influence the delivery plan and gain the help of other professionals and volunteers to enhance the work in which they are already engaged. They can train others to give parenting support, to be aware of signs and symptoms of postnatal depression, to recognise gastroenteritis and to be able to give correct advice in the treatment of diarrhoea and vomiting. This can only happen, however, if health visitors are not defensive about their professionalism and are willing to work in partnership with others in the community. Extra support can be given using community mothers (Suppiah 1994), Homestart volunteers, or grandparents as in the Transage Action volunteer scheme. Extra play opportunities can be provided using the skills of nursery nurses and mobilising the community to provide the often lacking and much-needed play space. Where there is obvious local unmet need then extra resources can be deployed to provide a service where none existed before. It is an opportunity to work in a more effective and coordinated way.

Not only does the Sure Start delivery plan meet the Sure Start national targets but it may also in the long term meet the local targets of the Health Improvement Plan. For example reducing the incidence of low birth-weight babies may in the long-term affect the amount of coronary heart disease, diabetes and hypertension seen in the community in later life (Acheson 1998) As the two principal determinants of a baby's weight at birth are the mother's pre-pregnant weight and her own birthweight, the need for policies to improve the health of future mothers and their children is obvious. Acheson (1998) also makes the point that where there are migrants moving from a poorly nourished community to a well-nourished community, there will be implications for foetal growth and adult health for more than one generation. This should be noted in areas where there are a high number of refugees and asylum seekers coming from third world countries.

Reducing the incidence of low birth-weight babies by 5% in three years may not be an achievable target in those designated as Sure Start areas. Acheson (1998) points out that many of the potentially beneficial interventions to reduce inequalities in health pertain to reducing the inequalities in mental and physical health of parents, particularly present and future mothers and children. He suggests that research shows that policies which reduce early adverse influences may result in multiple benefits, not only throughout the life-course of that child but to the next generation (Acheson 1998). Primary care groups would do well to note this and make it a priority to bring a Sure Start programme to their area

| BOX 12.20 | *Sure Start delivery plan (excerpt)* |

Public Service Agreement Target: All Sure Start programmes to have agreed and implemented in a culturally-sensitive way ways of identifying caring for and supporting mothers with postnatal depression (PND)

Start Point: Only 17 cases identified by health visitors in a year of approximately 450 new births. No agreed diagnostic criteria. No effective data collection. No agreed referral pathways. Scarce support other than medication.

Local Targets: Year 1: Baseline established for incidence of PND. Increased awareness of PND throughout Sure Start services. Establish level of need for group, family, and one-to-one support.

Activity:

- Raising awareness of PND and its causes
- Better methods of identification of PND
- Better recording of incidence, causes and effects of PND
- Provide effective referral pathways
- Provide emotional and practical support for all women with PND
- Provide home language support for non-English speaking and bilingual women with PND
- Offer training, support and consultation on PND for all Sure Start partners, workers, volunteers and resourceful friends. Train health staff in use of Edinburgh postnatal depression scale.
- Establish supervision consultation and continuing support for staff engaged in this work.
- Annual evaluation of diagnostic and referral processes.

Year 2: PND diagnosed in line with national average, i.e. 10% of postnatal women. A variety of support options offered within two weeks of identified need.

Year 3: 90% of all possible cases diagnosed and offered appropriate support.

Providers of Services: Health visitors, midwives, GPs, practice nurses, Homestart, Family Support, Child and Family Service, Resourceful Friends, Greek and Greek-Cypriot community, Turkish Cypriot Association

of deprivation. It is to be hoped that Sure Start will be evaluated not only in the short and medium term but also in the long term.

Box 12.20 shows an extract taken from one intervention from a Sure Start delivery plan. Health visitors have been hampered in this work with postnatal depression because of very large caseloads, in an area of deprivation with a highly mobile population living in temporary accommodation. Recruiting more health visitors with Sure Start funding should reduce caseloads and allow time for development of services for this client group. There will also be extra support given in a practical way through the work of trained volunteers. Ethnic minority community groups other than those mentioned may also become involved during the awareness-raising stage.

It will be seen from the intervention outlined in Box 12.20 that it is a whole-community approach where before only the health visitors were trying ineffectively to cope. It is now seen as a problem for the *whole* of the community in which the *whole* community must be involved. Sure Start makes people break out of the narrow confines of their own department or profession and engages with others to seek a solution. This must be the way forward. It is to be hoped that the lessons learned from the Sure Start programmes will be used to inform practice on a much larger scale in the future.

Also of paramount importance in the example above, is the interweaving of family support into the intervention. There is support for the mother in whichever way may be most appropriate, whether from a group or one-to-one. There may be support for the family in the form of childminding, befriending or practical help with household tasks. Finally, there is supervision and support for those people engaged in the treatment or support of those suffering from postnatal depression.

CONCLUSION AND IMPLICATIONS FOR PRACTICE

In this chapter we have seen how important family support is to family health, and therefore to public health. We have seen how new government policies encourage an enhanced role for health professionals working in the community, to provide family support in many dimensions. Finally, we looked in some depth at the new Sure Start programme which allows the enhanced role of community health visitors to be developed to the full. Sure Start offers a new way of working, a complete change in service delivery unlike anything we have known before. Let us make the most of this opportunity to make a real difference, in partnership with our communities, and evaluate and gather the evidence from practice that will be the basis of future service development.

Lack of support for families is clearly linked with poor health outcomes. Health visitors, school nurses and midwives can work together in teams, not only to provide the professional care that families need at crucial stages of their lives, but to lead others as part of that team to provide much needed support. Those 'others' could be other mothers, other fathers, grandparents, community mothers, nursery nurses, paediatric nurses and voluntary organisations and

DISCUSSION QUESTIONS

- How should health professionals resolve the difficulties of confidentiality of information within their extended role of partnership in care with other agencies and possibly volunteers?
- Can service providers break out of the narrow confines of their professionalism to work in true partnership with each other and with other agencies and community groups?
- If 'Sure Start' is a blueprint for delivery of services how will such services be funded in the future?
- Could there be a new broader service configured around the health needs of families with children? If so what would it look like?
- How are the new extended roles of health visitors, school nurses and midwives to be fulfilled in the light of the resource shortfall?

community groups. Clearly, the provision of services which support healthy living cannot be provided by one single service, the health service.

FURTHER READING

Community Practitioners and Health Visitors' Association 1999 Joined Up Working Community Development in Primary Health Care. CPHVA, London
A useful booklet detailing many examples of how health visitors have used a community development approach to their work.

Grimshaw R & McGuire C 1998 Evaluating Parenting Programmes, A Study of Stakeholders' Views. National Children's Bureau, London
This book examines open-access parenting programmes in depth and looks at the views and expectations of various stakeholders, from parents to funders and providers, as well as children themselves. Key principles are suggested for future development. For those who want to know more about fulfilling families needs, this is a useful text.

Holland S 2000 Promoting Mental Health. Community Practitioners and Health Visitors' Associations, London
This information pack and guide is an resource for all health visitors and others who are keen to develop their role in mental health promotion. It includes references to selected pieces of research on the promotion of mental health, highlighting their positive aspects and the pitfalls encountered. It also suggests a framework for translating aspects of this work into practice.

Jagger G & Wright C 1999 Changing Family Values. Routledge, London
This book was inspired by the last governments return to 'Family Values'. It asks, 'What does this mean?' It is informed by feminist insights and covers issues of the diverse realities of contemporary family life. It includes issues around single mothers, lesbian and gay families, the role of men and the changing family, the family in political theory and social policy and the future of the 'nuclear family'.

Pugh G, De'Ath E & Smith C 1994 Confident Parents, Confident Children. Policy and practice in parent education and support. National Children's Bureau, London
A book that looks at the challenges facing parents today. It examines the changes in society and in family patterns and at the skills involved in bringing up children and what can be done to make parenting more enjoyable, more satisfying and better-supported. The book presents a national overview of what is available to parents and identifies the substantial gaps and lack of coherence and coordination. It details an agenda for change, calling on communities to support parents with a stronger commitment to preventative rather than crisis work with families.

Smith C 1997 Developing Parenting Programmes. National Children's Bureau, London
One of the first books to summarise the availability of parenting programmes and support and to identify the gaps in service provision.

REFERENCES

Acheson D 1998 Independent Inquiry into Inequalities in Health. The Stationery Office, London

Barker D 1998 Mothers, Babies and Health in Later Life. Churchill Livingstone, Edinburgh

Bidmead C 1999 Bidding for success: making a Sure Start application. Community Practitioner 72(6):166–167

Breen S, Mattison K, McAlliser F & Roberts K 1998 One plus one information pack, 2nd edn. One plus One, London

Cockett M & Tripp J 1994 Children Living in Reordered Families, No. 45. Joseph Rowntree Foundation, York

Community Practitioner 1999 News Feature. Community Practioner 72(9):275

Community Practitioners and Health Visitors' Association 1998 Research Omnibus, Autumn 1998. Community Practitioners and Health Visitors' Association, London

Community Practitioners and Health Visitors' Association 1999 Response to Supporting Families. March 1999 Available from Community Practitioners and Health Visitors' Association Library and Information Service, London

Cowley S 1999 Early interventions: evidence for implementing Sure Start. Community Practitioner 72(6):162–163

Department for Education and Employment 1999a Sure Start: A Guide for Trailblazers. Department for Education and Employment Publications, Suffolk

Department for Education and Employment 1999b Sure Start: Drawing up Delivery Plans. Department for Education and Employment Publications, Suffolk

Department of Health 1995 Making it Happen, Public Health – the contribution, role and development of nurses midwives and health visitors. Report of the SNMAC. Department of Health, London

Department of Health 1999a Saving Lives, Our Healtheir Nation. The Stationery Office, London

Department of Health 1999b Making a differences: strengthening the nursing, midwifery and health visiting contribution to health and healthcare. Department of Health, London

Department of Health 1999c Non-Medical Workforce Census (NMWC). Department of Health, London

Evans G, Grant L, 1995 Moyenda Project Report 1991–1994 Exploring Parenthood. British Library Cataloguing in Publication Data, London

Farrington D, 1995 Intensive health visiting and the prevention of juvenile crime. Health Visitor 68(3):100–102

Japal C 1997 Parenting in Practice – A Parent's Perspective, Families Come First, Conference Proceedings October 1997, Profile Productions Ltd for the CPHVA 22

Labour Party Public Information Service 1996a Parenting. Labour Party, London

Labour Party Public Information Service 1996b Early Excellence: a head start for every child. Labour Party, London

Leith J 1997 Parenting in Practice - A Parent's Perspective, Families Come First, Conference Proceedings October 1997, Profile Productions Ltd for the CPHVA 23

Luck M & Jesson J 1996 Evaluation of community health development. Community Health UK, Bath

Mental Health Foundation 1999 Bright Futures Report. Mental Health Foundation, London

Ministerial Group on the Family 1998 Supporting Families. The Stationery Office, London

Murray L 1997 Postpartum depression and child development. Psychological Medicine 27:253–260

Oakley A, Rigby A & Hickey D 1994 Life stress, support and class inequality. European Journal of Public Health 4:81–91

One plus One 1998 Family Support Project. Bulletin Plus 2:4

Pugh G, De'Ath E & Smith C 1994 Confident Parents, Confident Children. Policy and practice in parent education and support. National Children's Bureau, London

Quinn M 1997 How can Professionals Help to create Parent-Friendly Communities? Families Come First, Conference Proceedings October 1997, Profile Productions Ltd on behalf of the Community Practitioners and Health Visitors' Association 17–19

Roberts I 1996 Family Support and the Health of Children. Children and Society 10:217–224

Russek L & Schwartz E 1997 Perceptions of parental caring predict health status in midlife: a 35-year follow-up of the Havard Mastery of Stress Study. American Journal of Psychosomatic Medicine 59:144–149

Seeley S, Murray L & Cooper P 1996 Post-natal depression: the outcome for mothers and babies of health visitor intervention. Health Visitor 69(4):135–138

Siddall R 1995 Journey's End. Community Care July: 26–27

Smith R 1997 Parent education: empowerment or control? Children and Society 11:108–116.

Suppiah C 1994 Working in partnership with community mothers. Health Visitor 67(2):51–53

Turner T 1999 Promoting public health. Community Practitioner 72(8):238–240

UNICEF 1990 United Nations Convention on the Rights of the Child, Sept. 1990. http://www.unicef.org./crc/crc/htm

Utting D, Bright J & Henricson C 1993 Crime and the Family, Improving Child-rearing and Preventing Delinquency. Family Policy Studies Centre, London

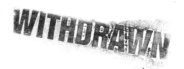

Index

Note: Page numbers referring to boxed material, tables and figures are in bold.

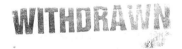